CORE CURRICULUM FOR CASE MANAGEMENT

CMSA
CASE MANAGEMENT SOCIETY OF AMERICA

CORE CURRICULUM FOR CASE MANAGEMENT

SUZANNE K. POWELL, RN, MBA, CCM, CPHQ
Director of Case Management/CQI
Health Services Advisory Group, Inc.
Phoenix, Arizona

DONNA IGNATAVICIUS, MS, RN, Cм
President
DI Associates, Inc.
Hughesville, Maryland

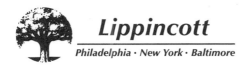

Lippincott
Philadelphia · New York · Baltimore

Acquisitions Editor: Jennifer Brogan
Editorial Assistant: Susan Barta Rainey
Senior Project Editor: Tom Gibbons
Senior Production Manager: Helen Ewan
Production Coordinator: Pat McCloskey
Design Coordinator: Brett MacNaughton
Manufacturing Manager: William Alberti
Indexer: Nancy Newman
Compositor: Peirce Graphic Services
Printer: R. R. Donnelley—Crawfordsville
Interior Design: Joan Wendt
Cover Design: Deborah Lynam

9 8 7 6 5 4 3 2

Library of Congress Cataloging-in-Publication Data

CMSA's core curriculum for case management / [edited by] Suzanne K. Powell,
Donna Ignatavicius.
p. ; cm.
Includes bibliographical references and index.
ISBN 0-7817-2454-6 (paper. : alk. paper)
1. Nursing care plans—Outlines, syllabi, etc. 2. Primary nursing—Administration—Outlines, syllabi, etc. 3. Hospitals—Case management services—Outlines, syllabi, etc.
I. Title: Core curriculum for case management. II. Powell, Suzanne K. III. Ignatavicius, Donna D. IV. Case Management Society of America.
[DNLM: 1. Case Management—Outlines. 2. Nursing Care—organization & administration—Outlines. WY 18.2 C649 2001]
RT90.7 .C636 2001
362.1'73'068—dc21

00-044815

Care has been taken to confirm the accuracy of the information presented and to describe generally accepted practices. However, the authors, editors, and publisher are not responsible for errors or omissions or for any consequences from application of the information in this book and make no warranty, express or implied, with respect to the content of the publication.

The authors, editors, and publisher have exerted every effort to ensure that drug selection and dosage set forth in this text are in accordance with the current recommendations and practice at the time of publication. However, in view of ongoing research, changes in government regulations, and the constant flow of information relating to drug therapy and drug reaction, the reader is urged to check the package insert for each drug for any change in indications and dosage and for added warnings and precautions. This is particularly important when the recommended agent is a new or infrequently employed drug.

Some drugs and medical devices presented in this publication have Food and Drug Administration (FDA) clearance for limited use in restricted research settings. It is the responsibility of the health care provider to ascertain the FDA status of each drug or device planned for use in his or her clinical practice.

Dedication

To case managers everywhere. . . and their patients

Contributors

SHERRY ALIOTTA, RN, BSN, CCM
President/CEO
S. A. Squared, Inc.
Las Alamitos, California

JANICE BENJAMIN, RN, MS, LAc
Nurse Acupuncturist
Faculty, The Southwest College of Naturopathic Medicine and Health
   Sciences
Tempe, Arizona

SHARON BRIM, RN, BSN, CCM
Medical Coordinator
Dodson Group
Kansas City, Missouri

PENNY BURMAN, RN, BSN, CCM
Supervisor, Case Management
Blue Cross/Blue Shield of North Dakota
Fargo, North Dakota

CAROL CANADA, RN, CCM
CMSA National Chairperson for Public Policy/Government Affairs
   (1997–1999)
Past President, Central Arizona Chapter CMSA
Director of Professional Community
CaregiverZone.com
Berkeley, California

NANCY CLAFLIN, RN, MS, CCRN, CPHQ
Carl T. Hayden Veterans Administration Medical Center
Phoenix, Arizona

LORI A. DAVIS, RN, CCM
Case Manager and Legal Nurse Consultant
www.MEDLEGALNURSE.com
Birmingham, Alabama

DEBORAH DiBENEDETTO, MBA, RN, COHN-S, ABDA
President, DV DiBenedetto & Associates, Ltd.
Yonkers, New York
President, The American Association of Occupational Health Nurses
Atlanta, Georgia
Instructor, Pace University School of Continuing Education
Lienhard School of Nursing
New York, New York

MARTHA EGGLESTON, MED, CRC, CCM, CDMS, PAHM
Rehabilitation Executive
General Reinsurance Corporation
Atlanta, Georgia

SUSAN GREGORY, RN, BSN, CCM, ABQAURP
Owner, Professional Quality Analysts, Inc.
Castleberry, Florida

RUFUS S. HOWE, FNP
Vice-President, Clinical Application Development
Click 4 Care
Columbus, Ohio

DONNA IGNATAVICIUS, MS, RN, CM
President
DI Associates, Inc.
Hughesville, Maryland

CHERI LATTIMER, RN
Vice-President, Utilization Management Programs
McKesson HBOC
Access Health Group
Broomfield, Colorado

LYNN MULLER, JMC, RN, JD, CDMS, CCM
Nurse-Attorney/Municipal Court Judge
Partner, Muller & Muller
Bergenfield, New Jersey

PATRICIA ORCHARD, CPHQ
Assistant Vice-President, Case Management
Virtua–West Jersey Hospital
Voorhees, New Jersey

PATRICIA M. PECQUEUX, RN, MS, CCM
Project Leader
Health Services Advisory Group
Phoenix, Arizona

SUZANNE K. POWELL, RN, BSN, CCM, CPHQ
Director of Case Management/CQI
Health Services Advisory Group, Inc.
Phoenix, Arizona

LINDA N. SCHOENBECK, RN, BS,C, CCM
Manager, Utilization, Quality, and Case Management
Health Services Advisory Group, Inc.
Phoenix, Arizona

MARLYS A. SEVERSON, RN, BSN, CCM
President/CEO
SCM Associates, Inc.
Bellflower, California

PAT STRICKER, RN, MEd
Director of Clinical Education
McKesson HBOC
Rancho Cordova, California

NANCY N. WHIPPLE, RN, BSN, MSCS
McKesson HBOC
Cambridge, Massachusetts

GARY WOLFE, RN, CCM
Case Manager, Continuous Learning (private practice)
San Francisco, California

LESLEY WRIGHT, MS, CRC, CCM, CDMS, CLCP, CDVC
Founder and President
The Wright Rehabilitation Service, Inc.
Roswell, Georgia

Reviewers

PENNY BURMAN, RN, BSN, CCM
Supervisor, Case Management
Blue Cross/Blue Shield of North Dakota
Fargo, North Dakota

SUSAN CASTON, MS, CRC, CCM,CDMS
Vice President/Director of Operations
The Wright Rehabilitation Service, Inc.
Roswell, Georgia

BARBARA ELLIS, RN, BA, CDMS, CCM, ABDA
Owner/President
Managed Care Strategies, Inc.
St. Louis, Missouri

CARRIE ENGEN, RN, BSN, CCM
President
Advocare, Inc.
Naperville, Illinois

KAY EVANS, RN, BSN
Organizational Development Specialist, Strategic Learning
Mercy Healthcare Sacramento
Sacramento, California

JUDY A. HARRIS, BSN, MS
Healthy Start, Nurse Abstractor
Tallahassee, Florida

TERRY KELLEY, RN, BSN, PHN, CCM
Manager, Health Care Services
Foundation Health Federal Services
Rancho Cordova, California

KAREN CHAMBERS KNIGHT, RN, CCM, CDMS
Director, Medical Management
Medical Services Department
GuideStar Health Systems, Inc.
Birmingham, Alabama

ANNE LLEWELLYN, RNC, BPSHSP, CCM, CRRn, CEAC
Owner, Educational Company
Staff Nurse—ER
Independent Case Manager
Plantation, Florida

SANDRA LOWERY, RN, BSN, CRRN, CCM
President and Senior Consultant
CCMI Associates
Francestown, New Hampshire

MINDY OWEN, RN, CRRN, CCM
Corporate Director
Complex Care Management
Glen Ellyn, Illinois

CYNTHIA A. PARKMAN, RN, BSN, MSN
Nursing Faculty (Instructor)
Division of Nursing
California State University—Sacramento
Sacramento, California

JULIA A. RIEVE, RN, BSHCM, CCM, CPHQ, FNAHQ
President
CQI: A Healthcare Management Services Company
San Diego, California

Foreword

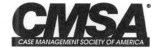

Case management is dynamic, requiring an ongoing study of the process, structure, and knowledge domains utilized by those of us who diligently practice in the fragile nucleus of patient-centered care. This core curriculum is a collaborative attempt by the Case Management Society of America (CMSA), the authors, and the editors to address an insatiable need to define the essential components of case management. It is an attempt to capture the essence of a practice that is rapidly evolving around the globe to meet the diverse and ever-changing needs of world health. It is a work in progress.

CMSA would like to acknowledge the dedication of Suzanne Powell and Donna Ignatavicius in pursuing our commitment as an organization to the ongoing education and advancement of case managers. Whether they are practitioners, engage in consulting, mentor colleagues, or instruct students, case management professionals collectively advance case management each time they pursue knowledge and excellence in practice.

In this spirit CMSA also acknowledges your commitment as the reader to pursue a greater understanding of perhaps the most evolutionary and revolutionary health care practice setting of the 20th century. As we embark on the 21st century, CMSA encourages you to share the vision and to be an active part of the dynamic case management culture—an advocacy culture that positively affects quality, cost-effective outcomes in health care worldwide.

Kathleen Moreo, RN, Cm, BSN, BPSHSA, CCM, CDMS, CEAC
1999–2000 CMSA President

Preface

Change. Perhaps the generation alive today knows more about this experience than at any previous time. In our own world of health care, professionals have seen the devastation of diseases that attack the core of human survival (the immune system); we have also seen health care "management" techniques that attack the core of the provider–patient relationship. The health care system rapidly and insidiously became more complex—so complex, in fact, that the average person could no longer navigate the course.

In the 1980s a group of health care professionals of various credentials intuitively knew that strict utilization review techniques were not addressing the major economic and ethical problems. The methods some organizations utilized to "review" for "medical necessity" became an additional barrier between the patient and his or her medical needs. So, in grassroots fashion and on a case-by-case basis, case managers began managing out-of-control resource utilization while helping to ensure quality of care and patient satisfaction. At this point, most case managers were learning the job through trial-and-error (or less eloquently, by the "seat of their pants"). There was a lack of published information to help chart the way.

Case management continued to grow and, realizing the fiscal possibilities, managed care organizations (MCOs) encouraged the concept. Case managers were now working throughout the continuum to coordinate patient care. Population-specific case management, or disease management, evolved case management from a case-by-case event to one in which entire groups of people could benefit.

Now there are many books and periodicals about various aspects of case management. Further, the *Case Management Society of America* (CMSA), founded in 1990, continues to promote the development of professional case management through annual conferences, through the development of the *Standards of Practice for Case Management* and the *Ethics Statement on Case Management Practice,* and through several critical task forces to enhance research and knowledge pertinent to the case management profession. *CMS International (CMSI)* communicates with members in Australia, New Zealand, Canada, the United Kingdom, Puerto Rico, South Africa, and Germany. Interested groups are forming in China, Japan, Singapore, and Spain.

This curriculum, sponsored by CMSA, represents a synthesis of the case management evolution. The chapters, which have been written by topic experts, identify and develop essential issues, such as:

- Introduction to Case Management Concepts
- The Case Management Process
- Disease Management
- The Health Care Delivery System and Managed Care (Insurance Issues)
- Utilization Management
- Legal Issues in Case Management
- Ethical Issues in Case Management
- Quality Reviews and Risk Management
- Credentials, Organizations, Guidelines, and Standards
- Case Management Technology, Tools, Pathways and Protocols
- Workers' Compensation Case Management
- Disability Case Management
- Occupational Health Case Management
- Behavioral Health Case Management
- Maternal-Infant Case Management
- Pediatric Case Management
- Geriatric Case Management
- Leadership Skills and Financial Management
- Outcomes Management
- Continuous Quality Improvement (CQI)
- Complementary and Alternative Medicine (CAM)

It is important to note that curricula are essentially an overview of each topic; although they are usually in an outline format, these chapters contain a great deal of useful information, charts, graphs, examples, tables, and supporting material for further study. The broad scope of pertinent case management issues lends itself to several useful purposes as a teaching tool and reference for

- College and university curriculum
- Orientation and training within an organization or facility
- Study parameters for various credentials
- Accreditation basics
- Self-orientation when beginning a "new" case management career

Case management is a major solution to a truly economic and humanitarian problem. It will continue to grow because it works! New additions to the second edition of the curriculum are already being planned. No longer do case managers have to learn their role by flying by the seat of their pants. We would like to thank CMSA and all the contributors for their expertise and dedication to this project. They are truly a group of special individuals who shared their knowledge for the greater growth of the case management profession.

Suzanne K. Powell
Donna Ignatavicius

Acknowledgments

The authors would like to thank the contributors who dedicated so much of their time and expertise to this important work. Your devotion to case management is evident in your work and we thank you!

We would also like to thank the Board of the Case Management Society of America for all of their input and encouragement throughout the writing process, and for putting their faith in us and our abilities.

Last, but certainly not least, we would like to thank Senior Editor Jennifer Brogan for all of her support and guidance during this project, and Editorial Assistant Susan Barta Rainey for coordinating this truly collaborative effort. Thank you!

Contents

■ Chapter **7** / Ethical Issues in Case Management   83

■ Chapter **8** / Quality Reviews and Risk
Management   89

■ Chapter **9** / Credentialing, Accreditation,
Standards, and Pathways in
Case Management   99

■ Chapter **10** / Case Management Tools and
Technology   115

■ Chapter 11 / Workers' Compensation Case Management   145

SHARON BRIM

■ Chapter **12** / Disability Case Management   181

LESLEY WRIGHT, MARTHA HEATH EGGLESTON,
DEBORAH V. DiBENEDETTO

■ Chapter **13** / Occupational Health Case
      Management   195

DEBORAH V. DiBENEDETTO

CHAPTER 1

Introduction to Case Management Concepts

MARLYS A. SEVERSON

LEARNING OBJECTIVES

Upon completion of this chapter, the reader will be able to:

1. Recognize the development of case management over the past century and identify the impetus for its rapid growth over the past two decades.
2. Differentiate the various models of case management and state the criteria for consideration prior to implementation.
3. List the purposes and goals of case management.
4. Define the domains of case management.
5. Identify the functions of case management.
6. Distinguish the job functions and activities of the case manager.
7. Describe the core competencies of case management.
8. Indicate the knowledge levels & skill sets necessary to practice case management.
9. List various disciplines of case management practitioners and the potential practice settings.

IMPORTANT TERMS AND CONCEPTS

American Nurses Association (ANA)
Case Management
Certification for Case Management
  (CCM)

Case Management Models
Case Management Process
Case Management Society of America
  (CMSA)

Commission for Case Management Certification	Foundation for Rehabilitation Education and Research
Core Competencies of Case Management	National Association of Rehabilitation Professionals in the Private Sector (NARPPS)
Domains of Case Management	

■ INTRODUCTION

A. Historical perspective
1. Early 1900s—Public health nurses and social workers coordinated services through the public health sector.
2. 1920s—Psychiatry and social work focused on long-term, chronic illnesses, managed in the outpatient, community setting.
3. 1930s—Public health visiting nurses used community-based case management approaches in their patient care.
4. 1943—Liberty Mutual used in-house case management/rehabilitation as a cost-containment measure for workers' compensation.
5. World War II—insurance companies employed nurses and social workers to assist with the coordination of care for soldiers returning from the war who suffered complex injuries requiring multidisciplinary intervention.
6. 1966—Insurance Company of North America (now CIGNA) led by George Welch developed an in-house program that incorporated vocational rehabilitation and case management, which later became known as Intracorp.
7. 1970s—Insurance companies used case management services with a focus on cost containment due to the double-digit inflation rate for medical costs.
8. 1971—Medicaid and Medicare demonstration projects employed social workers to arrange for and coordinate medical and social services to defined patient populations (low income, mentally ill, frail elderly).
9. 1980s—Types of case managers increased with focus varying depending on the type of organization, the target population, and the discipline of the case manager. Focus was on cost containment.
10. 1990s—Number of case managers increased to an estimate of greater than 100,000. Cost containment remained important, but the focus grew to include quality management issues.

B. Impetus for the explosive growth of case management
1. Cost of health care—Increasing amount of the gross domestic product (GDP) that goes toward health care, as compared with global competitors. In early 1990s, one-seventh of the United States GDP went toward the payment for health care (Cohen, 1996).
2. Increasing consumerism secondary to more accessible information, increased expectations of patient involvement on the part of health plans, and negative repercussions of managed care

3. New emphasis on complementary alternative medicine with limited reimbursement by health plans
4. Information explosion through technological, genetic, and medical advances
5. Emphasis on results and accountability
6. Changes in the health care delivery system and reimbursement for care
7. Increased fragmentation of care owing to the changes in health care delivery and reimbursement

■ KEY DEFINITIONS

A. *Case Management*

1. Case management is a system of health care delivery designed to facilitate achievement of expected patient outcomes within an appropriate length of stay. The goals of case management are the provision of quality health care along a continuum, decreased fragmentation of care across settings, enhancement of the client's quality of life, efficient utilization of patient care resources, and cost containment (ANA, 1988).
2. Case management is the process of getting the right service to the right client (Yee, 1990).
3. Case management is a health care delivery process whose goals are to provide quality health care, decrease fragmentation, enhance the client's quality of life, and contain costs (ANA, 1991).
4. Case management is a clinical system used for selected individuals who are chosen based on a particular diagnostic category or targeted within a diagnostic category because they represent a higher risk than the rest of the population within that category. Ideally, case management should be employed across the continuum of care—over a variety of settings and over time—to coordinate the delivery of care.
5. Medical case management is defined as the process of assessing, planning, coordinating, monitoring, and evaluating the services required to respond to an individual's health care needs to attain the goals of quality and cost effective care.
6. Case management is a collaborative process that assesses, plans, implements, coordinates, monitors, and evaluates the options and services required to meet an individual's health needs, using communication and available resources to promote quality and cost-effective outcomes (CCM/CMSA, 1993).
7. The purpose of care coordination is to work directly with clients and families over time to assist them in arranging and managing the complex set of resources that the client requires to maintain health and independent functioning. Care coordination seeks to achieve the maximum cost-effective use of scarce resources by helping clients get the health, social, and support services most appropriate for their needs at a given time. It guides the client and family through the maze of services, matches service needs with funding authorization, and coordinates with clinician and provider organizations (Williams & Torrens, 1993).

8. Case management is a method of managing the provision of health care to members with catastrophic or high-cost medical conditions. The goal is to coordinate the care so as to improve continuity and quality of care as well as lower costs (Kongsvedt, 1993).

9. Case management is a multidisciplinary clinical system that uses registered nurse case managers to coordinate the care for selected patients across the continuum of a health care episode (Frank & Strassner, 1996).

10. Nursing case management is an approach that focuses on the coordination, integration, and direct delivery of patient services and places internal controls on the resources used for care. . .A nursing care delivery system that supports cost-effective, patient outcome oriented care (Cohen & Cesta, 1997).

11. Case management is a coordination of a specific group of services on behalf of a specific group of people. Case management can also be defined by listing its component processes. By widespread agreement, these processes include screening or case finding; comprehensive multidimensional assessment; care planning; implementation of the plan; monitoring; and reassessment (Cesta, 1998; Kane, 1998; Powell, 2000).

B. *Case Management Domains*—The case manager's sphere of influence and activity. These domains, which were defined by a 1999 study completed by the Foundation for Rehabilitation Education and Research, are Processes and Relationships, Health Care Management, Community Resources and Support, Service Delivery, Psychosocial Intervention, and Rehabilitation Case Management (CCM, 1999).

C. *Case Management Model*—The organizational structure within which the case manager functions.

D. *Case Management Process*—The essential activities of case management

1. *Assessment*—Process of collecting in-depth information about a person's situation and functioning to identify individual needs in order to develop a comprehensive case management plan that will address those needs

2. *Planning*—The process of determining specific objectives, goals, and actions designed to meet the patient's needs as identified through the assessment process

3. *Implementation*—The process of executing specific case management activities or interventions, or both, that will lead to accomplishing the goals set forth in the case management plan

4. *Coordination*—The process of organizing, securing, integrating, and modifying the resources necessary to accomplish the goals set forth in the case management plan

5. *Monitoring*—The ongoing process of gathering sufficient information from all relevant sources about the case management plan and its activities or services to enable the case manager to determine the plan's effectiveness

6. *Evaluation*—The process, repeated at appropriate intervals, of deter-

mining the case management plan's effectiveness in reaching desired outcomes and goals (CMSA, 1999)

E. *Case Management Society of America (CMSA)*—A nonprofit, multidisciplinary, interdisciplinary, international society of case management and allied health care professionals with a mission of "Advancing Case Management. . .To promote the growth and value of case management and to support the evolving needs of the case management professional" (CMSA, 1999)

G. *Commission for Case Manager Certification*—Independent credentialing agency solely responsible for the CCM certification process

H. *Critical Paths*—A paper-and-pencil system for outlining the course of events for treating a particular DRG for each day of hospitalization (Cesta, 1998)

I. *Essential Job Functions*—Job activities essential for case management performance (Chan, 1999)

J. *Foundation for Rehabilitation Education and Research*—501-c-3 organization dedicated to research. They commissioned the 1999 study on Case Management Knowledge and Practice Domains.

K. *Managed Care*—"a set of techniques used by or on behalf of purchasers of healthcare benefits to manage healthcare costs by influencing patient care decision-making through case-by-case assessment of the appropriateness of care prior to its provision. The implementation of managed care strategies follows a series of other cost control measures including insurance benefit limitations and exclusions, prepaid health plans, prospective payment system and fee schedules" (Powell, 2000; Williams & Torrens, 1993).

L. *Practice Setting*—The organization in which the case manager is employed and functions

■ CASE MANAGEMENT MODELS

A. Types of models—Multiple case management models are described in the literature. They are broken down by a number of methodologies, such as setting, patient diagnosis, or payer source. The following models are organized by the practice setting in which the case manager works with examples of organizations that utilized that model.

    1. Acute Care Models—Acute care models are the most often cited models in case management literature. The focus of the case management services in the acute care setting is on one episode of care from admission to discharge. In many instances, it encompasses utilization management or discharge planning functions. Typically, registered nurses or social workers provide the case management services, and they may or may not function within a multidisciplinary environment or provide direct patient care. When possible, the facility that published the model was listed.

        a. Beth Israel Multidisciplinary Patient Care Model
          They used the concept of primary and team nursing to support the coordination and management of the care of patient from admis-

sion to discharge. No direct patient care services were provided, and the case managers used multidisciplinary action plans to record expected outcomes and progress. The program objectives were improved quality and satisfaction, decreased length of stay, and controlled resource utilization.

This type of model, in which the case manager is responsible for the management and coordination of patient care needs but provides no direct patient care, is also termed a "Leveled Practice Model."

b. Dyad model
   Case management functions are provided by a nurse or a social worker, depending on the needs of the patient served.

c. Hermann Hospital—Houston, TX
   Another primary case management model, with the case managers being unit based, using care plans as the tool to monitor and evaluate care.

d. Long Island College Hospital—Brooklyn, NY
   Their model was essentially the same as that of Beth Israel, but they used clinical nurse specialist to perform the functions of case management.

e. New England Medical Center—Boston, MA
   Primary Nurse Case Management Model—The case managers carried a core group of patients for whom they provided direct patient care. The process was outcome driven, using case management plans, critical path reports, and variance analysis to manage, document, and evaluate care and outcomes.

f. Social work case management
   The focus of service delivery is on social, financial, and discharge needs of the client.

g. St. Joseph Mercy Hospital's Pontiac Project
   A collaborative practice model in the medical-surgical unit that used critical paths and patient care teaching plans to focus care and resources for high-risk clients.

h. St. Michael Hospital- Milwaukee, WI
   Expanded the practice concepts used at New England Medical Center and coordinated care through the use of critical paths and a comprehensive variance analysis system.

i. Tucson Medical Center Case Management Model
   Collaborative nursing case management. Incorporated elements of the New England Medical Center's model. Focused on standardizing resource use and service delivery for selected Diagnostic Related Groups (DRGs) through the use of collaborative case management plans that identified the contributions to all health care providers and supported a unit-specific standard of patient care.

j. Utilization review nurse case manager
   The traditional utilization view role is eliminated, and the staff are converted to the position of case managers. Utilization review is changed to utilization management, and the discharge planning function is added.

2. Community-Based Models—Community-based models can provide case management services throughout the continuum of care or at a specific practice setting. Additionally, it can be in either a provider or payer setting.
   a. Carondelet St. Mary's Health Care—Tucson, AZ
      Initially, this model was designed as acute care case management model, but the case manager was responsible for management along the continuum. The population serviced initially was high risk but later moved to moderate risk and low risk. Services were provided in nurse-managed and neighborhood-accessible community health centers. This was the first funded community nursing organization—a risk-adjusted, capitated, nurse-managed ambulatory system of care. In 1989, they developed a nursing HMO (1989) to provide health care and support services to elderly, chronically ill, and disabled individuals within a Medicare Senior Plan Contract.
   b. Community-Based Case Management
      The focus of the program is on primary care and primary prevention. It serves well individuals who are at risk and have the potential for needing health care services.
   c. Mercy Hospital's Port Huron Project
      Case management was incorporated into the community health care system through collaborative practice arrangements. Preventive education program and outpatient services such as home care and respite were incorporated into the system.
   d. Primary Care Case Management
      The focus is on the role of gatekeeper, focusing on the treatment of health problems, maintaining the individual in the lowest level of care possible. The case manager is either a physician or an advanced practice nurse.
   e. Silver Spring Community Nursing Center; University of Wisconsin-Milwaukee
      This was a family-oriented model whose goal was to support and empower individuals and families to use their personal and community resources to achieve an optimal level of health and well-being for all family members (Cohen, 1996).
   f. Saint Joseph Medical Center's Community-based Nursing Case Management—Wichita, KS
      This organization developed a multidisciplinary, multiservice model that focused on coordination of services and management of the patient. It collaborated with a local school of nursing on educational issues and on the incorporation of other disciplines into the model.
3. Geriatric Care Management
   a. Medical-Social Case Management
      Team approach focusing on the long-term-care population. Coordinates services that are usually not covered by insurance plans to prevent institutionalization.
   b. Private Geriatric Case Management

Provides social and health access and coordination to the elderly, with an emphasis on long-term-care issues, maintaining them in the lowest level of care.

4. Independent Case Management/Entrepreneurial Models
   The practitioner practices either independently or under the auspices of a case management firm. Case management inventions are provided throughout the continuum of care to reach mutually agreed-on outcomes. There is no provision of direct patient care. The focus is on enabling the patient to make the needed transitions through the health care delivery system, monitoring resource utilization, managing costs, and providing quality services.

5. Integrated Delivery System Model—Systems Model
   The case manager is assigned to the case at one of seven defined access points, depending on where services were provided. The responsibility for case management resides at the location where the patient is receiving care, and continuity is maintained by providing referral and tracking services.

6. Long-Term or Chronic Care Case Management Model
   Much like geriatric case management, long-term or chronic care case management provides for social and health needs but serves other populations with long-term care and chronic care needs.

7. Managed Care Model
   The main objective of the model is to contain costs by controlling utilization and coordinating care. Two types of case managers are described:
   a. Financial case manager—functions in a traditional utilization management model, and the role is high volume/low intensity
   b. Clinical case manager—the focus is on high-intensity/low-volume interventions with high-risk patient populations (Cesta, 1998).

8. Provider-Based Case Management Models
   Provides coordination and management services to patients service by the agency. Role can be seen in home health, durable medical equipment, or home infusion companies. This role becomes paramount in capitated reimbursement systems. It may or may not include direct staff supervision.

9. Others
   a. Weil and Karls (1985)—Describe three case management models:
      (1) Generalist case manager or broker model
          Structured to provide direct service, access, planning, and monitoring activities to patients. The case manager acts as a broker and is involved in the intake, coordination, and evaluation of care provided.
      (2) Primary therapist as case manager model—Emphasizes a therapeutic relationship between the case manager and the patient. The case manager is required to have a master's degree and training in psychology, social work, psychiatry, or psychiatric clinical nursing specialties.

(3) Interdisciplinary team model—Focuses on providing case management services through a collaborative team approach. Responsibilities and functions are divided among the team members according to their area of specialization. One team member is responsible for maintaining overall service coordination and evaluation (Cohen, 1996).

B. Selecting the most effective model

There are multiple considerations when adapting a case management model. They include the elements of the patient population served, issues surrounding the organization providing case management, and the funding source.

1. Patient Population
    a. Age
    b. Educational level
    c. Financial resources
    d. Most frequent diagnoses
    e. Geographic location—rural versus suburban
    f. Recidivism
2. Organizational Issues
    a. Mission
    b. Vision
    c. Long-term and short-term goals of the organization
    d. Organizational structure
    e. Strengths
    f. Human resources
3. Funding Source
    a. Reimbursement system
    b. Regulatory agencies

■ TARGET PATIENT POPULATIONS

A. Diagnostic category (DRG)
1. Acute injury or illness
2. Chronic illness
3. Complex treatment plan

B. Potential for large consumption of resources
1. Financial
2. Community

C. Frail and elderly

D. Hospitalized

E. Procedure (e.g., chest physiotherapy [CPT])

■ CASE MANAGEMENT PHILOSOPHY

"All individuals, particularly those suffering from catastrophic and/or high risk or costly injuries or illnesses, should be afforded the services of a case manager regardless of the client's ability to pay" (CMSA, 1995).

■ CASE MANAGEMENT ROLE

A. Collaborate, through the case management process, to meet the health needs on an individual basis (CMSA, 1995).

B. May include the arena of job modification and assistance with transitional return-to-work programs (Siefker, 1998).

C. Facilitate the delivery of cost-efficient, individualized, and coordinated care to patients and patients with chronic illnesses and disabilities (Chan et al., 1999).

■ PURPOSE AND GOALS OF CASE MANAGEMENT

A. Purposes

1. Interject objectivity and information where it is lacking
2. Maximize efficiency in use of available resources
3. Work collaboratively with patient, physician, family/significant other, and the health care provider to implement a plan of care that meets the individual's needs.
4. Promote the optimal allocation of health dollars through effective and efficient use of resources (CMSA, 1995).

B. Goals

1. Through early assessment, ensure that services are generated in a time and cost-effective manner
2. Assist patients to achieve an optimal level of wellness and function by facilitating timely and appropriate health services
3. Assist patients to self-direct care appropriately, self-advocate, and make informed decisions to the degree possible
4. Maintain cost effectiveness in the provision of health services
5. Appropriate expenditure of claims dollars and timely claim determinations
6. Enhance employee productivity, satisfaction, and retention, when applicable (CMSA, 1995)
7. Resolve medical issues
8. Empower the patient to make informed decisions
9. Return the patient to work or assess the patient's ability to return to work and develop a plan that will assist the patient in returning to work or becoming employable.
10. Enhancement of quality of care (Siefker et al., 1995)

■ CASE MANAGEMENT FUNCTIONS

The Standards of Practice for Case Management describe four case management functions.

A. Assessor

Obtaining and evaluating relevant information (medical, psychosocial, functional, vocational and financial) through interviews with all parties

B. Planner

From the information gathered, a needs list is developed and prioritized, with input from all parties. The patient and family are active decision makers in the process. Contingency plans are developed and instituted as necessary.

C. Facilitator

The focus is on communication and collaboration with all parties to enhance patient care and maximize outcomes.

D. Advocate

Until the patient is able, the case manager advocates for the services and funding necessary to meet the established goals. Education and support is provided to encourage patient empowerment and self-reliance. Throughout this process, the patient's best interests remain paramount.

■ ESSENTIAL JOB ACTIVITIES

In 1999, the Foundation for Rehabilitation Education and Research commissioned a study looking at case management essential job activities. They are ranged in their order of importance based on study results. As the list is so inclusive and all encompassing, it is listed in its entirety.

A. Very important to extremely important job functions

1. Conducting assessment of the patient (medical, psychological, social, environmental, vocational, financial)
2. Synthesizing assessment information to prioritize care needs and develop treatment plans
3. Conducting and performing medical case management functions
4. Communicating with clients, family, treating physicians, other service providers, attorneys, and payors
5. Monitoring and evaluating the patient's response to treatment and revising treatment plans as needed
6. Researching alternative treatment options and selecting and locating appropriate providers
7. Providing education, information, direction, and support related to care goals of clients
8. Acting as an advocate for the patient and family with third-party payors and service providers
9. Implementing care and treatment plans
10. Performing case management functions (e.g., coordinating community resource services, documentation, and functional assessments)

11. Performing case recording, documentation, and report writing functions
12. Coordinating acquisition of medical equipment (including assessment, negotiation, proper use, and follow-up)
13. Engaging in professional development activities to keep abreast of state of the art case management practices
14. Implementing conflict resolution strategies with client
15. Performing case identification, selection, and outreach functions
16. Performing advocacy and intervention functions
17. Preparing discharge plan

B. Important job functions
1. Reviewing and coordinating health care, worker's compensation, and government insurance benefits related to care needs of clients
2. Reviewing medical records and employment-related information
3. Performing return-to-work functions
4. Researching and securing funding, community resources, and support needed for community reentry
5. Conducting home visits and on-site visits with employers and physicians; inspecting and selecting facilities that provide specialized care services for clients
6. Evaluating, purchasing, and coordinating the acquisition of appropriate assistive technologies for adaptive, accommodative, or job modification purposes
7. Performing early intervention functions with disabled workers, treating physicians, and others to meet safe and timely return to work objectives
8. Educating other stakeholders regarding the role and value of case managers in health care
9. Monitoring and evaluating the impact of case management outreach, community living, return-to-work, and overall program outcomes
10. Developing methodologies to measure case management outcomes meaningful to the payor (e.g., return-to-work rate, improved functional work status, improved health status, disability cost reduction, reduced lost time, disability cost savings, and worker and employer satisfaction)
11. Attending team conferences
12. Networking for relationship building and resource development
13. Negotiating cost-effective rates for services purchased
14. Performing program evaluation and research functions to document improvements in patient outcomes, cost savings, patient compliance, and return to productivity
15. Coordinating and facilitating health promotion, illness and disability prevention, and health education activities
16. Performing prevention and wellness program functions (e.g., health counseling and health education)

17. Preparing a life care plan
18. Conducting job analyses and job accommodation activities to facilitate prevention of disability or injury

C. Less than important job functions
1. Performing administrative and coordination functions related to the operation of a case management program
2. Promoting and marketing the case management program
3. Performing job placement or out-placement services
4. Performing utilization review functions (Chan et al., 1999)

■ CORE COMPONENTS OF CASE MANAGEMENT—CASE MANAGEMENT DOMAINS

A. Processes and relationships
1. Interpersonal communication skills
2. Interpersonal relationship skills
3. Case recording and documentation
4. Clinical problem-solving and critical-thinking skills
5. Case management process and tools
6. Basic interviewing skills
7. Negotiation and conflict resolution strategies

B. Health care management
1. Medical case management
2. Medical aspects of acute and chronic illness and disability
3. Goals and objectives of case management
4. Health care ethics
5. Assessment of physical functioning
6. Legal aspects of case management
7. Medical and allied health professions
8. Clinical pharmacology

C. Community resources and support
1. Levels of care (e.g. hospital, extended care facility, subacute facility, home)
2. Community resources and support programs
3. Rehabilitation service delivery systems
4. Public benefit programs (e.g., SSI, SSID, Medicare, Medicaid)
5. Assistive technology

D. Service delivery
1. Managed care concepts
2. Cost-containment procedures and strategies
3. Health care benefits
4. Critical pathways, standards of care, practice guidelines
5. Health care delivery systems

    6. Health care and disability related legislation
    7. Cost-benefit analysis
    8. Wellness and illness prevention concepts and strategies
    9. Case management models
   10. Utilization management
   11. Program evaluation and research (e.g., outcomes and satisfaction)
   12. Risk management and insurance principles
   13. Integrated benefits systems

E. Psychosocial intervention
    1. Family dynamics
    2. Multicultural issues and health behavior
    3. Psychosocial aspects of chronic illness and disability
    4. Psychological and neuropsychological assessment
    5. Mental health and psychiatric disability concepts
    6. Substance use, abuse, and addiction
    7. Managed behavioral health care

F. Rehabilitation case management
    1. Disability compensation systems (e.g., worker's compensation, auto insurance, LTD, STD, accident and health)
    2. Job analysis, job modification, job accommodation
    3. Work adjustment and work transition
    4. Vocational aspects of chronic illness and disability
    5. Work-hardening resources and strategies
    6. Ergonomics
    7. Vocational assessment
    8. Job development and placement
    9. Barrier-free architectural design
   10. Life care planning (CCM, 1999)

■ CASE MANAGEMENT KNOWLEDGE AREAS

The same previously mentioned study conducted by the Foundation for Rehabilitation Education and Research also evaluated case management knowledge areas. They are ranged in their order of importance based on study results. Because the list is so inclusive and all-encompassing, it is listed in its entirety.

A. Very to extremely important
    1. Medical case management
    2. The goals and objectives of case management
    3. Medical aspects of acute and chronic illness and disability
    4. Assessment (physical status, psychosocial adjustment, and vocational functioning)
    5. Communication skills (oral and written)
    6. Legal aspects of case management

7. Health care ethics
8. Case recording and documentation
9. Health care terminology
10. Basic interpersonal communication skills
11. Case management process and tools
12. The definition, philosophy, and values of case management
13. Negotiation and conflict resolution strategies
14. Clinical problem-solving and critical thinking skills
15. Interpersonal relationship skills
16. Psychosocial aspects of chronic illness and disability
17. Medical aspects of chronic illness and disability
18. Levels of care (e.g., hospital, extended care facility, subacute facility, and home)
19. Community resources and support programs
20. Basic interviewing skills
21. Knowledge of medical and allied health professions
22. Managed care concepts
23. Health care benefits
24. Psychosocial aspects of chronic illness and disability
25. Health care, employment, disability-related legislation (e.g., ADA, EEOC, FMLS, ERISA) compliance strategies, and program interventions.
26. Family dynamics

B. Important
1. Critical pathways, standards of care, practice guidelines
2. Theory and techniques of case management and case load management
3. Advocacy, negotiation, and conflict resolution techniques
4. Multicultural issues and health behavior
5. Managed health care, managed behavioral health care, and managed care worker's compensation systems (including utilization review and quality assurance)
6. Assistive technology for people with disabilities
7. Public benefit programs (e.g., SSDI, SSI)
8. Rehabilitation service delivery systems
9. Risk management and insurance principles
10. Cost-containment procedures, strategies, and analysis
11. Cost–benefit analysis
12. Wellness and illness prevention concepts and strategies
13. Case management models
14. Integrated benefits systems
15. Mental health and psychiatric disability concepts (e.g., stress management in the workplace, accommodating psychiatric disabilities)
16. Job analysis, job modification, and job accommodation

17. Health care economics
18. Theory and techniques of counseling
19. Health care and disability and rehabilitation systems
20. Vocational aspects of chronic illness and disability
21. Clinical pharmacology
22. Program evaluation and research (e.g., outcomes and satisfaction)
23. Vocational rehabilitation systems (public and private)
24. Substance use, abuse, and addiction
25. Occupational rehabilitation (e.g., work adjustment, work transition, and work-hardening resources and strategies)
26. Organizational consulting intervention skills
27. Teaching, training and presentation techniques
28. Utilization management
29. Vocational rehabilitation concepts
30. Health care information systems
31. Ergonomics
32. Job placement and job development

C. Important
1. Utilization review
2. Financial counseling
3. Labor market information (Chan et al., 1999)

■ CASE MANAGEMENT SKILL SET

The role of the case manager is a complex and demanding one. A variety of skills are necessary to accomplish the outcomes that are being demanded.

A. Apply problem-solving techniques to the case management process.

B. Assess variables that affect health and functioning.

C. Interpret clinical information and assess implications for treatment.

D. Develop an individualized case management plan that addresses the patient's physical, vocational, psychosocial, financial, and educational needs.

E. Negotiate competitive rates to maximize available funding for an individual's care.

F. Understand the language used in insurance policies.

G. Present various health care options.

H. Document case management activities.

I. Maintain confidentiality regarding the release of information according to legal and ethical requirements and guidelines.

J. Maintain familiarity with disease processes, available resources, and treatment modalities, assessing their quality and appropriateness for specific disabilities, illnesses, and injuries (Chan et al., 1999).

K. Positive relationship building.

L. Effective written/verbal communication.

M. Ability to effect change.

N. Perform critical analysis.

O. Plan and organize effectively.

P. Promote client/family autonomy (CMSA, 1995).

Q. Assessment skills.

R. Teaching.

S. Discharge planning.

T. Team work (Powell, 2000).

U. Business skills.

■ PRACTICE SETTINGS

Case management is now practiced in a multitude of service settings. In almost any organization that provides or reimburses health care, case managers can be found. The following list is by no means all-inclusive:

A. Institutional care
  1. Acute care
  2. Subacute
  3. Skilled nursing facility

B. Insurance
  1. Public insurance
    a. Medicaid
    b. Medicare
  2. Private insurance
    a. Long-term care
    b. Disability
    c. Liability
    d. Casualty
    e. Auto liability
    f. Accident and health

C. Management care organizations
  1. Preferred Provider Organizations (PPO)
  2. Health Maintenance Organizations (HMO)
  3. Exclusive Provider Organizations (EPO)
  4. Physician Hospital Organizations (PHO)

D. Third party payors

E. Physician groups
  1. Independent Practice Associations (IPA)

2. Medical Group Practice
3. Medical Service Organizations (MSO)

F. Employer based/corporations

G. Independent case managers or case management companies

H. Government-sponsored programs

I. Provider agencies and facilities
1. Mental health
2. Home health
3. Hospice
4. Durable medical equipment
5. Home infusion

■ CASE MANAGEMENT PRACTITIONERS

Case management is an interdisciplinary and multidisciplinary process. As such, there are myriads of practitioners who provide case management services. Some of the more common are the following:

A. Disciplines of case management
1. Nurses
2. Social workers
3. Therapists
   a. Physical
   b. Occupational
   c. Respiratory
4. Physicians
5. Rehabilitation counselors
6. Dieticians

B. Determining which discipline is best
1. Population being served
   a. Most common diseases seen
   b. Needs of the population
   c. Types of services most required

REFERENCES

Case Management Society of America. (1999) The case report. *CMSA*, December.
Cesta, T., et al. (1998). *The case manager's survival guide*. St. Louis: Mosby.
Chan, F., et al. (1999). Foundational knowledge and major practice domains of case management. *The Journal of Care Management*, 5(1), 10–11, 14, 17–18, 26–28, 30.
Cohen, E. (1996). *Nurse case management in the 21st century*. St. Louis: Mosby.
Commission for Case Manager Certification. (1999) *CCM update*. Summer.
Mullahy, C. (1998). *The case manager's handbook*. Gaithersburg, MA: Aspen.
Powell, S. (2000). *Case management: A practical guide to success in managed care*. Philadelphia: Lippincott Williams & Wilkins.
Siefker, J.M. et al. (Eds.) (1998). *Fundamentals of case management*. St. Louis: Mosby.
Standards of practice for case management. (1995). Little Rock, AR: Case Management Society of America.

CHAPTER 2

. . . .

The Case Management Process

PATRICIA M. PECQUEUX

LEARNING OBJECTIVES

Upon completion of this chapter, the reader will be able to:

1. Describe the case selection process and the importance of this stage to the entire case management process.
2. Discuss the difference between the case selection process and the assessment/problem identification process.
3. Explain the major steps in the development and coordination of the case plan.
4. Discuss the differences in implementing a case management plan as an internal and external case manager.
5. Discuss the importance of the evaluation and follow-up stage of the case management process and how it relates to the development of outcomes.
6. Explain the significance of the continuous monitoring, reassessing, and re-evaluating stage of case management and how it differs from the evaluation and follow-up stage.

IMPORTANT TERMS AND CONCEPTS

Assessment
Case Identification and Selection
Continuous Case Management
Coordination and Development of the
    Treatment/Discharge Plan

Final Evaluation or Post-discharge
    Follow-Up
Implementation of the Final Plan
Problem Identification

■ INTRODUCTION

A. Each patient is unique, and the case management process needs to take into consideration the individual needs of the patient.

B. Each case manager has his or her own unique style of case management based on his or her experience, education, and creativity.

C. Some stages of the case management process may vary significantly based on the case management setting and the population served. Stages that may vary based on these variables are case selection, implementation of the plan, and evaluation and follow-up.

D. Other stages of the case management process have universal principles that apply to several types of case management. These stages are assessment/problem identification, development and coordination of the case plan, and continuous monitoring, reassessing and re-evaluation.

E. The process of case management is much broader than the nursing process. The nursing process assesses the patient for changes in the physical, medical, psychosocial and safety needs; plans how to meet these needs; implements these plans; and evaluates the results of these plans. The case management process includes collecting assessment data before the onset of the current illness; assessing the environmental, financial, and support system available to meet the identified needs; and planning future care.

■ KEY DEFINITIONS

A. Assessment—The process in which the case manager obtains factual information about the patient and family. The scope of the assessment should be broad, covering personal and environmental factors as well as medical information (Satinsky, 1995).

B. Case Selection—The first step in the case management process in which the case manager appraises the need for patient intervention through gathering relevant data and the critical, objective evaluation of those data (Case Management Society of America [CMSA], 1995).

C. Continuous Case Management—The case manager uses a method of checking, regulating, and documenting the quality of care, services, and products delivered to the patient to determine if the goals of the care plan are being achieved or if those goals remain appropriate and realistic. This part may also be called the monitoring, reassessing, and re-evaluating phase of case management (CMSA, 1995).

D. Coordination and Development of the Treatment/Discharge Plan—The case management plan identifies immediate, short-term, and ongoing needs, as well as where and how these care needs can be met. The plan sets goals and time frames for achieved goals that are appropriate to the individual and his or her family, and are agreed to by the patient or family and treatment team. The case manager also ensures that funding or community resources, or both, are available to implement the plan (CMSA, 1995).

E. Final Evaluation or Post-discharge Follow-up—The case manager employs a methodology designed to measure the patient's response to the health care services and products being delivered, while also measuring the effectiveness, necessity, and efficacy of the care plan itself, and the quality of the services and products from the providers (CMSA, 1995).

F. Implementation of the Final Plan—In this phase of case management, the patient's assessed needs have been linked up with private and community services, gaps are filled, there is no duplication of services, and the patient and support systems are in agreement with the plan. The goal of this phase is to maximize the safety and total well-being of the patient (Powell, 2000).

G. Problem Identification—Utilizing objective data gathered through careful assessment and examination of the potential for effective intervention, the case manager selects a caseload reflecting practice patterns and trends wherein patient outcome can be positively influenced (CMSA, 1995).

■ STAGES OF THE CASE MANAGEMENT PROCESS

A. Case Selection
1. A process of evaluating individuals referred for case management services based on an established set of criteria.
2. Criteria enable case manager to determine whether the patient needs case management services and the services that will be needed.
3. No single condition or diagnosis, with the exception of reportable events, is automatically a problem that necessitates full case management services.
4. An essential aspect of the case management process that enables a case manager to reduce systematically the number of cases in his or her caseload.
5. Identifies specific needs of a patient and matches those needs with specific skills of the case manager
6. Determines the need for case management
    a. Requires at least a cursory assessment to determine needs of patient
    b. All patient do not need a case manager.
    c. Case management may not be necessary if
        (i) Patient meets intensity of services or severity of illness criteria
        (ii) No major discharge barriers are identified
        (iii) If readmission is not a concern
        (iv) There are no financial barriers present
    d. Case management may be necessary when there are
        (i) Complex medical issues or comorbidities
        (ii) Complex discharge needs
        (iii) Complex social issues
7. Establishing selection criteria
    a. May be specific to the goals of the organization (i.e., rehabilitation potential, ventilator dependent)
    b. Ideally should be based on the anticipated needs of the patient
    c. Avoid exclusively using length-of-stay and claims data as selection criteria. These criteria are late indicators of case management needs. By the time the patient has exceeded the established length of stay

and maximum dollar expenditure for the diagnosis, much case management intervention could have already taken place.

   d. Criteria to be used with caution or in conjunction with other criteria include but are not limited to the following items:

     (i) Lives alone or with someone with a disability

     (ii) Age over 65 years

     (iii) Payor source

     (iv) Readmission within 15 days

     (v) Physicians

     (vi) Diagnosis or diagnosis-related group (DRG)

     (vii) Overdose (unintentional)

     (viii) Overdose (intentional)

     (ix) Alcohol and drug abuse

     (x) Eating disorder (e.g., bulimia, anorexia nervosa, failure to thrive)

     (xi) Chronic mental illness

     (xii) Alzheimer's dementia

     (xiii) Noncompliance

     (xiv) Uncooperative, manipulative, or aggressive behavior

     (xv) Miscellaneous conditions (Munchausen's syndrome)

     (xvi) Socioeconomic indicators

       (a) Suspected child abuse and neglect

       (b) Suspected elder abuse and neglect

       (c) Victim of violent crime

       (d) Homelessness

       (e) Poor living environment

       (f) No known social or family support system

       (g) Admission from an extended care facility (ECF) or sheltered living arrangement

       (h) Need for transitional care in an ECF or sheltered living arrangement

       (i) Out-of-state or out-of-country residence

       (j) Residence in rural community with limited or nonexistent services

       (k) Limited or no financial resources

       (l) No or inadequate health insurance

       (m) Single parent

       (n) Dependent in activities of daily living

       (o) Repeated admissions to acute care

       (p) Frequent visits to the emergency room (ER), family physician, or clinic

       (q) Disruptive or obstructive family member or significant other

B. Assessment or Problem Identification

1. Process that begins after the completion of the case selection process.
2. A thorough assessment must be done at this point in order to determine the needs of the patient, particularly as they relate to the discharge plan.
3. An inaccurate or poor assessment can lead to an unsafe discharge plan.
4. Identification of actual and potential problems are identified and goals are established.
5. Sources of assessment data:
   a. Patient
   b. Family physician
   c. Office and hospital medical records
   d. Ancillary staff
   e. Family
   f. Employer
6. Patient data to be collected
   a. Patient history and demographics
   b. Current medical status
   c. Nutritional status
   d. Medication assessment
   e. Financial assessment
   f. Functional assessment: environmental factors
      (i) Home environment assessment
      (ii) Activities of daily living (ADLs) assessment
   g. Psychosocial assessment
   h. Cultural and religious diversity
7. Screening and assessment tools
C. Development and Coordination of the Case Plan
1. Establishing goals
2. Prioritizing needs and goals
3. Service planning and resource allocation
D. Implementation of the Plan
1. Case managers within a facility (internal)
   a. Before discharge
   b. The day of discharge
2. Case managers outside of the facility (external)
   a. Initial checks
   b. Intermediate checks
   c. Case closure
3. Family needs:
   a. Must be assessed by the case manager and addressed with the patient's family members to help them cope with illness and hospitalization
   b. Specific needs of the family have been identified in numerous research studies (Hickey, 1990; Kleinpell, 1990; Molter, 1979).

c. The need for hope and the need for information about their family member's condition were seen as the most important of all the needs identified.

d. A key role of the case manager is communicating accurate information to the family to enable then to make informed decisions, thereby assisting them to gain understanding and a feeling of control over a difficult situation (Powell, 2000).

E. Evaluation and Follow-Up

1. Depends on the type of case management employed

2. Case evaluation

3. Case management outcomes

F. Continuous Monitoring, Reassessing, Re-evaluation

1. Frequency depends on the site where case management is provided (i.e., case management in a hospital may require more frequent follow-up than for an individual in a private home or ECF).

2. Changes in medical status

3. Changes in social stability of the patient

4. Quality of care

5. Changes in functional capacity and mobility

6. Evolving educational needs

7. Termination of case management services

REFERENCES

Blancett, S. S., & Flarey, D. L. (1996a). *Handbook of nursing case management.* Gaithersburg, MD: Aspen Publishers.

Blancett, S. S., & Flarey, D. L. (1996b). *Case studies in nursing case management.* Gaithersburg, MD: Aspen Publishers.

Case Management Society of America (1996). *Code of professional conduct for case managers.* Rolling Meadows, IL: Commission for Case Management Certification.

Case Management Society of America (1995). *Standards of practice for case management.* Little Rock, AR: Case Management Society of America.

Cohen, E. L. (1996). *Nursing case management in the 21st century.* St. Louis: Mosby.

Cohen, E. L., & Cesta, T. G. (1993). *Nursing case management: From concept to evaluation.* St. Louis: Mosby.

Donovan, M. E., & Matson, T. A. (Eds.) (1994). *Outpatient case management.* Chicago: American Hospital Publishing, Inc.

Etheredge, M. L. S. (1989). *Collaborative care: Nursing case management.* Chicago: American Hospital Publishing, Inc.

Hickey, M. (1990). What are the needs of families of critically ill patients? *Heart and Lung, 19*(4), 401–415.

Kleinpell, R.M. (1990). Needs of families of critically ill patients: A literature review. *Critical Care Nurse, 11*(8), 34–40.

Kongstvedt, P. R. (1993). *The managed care handbook* (2nd ed.). Gaithersburg, MD: Aspen Publishers, Inc.

Molter, N. (1979). Needs of the relatives of critically ill patients: A descriptive study. *Heart and Lung, 8*(2), 332–339.

Mullahy, C. M. (1995). *The case manager's handbook.* Gaithersburg, MD: Aspen Publishers, Inc.

Powell, S. K. (2000). *Case management: A practical guide to success in managed care.* Philadelphia: Lippincott Williams & Wilkins.

Raymond, A. G. (1994). *The HMO health care companion.* New York: Harper Perennial.

Satinsky, M. A. (1995). *An executive guide to case management strategies.* Chicago: American Hospital Publishing, Inc.

Todd, W., & Nash, D. (1996). *Disease management: A systems approach to improving patient outcomes.* Chicago: American Hospital Publishing, Inc.

CHAPTER 3

. . . .

Disease Management

SUZANNE K. POWELL

LEARNING OBJECTIVES

Upon completion of this chapter, the reader will be able to:

1. Determine the similarities and differences between case management and disease management strategies.
2. Define important terms and concepts relative to disease management.
3. List the driving forces that lead to disease management programs.
4. Discuss important components to building a successful disease management program.
5. Describe factors that are important to the development and design of a disease management program.
6. Identify the stages of the case management or disease management process.

IMPORTANT TERMS AND CONCEPTS

"At-Risk" Member
Best Practices
Component Management Model
Continuous Quality Improvement (CQI)
Cross-Functional Team
Demand Management
Disease Management Model
Disease Management Society (DMS)
Disease State Case Management (DSCM)
Disease State Management
Evidenced-Based Guidelines
Health Plan Employer Data and Information Set (HEDIS)
Multidisciplinary Team
National Committee for Quality Assurance (NCQA)

Outcomes Measurement	Practice Parameters
Pilot Project	Quality Indicators (QI)
Practice Guidelines	Report Card

■ INTRODUCTION

A. Case management as a component of disease management versus disease management as a component of case management

B. Case management: use of an *individual*-based approach; disease management: use of a *population*-based approach

■ KEY DEFINITIONS

A. *Disease State Management and Disease State Case Management (DSCM):*

1. Disease management uses a set of prospectively determined interventions with the intent of altering the course of the disease, improving clinical and financial outcomes as well as quality of life, while reducing health care costs. The goal is prevention of exacerbation of illness and reduction of the effects of co-morbidities, thereby avoiding or delaying the onset of acute episodes of illness (Powell, 2000b).

2. Disease management brings together outcomes research and clinical management of diseases to provide efficient care to patient populations in a continuous quality improvement environment. Furthermore, disease management is a continuous process focused on efficiency and is applied to selected patient populations (Nash & Todd, 1997).

3. Disease management is a comprehensive, integrated approach to care and reimbursement based on a disease's natural course, focusing on clinical and nonclinical interventions when and where they are most likely to have the greatest impact. Ideally, disease management prevents exacerbation of a disease and use of expensive resources, making prevention and proactive case management two important areas of emphasis (Rieve, 1998).

4. *The Disease Management Society (DMS)* definitions:

   a. The "ideal" definition: A clinical management process of care that spans the continuum of care from primary prevention to ongoing long-term maintenance for individuals with chronic health conditions or diagnoses.

   b. The "working" definition: The process of caring for patients using standardized treatment strategies that ensure appropriate utilization and high-quality care across the continuum.

5. Disease state case management (DSCM) is a population-based approach that identifies individuals with chronic diseases, assesses their health status, develops a program or plan of care, and collects data to evaluate the effectiveness of the process. DSCM proactively intervenes with treatment and education so that the individual with a chronic disease can maintain optimal function with the most cost-effective and outcome-effective health care expenditure. The goal of DSCM is to

manage at-risk populations across the entire continuum of care (Levitt et al., 1998).

B. *Component Management Model*—In this model, the "components" are the various providers that a patient may require along the continuum. Each component, separately and episodically, may strive for cost-effective, quality care.

C. *Disease Management Model*—The disease management model is a more holistic model, in which all the components are (ideally) working toward the good of the *population*, or patients with a particular disease state.

D. *Disease Management Society (DMS)*—An organization sponsored by the National Managed Health Care Congress (NMHCC), whose mission is to "provide health care professionals with vehicles for information sharing that will help them in the development, implementation, assessment and improvement of disease prevention and management strategies. . .(and) provide members with information on current research, partnerships and processes that underscore the delivery of cost effective, quality care" (DMS)

E. *Demand Management*—"The use of self-management and decision support systems to enable, educate, and encourage people to improve their health and make appropriate use of medical care" (Nash & Todd, 1997, p. 331).

F. *Best Practices*—Practices that have been determined to produce the most favorable outcomes; these practices have been gleaned from comparative quality measurements.

G. *Evidenced-Based Guidelines, Practice Guidelines, Practice Parameters, and Clinical Practice Guidelines*—defined by the Institute of Medicine as "systematically developed statements to assist practitioner and patient decisions about appropriate healthcare for specific clinical circumstances."

H. *Report Cards and Performance Indicators*—Measures that can be used to rate providers, insurers, or health care plans according to their performance along several criteria. Common indicators include mortality rates, cost, rates of specific procedures, or rates of hospitalization for preventable diseases.

I. *Outcomes Measurement*—Seeks to produce desirable outcomes in a clinical setting, and is the application of outcomes research into practice.

■ DRIVING FORCES THAT LEAD TO DISEASE MANAGEMENT PROGRAMS

A. Fragmentation of Care

  1. In part due to the "Component Management Model" of health care

    a. The "components" are the various providers that a patient may require along the continuum, with each component, separately and episodically, striving for cost-effective, quality care.

    b. Usually does not support education or preventive elements with which hospitalizations and emergency care can be reduced

    c. Studies have shown that optimizing any component of care sepa-

rately from other components often generates higher system-wide costs (Nash & Todd, 1997).
   2. The "Disease Management Model" as an antidote to fragmentation of care
B. Financial Pressures
   1. Cost pressures: Disease-specific health care spending
   2. Risk sharing: Financial risk being transferred from the insurance company as the sole payor to the provider sector, thus sharing the risk
C. Quality Improvement Projects Showing Outcomes of Care
   1. Importance of quality improvement projects
      a. Early projects often demonstrated poor quality of care.
      b. Variations of practice patterns for the same disease state or procedure (e.g., prostate cancer or total hip replacement) is a concern among providers and health care payers.
   2. Quality improvement projects assist in development of "best practice" guidelines.
   3. "Best practice" clinical guidelines support strong disease management programs.
D. Accreditation programs that help ensure quality of care in disease management programs:
   1. The National Committee for Quality Assurance (NCQA)
   2. Health Plan Employer Data and Information Set (HEDIS)
   3. National Association for Healthcare Quality (NAHQ)
   4. Healthcare Quality Certification Board (HQCB)
   5. Joint Commission on Accreditation of Healthcare Organizations (JCAHO)
   6. Quality Improvement System for Managed Care (QISMC)
   7. The ORYX Initiative
E. Computer Systems
   1. Computer and information technology as a *driving force* in disease management
      a. Sophisticated software assists the disease management steps of patient identification, assessment, planning, and outcomes.
      b. Disease-specific decision trees are available and used by telephone triage nurses and demand management companies.
      c. The crucial outcome measurement element that is responsible for continuous improvement in the management of disease would be impossible without sophisticated and integrated computer systems.
   2. Computer and information technology as a *barrier* to disease management
      a. There is an abundance of information; however, putting it together into a useful whole is cost prohibitive and will require collaborative efforts.
F. Informed Consumers

1. Consumers are demanding good care.
2. Health care information is relatively easy to acquire:
   a. HEDIS report cards and major magazines compare plans.
   b. Internet users find disease-specific protocols easily.
   c. Pharmacies pass out free literature about disease, health, and prevention.
   d. Prime-time commercials inform the public of drug uses and side effects.
   e. Magazines, newspapers, and television regularly carry information about new treatments for cancer, human immunodeficiency virus (HIV), and other conditions.
   f. Health fairs saturate the public with important topics.
3. The case manager as an informational resource: An important role of the case manager is to ensure that the patients in their charge get the most accurate information for their health and disease prevention.

■ COMPONENTS OF A SUCCESSFUL DISEASE MANAGEMENT PROGRAM

A. Understanding the Course of the Disease and Practice Guidelines
   1. Disease-specific clinical excellence is required in every aspect of management of the disease.
   2. Case managers examine strategic data to delineate issues such as what the cost and quality drivers, causes, and patterns of symptom manifestation may be in any given disease.
   3. Judicious use of primary care physicians and specialists for disease-specific care
   4. Prevention of exacerbations of diseases
   5. Preventive measures to avoid disease-specific conditions
   6. Use of evidenced-based practice guidelines
   7. Complementary and alternative medicine (CAM) as it relates to disease-specific conditions

B. Targeting Patients Likely to Benefit From Intervention
   1. Evaluation of members most likely to benefit from a given disease management program

C. Focusing on Prevention: Prevention of acute episodes is an essential function of disease management.
   1. Educational efforts as an important component of preventative care
   2. Use of demand management as an educational method and as a system to use medical resources wisely
   3. Judicious use of CAM modalities for prevention

D. Increasing Patient Compliance Through Education and Support Groups
   1. Patient educational component should, at the minimum, include
      a. Etiology and progression of the disease—instruction in how to monitor the disease to avoid exacerbation

      b. Precipitating reasons and signs and symptoms of impending problems

      c. Medication time tables, dosages, side effects, what to do about various side effects

      d. Dietary considerations and other lifestyle modifications

      e. A discussion about compliance with physician and clinic appointments

  2. Reimbursement is limited for counseling, support groups, education, and many forms of preventative therapy.

  3. Case management creativity is essential.

E. Providing Care Across the Continuum

  1. Integration of health care in organizations through

      a. Mergers

      b. Partnering with other companies

      c. Carve-outs for specific treatments or diseases.

  2. The continuum of care must be geographically convenient to provide access to care and preventive services.

  3. Use of case or disease managers throughout the continuum.

F. Establishing Integrated Data Management Systems for Outcome Measurements

  1. Measuring outcomes is important, because outcomes point the direction toward change; they show what works and what needs improvement.

  2. Sophisticated software systems that integrate care based in inpatient and outpatient settings are necessary to elicit the information necessary for a well-developed disease management program.

  3. Barriers to care

      a. Cost to integrate computer systems across the continuum

      b. Time consuming to input all the details necessary for good data

■ DEVELOPMENT AND DESIGN OF A DISEASE MANAGEMENT PROGRAM

A. Define the Target Population (decide which diagnosis or diagnoses to target)

  1. Consider your organization's case mix and location.

  2. Evaluate criteria for the selection of conditions; decide which criteria will elicit the most accurate data.

  3. Evaluate the organization's current processes and programs that are in place.

  4. Common diseases and conditions targeted for disease management programs include

      a. Asthma

      b. Cancer (various types)

      c. Cardiovascular diseases (congestive heart failure, coronary artery disease)

    d. Chronic obstructive pulmonary disease (COPD)

    e. Depression and mental health disorders

    f. Diabetes

    g. High-risk pregnancy/neonates

    h. HIV or acquired immunodeficiency syndrome (AIDS)

    i. Hypertension

    j. Pain management

    k. Pneumonia and infectious diseases

    l. Renal failure and hemodialysis

    m. Transplants

B. Organize a Multidisciplinary, Cross-Functional Team

    1. Determine the goals, objectives, and expected outcomes for the team.

    2. Determine who will be on the team.

    3. Team tasks include

        a. Examination and evaluation of data

        b. Ongoing training required for team members and for those who will manage and implement the disease management program

        c. May require development of clinical pathways, admissions, or discharge orders

    4. Assess barriers to a successful disease management program:

        a. System barriers

        b. Patient or provider barriers

        c. Economic barriers

        d. Regulatory barriers

C. Define Core Components, Treatment Protocols, and Monitoring and Evaluation Methods

    1. Determine how to monitor and evaluate the outcomes.

    2. Design a continuous approach to quality improvement.

    3. Base the disease management program on "best practices" and current *evidence-based guidelines.*

    4. Consider a well-respected physician "champion" to direct the disease management effort; this person would facilitate the medical advisory team.

    5. Determine goals and objectives

        a. Organizational goals and objectives

        b. Clinical goals and objectives

        c. Financial objectives

D. Pilot the Program

    1. Initially, conduct the program on a small scale.

    2. Incorporate training when required.

E. Measure the outcomes of the *pilot* disease management program.

    1. Examine

a. Clinical Outcomes

b. Humanistic (patient and provider satisfaction) outcomes

c. Financial outcomes

2. Understand quality indicators as a measurable method of determining outcomes.

3. Determine whether the pilot disease management program was successful.

a. The program was successful, or

b. The program requires revisions

F. Implement the Disease Management Program And Plan Continuous Improvement (CQI)

■ THE CASE MANAGEMENT AND DISEASE MANAGEMENT PROCESS

A. Identification of At-Risk Members

1. Use criteria to evaluate high-risk members for the chosen disease

2. Potential sources to identify high-risk members

a. Encounter data

b. Hospital and outpatient utilization patterns

c. Pharmacy data

d. Claims and billing data

e. Case manager's knowledge of particular members or population

B. Assessment and Evaluation of Members and Patients

1. Psychosocial issues

2. Financial issues

3. Individual motivational factors

4. Competency barriers to optimal self-care behavior

5. Disease-specific clinical details

a. Physical signs and symptoms

b. Knowledge deficits

6. Assess for severity of target disease state

a. Priority 1—Patients who have a significant potential for exacerbations and emergency room visits or rehospitalizations (high risk)

b. Priority 2—Patients whose needs must be monitored on a regular basis, but can often be managed telephonically (moderate risk)

c. Priority 3—Patients requiring minimal attention, whose sole need may be education about the disease (low risk)

7. Assess available health care benefits

C. Development and Coordination of Disease Management Plans

D. Implementation of Disease Management Plans

1. Involvement of the patient and family in the disease management program and plans

E. Evaluation—Outcome Measurements
1. Clinical outcomes
   a. Use of quality indicators
2. Humanistic (patient and provider satisfaction) outcomes
   a. For patients, *The Health Status Survey (SF-12 or SF-36)* is a patient's self-assessment of perceived quality-of-life issues and has been proved to be a predictive tool that may indicate the member has a potential for a hospital admission in the next 6 to 12 months.
   b. Provider satisfaction tools
   c. Use of quality indicators
3. Financial outcomes
   a. Use of quality indicators

REFERENCES

Goldstein, R. (1998). The disease management approach to cost containment. *Nursing Case Management, 3*(3), 99–103.

Kozma, C., Kaa, K., & Reeder, C. E. (1997). A model for comprehensive disease state management. *The Journal of Outcomes Management, 4*(1), 4–8.

Levitt, D., Startz, T., & Higgins, R. (1998). Disease state case management in an academic medical center utilizing osteoarthritis-of-the-knee model. *The Journal of Care Management, 4*(5), 45–55.

Minerd, R., & Lee, S. (1997). Using business process reengineering to develop disease management programs. *Inside Case Management, 4*(9), 8–9.

Nash, D., & Todd, W. (Eds.) (1997). *Disease management: A systems approach to improving patient outcomes.* Chicago: American Hospital Publishing, Inc.

Powell, S. K. (2000a). *Case management: A practical guide to success in managed care.* Philadelphia: Lippincott Williams & Wilkins.

Powell, S. K. (2000b). *Advanced case management: Outcomes and beyond.* Philadelphia: Lippincott Williams & Wilkins.

Rieve, J. (1998). Disease management concerns. *The Case Manager, 9*(2), 34–36.

Schofield, G. (1998). Developing a disease management program to improve outcomes and efficiencies. *Health Care Innovations, 8*(1), 11–29.

Ward, M., & Rieve, J. (1995). Disease management: Case management's return to patient-centered care. *Journal of Care Management, 1*(4), 7–12.

CHAPTER 4

· · · · · · · · · · · · · ·

The Health Care Delivery System and Managed Care

PENNY M. BURMAN

LEARNING OBJECTIVES

Upon completion of this chapter, the reader will be able to:

1. Define important terms and concepts related to the health care delivery system and managed care.
2. Name the major components of managed care.
3. Name four types of health care delivery systems.
4. Name the major issues facing managed care and health care delivery system.
5. Name the different types of reimbursement methods.
6. Name the types of insurance.

IMPORTANT TERMS AND CONCEPTS

Access
Acute Care
Adjudication
Allied Health Professional
Allowable Charge
Application
Assignment of Benefits
Average Wholesale Price (AWP)
Beneficiary
Benefit Period

Capitation
Coinsurance
Concurrent Review
Consolidated Omnibus Budget
   Reconciliation Act (COBRA)
Contract Number
Coordination of Benefits
Copayment Amounts
Credentialing
Deductible

Employment Retirement Income Security Act (ERISA)
Exclusive Provider Organization (EPO)
Fee for Service
Fee Schedule
Health Maintenance Organization (HMO)
Lifetime Maximum
Loss Ratio
Network
OBRA
Per Diem
Preferred Provider Organization (PPO)
Preauthorization
Primary Care Physician (PCP)
Prior Approval
Risk Sharing Arrangements
Self-Funded or Self-Insured
Stop Loss
Target
Third Party Administrator (TPA)
Utilization Review and Utilization Management

■ INTRODUCTION

A. Managed care encompasses a wide variety of terms and concepts, from the organization itself to the tools used in a health care delivery system or insurance plan.

B. Managed care is a continually evolving and changing process.

C. Differences between the types of health care delivery systems are becoming less distinct. Health care systems and health insurance are using similar processes to manage care and costs.

■ KEY DEFINITIONS

A. Managed Care
   1. "A system of health care delivery aimed at managing the cost and quality of access to health care" (Mullahy, 1998, p. 556).
   2. May mean just the financing of health care and the delivery of (i.e., HMO).
   3. The term can also mean the tools used to manage health care (i.e., utilization management).

B. Health Care Delivery System
   1. A model or system used in the delivery of health care, for example, Independent Practice Association (IPA), Integrated Delivery System (IDS), or Preferred Provider Organization (PPO).

C. Capitation
   1. A fixed dollar amount paid for services to a provider for each person regardless of the actual number or types of services provided. The rate may be fixed or adjusted based on the age and sex of the members and is based on utilization projections done by an actuarial department.

D. Underwriting
   1. Process of calculating a person's risk of predictable loss. Used to determine a group of member's premium
   2. Factors in risk assessment

      a. Group size

      b. Group composition (i.e., age, gender)

      c. Level of participation

      d. Level of benefits

      e. Occupational hazards

      f. Geographic location (Mullent, 1995, p. 11)

E. Cost Share Amounts

  1. Coinsurance

      a. A percentage of the allowed charges of a covered service a member is responsible for.

  2. Deductible

      a. A specified dollar amount of the covered services that a member must pay before the insurer will pay benefits.

  3. Copayment Amount

      a. A predetermined dollar amount a member is responsible for each time a specific service is rendered, that is, for office visits, emergency room visits, or prescriptions.

  4. Out of Pocket Maximum

      a. A maximum dollar amount per calendar year a member is responsible for. Coinsurance and deductibles accumulate toward this maximum.

F. Network

  1. A group of physicians and related health care providers contracted with a health plan from which a member should seek services from for either full coverage or partial coverage of benefits from the insurer. Benefits may be lower or nonexistent if a member is seen by a provider who is not in the network.

G. Actuarial

  1. Process of establishing premium rates through research and statistical analysis. Does research to predict mortality and morbidity, establishes guidelines for predicting risk, and helps predict profitability (Huggins & Laud, 1992, p. 90).

H. Reinsurance

  1. Insurance taken out by plans and self-funded employer groups to cover any losses incurred while covering claims that exceed a specified dollar threshold (stop-loss).

I. Stop-Loss Amount

  1. Dollars that need to be paid by a plan in benefits before reinsurance takes over.

J. Closed Panel

  1. Physicians are employees of or part of a group that contracts with a Managed Care Organization (MCO). Physicians see only those members who are part of the MCO. No benefits are allowed to members for providers outside of the Panel.

K. Open Panel
1. Any doctor meeting the MCO's standards or credentialing process may be contracted with to provide services. Physicians will see any patient, not just those members of a particular MCO.

■ DRIVING FORCES BEHIND MANAGED CARE

A. Increased technology
B. Increased aging population
C. Increased pharmaceutical cost and use
D. Increased durable medical equipment (DME) costs
E. Increased consumer demand
F. Increased malpractice claims
G. Increased insurance premiums

■ COMPONENTS OF MANAGED CARE

A. Accessibility
1. Utilization management—Preauthorization/concurrent review. Case managers should be aware of their patients' (members') insurance plan's or MCO's requirements.
2. Affiliation—Members must choose a select group of contracted providers (a network).
B. Reimbursement Mechanisms:
1. Reimbursement for services is outlined in the contract between the plan or MCO and providers. Case managers should know the type of reimbursement methods being used for cost—benefit analysis.
C. Quality of Care and Quality Management
1. Healthplan Employer Data Information Set (HEDIS)
   a. Set of data reporting standards
   b. Performance standards for reporting for financial, utilization, membership, and clinical data
   c. Allows for comparison between plans
   d. Developed by NCQA
2. NCQA (National Committee on Quality Assurance)
   a. Not-for-profit organization
   b. A quality-oriented accreditation for HMOs
3. Joint Commission on Accreditation of Healthcare Organizations (JCAHO)
   a. Also known as Joint Commission
   b. Nonprofit organization
   c. Accreditation primarily done on hospitals, outpatient facilities, and other institutional facilities.
4. American Accreditation HealthCare Commission (URAC)

      a. Nonprofit organization

      b. Accreditation primarily done on utilization management, health plans, and PPOs

      c. Accreditation standards for case management recently developed

D. Credentialing

    1. Generally done when recruiting a physician to join a health care system and then periodically thereafter.

    2. For some managed care organizations, credentialing verification organziations (CVOs) do the initial credentialing, and then HMOs and PPOs can access that information (Kongstvedt, 1996, p. 112).

    3. Looks at the areas of training, current medical license, Drug Enforcement Agency (DEA) number, hospital privileges, malpractice insurance and history, Social Security number, National Practitioner Data Bank status, limitations of privileges, and felony conviction.

E. Medical Management

    1. Case management

    2. Disease management

    3. Utilization management

      a. Prior approval requirements for certain procedures considered cosmetic or high cost (e.g., transplants).

      b. Precertification for inpatient hospital admissions to determine medical appropriateness and necessity. Some plans may have requirements for other outpatient procedures.

      c. Concurrent review done to monitor a length of stay for medical appropriateness and necessity and for discharge planning.

F. Data reporting

    1. Necessary and useful tools

    2. Helps show those plans or delivery systems that do well or not so well

    3. Gives feedback to show areas that need improvement within a system

G. Pharmaceutical Services

    1. Mail-order pharmacy programs offer prescription drugs via mail order at a reduced cost.

    2. Drug card programs (or pharmacy benefit management) offer prescription drugs that are considered preferred therapy (formulary list) to managed care organizations members (Academy for Healthcare Management, 1997). Members generally are responsible for a copay or coinsurance, or both.

■ **HEALTH CARE DELIVERY SYSTEMS**

A. Health Maintenance Organizations (HMOs)

    1. A set of designated health care providers available in a specific area for a group of people for a predetermined payment

      a. Focus on limiting access to specialists to prevent overutilization of specialty care

    b. The primary care physician (PCP) serves as gatekeeper

    c. No coverage for services received out of network

    d. A combination of healthcare delivery system and a health plan (Kongstvedt, 1996, p. 34)

2. Previously called a prepaid health plan

3. Responsible for being health insurer or financier and healthcare delivery system, providing a broad range of services

4. Reimbursement based on a variety of methods

5. Utilization management is a component

6. Types of HMOs:

    a. Staff model

        (i) Salaried physicians and HMO-owned facilities

        (ii) Monetary incentives may exist that are dependent on performance and productivity

        (iii) Also called a closed-panel HMO

        (iv) Provides comprehensive services at one site

    b. Group practice model

        (i) Physician services are provided via group practices independent of an HMO (Siefker et al., 1998, p. 22). Services are contracted and paid at a negotiated rate.

        (ii) Also called a closed-panel HMO.

        (iii) Limited choice of physicians.

        (iv) Two types: Captive group is a group practice that forms to service only HMO members through contractual arrangement, and an independent group is an existing group practice that is contracted with to serve HMO members but may also serve non-HMO members.

    c. Network model

        (i) Similar to a group model, except the HMO contracts with more than one physician group.

        (ii) May be considered either closed or open panel, depending on how many group practices or specialties are contracted with.

    d. Independent practice association (IPA)

        (i) Services provided through an association of independent physicians. Services are contracted either by negotiated per capita, flat retainer, or negotiated fee for services (Siefker et al., 1998, p. 22).

        (ii) Physicians see both HMO and non-HMO members.

        (iii) Considered an open-panel HMO.

    e. Mixed model or direct contact

        (i) Contracts directly to physicians (both PCP and specialties)

        (ii) Similar to IPA

        (iii) Reimbursement is generally either capitation or fee for service

B. Preferred Provider Organization (PPO)

1. Group of hospitals and physicians contracted with an insurance carrier, TPA, or others to furnish comprehensive care (Siefker et al., 1998, p. 23)
2. Considered a "limited provider panel" of providers who are chosen for their cost-effective practice style (Mullahy, 1998, p. 25). Providers are chosen for the comprehensive services and the quality of care they provide.
3. Services may be received outside the network at a reduced level. Services within the network are generally paid at 100% or at a reduced cost share amount.
4. May also be called professional provider arrangements (PPA).
5. Reimbursement is generally a negotiated rate.
6. Utilization management is a component.
7. Considered to be a type of health care delivery system only.

C. Point of Service (POS)
   1. Combination of HMO and traditional indemnity. Services received within the network are paid at a higher level. Any service received by the member outside the network is paid at a lesser level when performed without a referral.
   2. Reimbursement for in-network providers is generally at a capitated rate.
   3. PCP may act as a gatekeeper for services.

D. Exclusive Provider Organization (EPO)
   1. A combination of HMO and PPO but not an insurance plan. Has a network of physicians and hospitals. Members are required to go there for health care services, otherwise no coverage is provided (Siefker et al., 1998, p. 24).
   2. Uses gatekeeper approach for non-PCP services.
   3. Utilization management is a component.

E. Integrated Delivery System (IDS)
   1. A partnership formed between physicians, physician groups, hospitals, and other providers (Siefker et al., 1998, p. 24).
   2. "A system of health care providers organized to span a broad range of healthcare services" (Mullahy, 1998, p. 26).
   3. IDSs try to "optimize cost and clinical outcomes, accept and manage a full range of financial arrangements to provide a set of defined benefits to a defined population" (Kongstvedt, 1996, p. 996).
   4. Encourage decrease of use of specialty physicians.
   5. Reasons for the development of IDSs:
      a. Competition
      b. Market niche
      c. Decreased hospitalizations
      d. Economies of scale (Siefker, p.24)
   6. Other names for IDSs:
      a. Integrated delivery network (IDN)

b. Integrated delivery and financing system (IDFS)

c. Integrated delivery and financing network (IDFN)

7. Three types of IDSs:

a. Integrated physicians

b. Integrated physicians and hospitals

c. Systems with insurance functions

8. IDS—physician practice management organization

a. Provide physician management for support functions (i.e., contracting and billing) and are uninvolved in clinical aspects

b. Generally for-profit organizations

9. IDS—group practice without walls

a. Group of physicians in practice at different locations form a legal entity.

b. Income can be affected by practice patterns, and peer pressure can affect this.

10. IDS—consolidated medical group

a. Physicians occupy the same facility and own the group practice.

b. Generally independent of a hospital.

11. IDS—physician hospital organization (PHO)

a. May only oversee the relationship between the hospital, physicians and the insurers.

b. Hospitals and physicians may choose to negotiate with insurers directly.

12. IDS—managed service organization (MSO)

a. Developed from a PHO

b. Provides more services to physicians by negotiating contracts and providing support services (i.e., billing)

c. May purchase the physician's assets (i.e., office equipment)

13. IDS—foundation model

a. Hospital creates a nonprofit foundation that purchases physician practices.

b. Physicians generally exclusively work for the foundation.

14. IDS—staff model

a. Owned by an IDS, not an HMO; the difference is whether the primary business owner is a licensed entity or a provider of care primarily.

b. Health system that employs physicians directly.

15. IDS—physician ownership model

a. Requires a large amount of capital to operate

b. Physicians hold a large portion of ownership in the system

c. May contract directly with the hospital

F. Independent Practice Arrangement (IPA)

1. A group of physicians who have contracted with a managed care plan

to provide services for a single capitated rate. The IPA contracts with individual providers to deliver the services. All specialties are generally provided (Mullahy, 1998, p. 25).

■ REIMBURSEMENT METHODS

A. Fee for Service
   1. Traditional approach
   2. Providers (e.g., physicians and hospitals) are paid a set "fee for service"
   3. No discounts are given

B. Discounted Fee for Service
   1. Providers are paid a set fee for a specific service but at a previously agreed-on discount percentage.

C. Sliding Scale Discount on Charges
   1. The percent of discount given depends the volume of admissions and outpatient procedures for a specified time period (usually yearly).
   2. A settlement is made at the end of the year, with an interim discount percent used until settlement time.

D. Per Diem Arrangements
   1. All services are provided for a specific amount per day regardless of actual costs.
   2. Based on averaging costs and number of days.

E. Differential by Day Inpatient
   1. Based on theory that a first-day inpatient is more costly.
   2. Similar to per diem.
   3. A first-day inpatient is paid at a higher rate than subsequent days.

F. Percentage of Revenue
   1. A fixed percentage of premium revenue paid to hospitals to cover all services.
   2. Percent may vary with premium rate charged.
   3. Revenue is dependent on premium yields and revenue.

G. Risk Sharing
   1. A target dollar amount is set for health care costs per member per month between the plan and the network.
   2. At year-end, costs are figured. If costs are less than the target, the plan and the network or provider share the gains. If costs are higher than the target, the costs are also shared between the plan and the network/provider.

H. DRG (Diagnosis Related Group)
   1. Specific dollar amount paid based on classification of illness or diagnosis
   2. Audits required to verify coding practices

3. Used by Medicare

I. Resource-Based Relative Value Scales (RBRVS)
   1. A weighted value is given to a service, and the value is then multiplied by a set dollar amount.
   2. The value takes into consideration all of the things or services needed to provide care, with the idea that more complicated procedures are given a higher value.

J. Per Discharge Payment
   1. Set amount for each member's hospital stay regardless of the diagnosis or length of stay.
   2. Also called service—related case rates.

K. Per Capita Payment and Capitation
   1. Set amount per year or per month per member, no matter what care is provided or not provided.
   2. Rates vary with age and sex of members

L. Bed Leasing
   1. Plan leases beds from a facility regardless if beds are used.
   2. Ensures revenue to a facility and is budgetable for the plan

M. Periodic Interim Payments/Case Advances
   1. Plan advances cash to hospital to cover expected claims.
   2. Cash "fund" is periodically replenished.

N. Performance-Based Reimbursement
   1. A form of capitation.
   2. Penalties and withholdings are built into the contract with the hospital.
      a. Goals for utilization management are set each year. If the goals are met, a bonus is paid to the hospital. If the goals are not met, penalties or withhold amounts are applied to the hospital or deducted from the payments to the hospital.

O. Global Payment and Package Pricing
   1. Combines reimbursement for both institutional and professional services into one lump payment
   2. Commonly done for transplants but has been done for other services and procedures such as cardiac bypass surgery and maternity care
   3. Usually includes both preoperative and postoperative care (Kongstvedt, 1997; Siefker et al., 1998, p. 23)

■ OBJECTIONS TO MANAGED CARE

A. Financial
   1. Incentives may compromise the quality of care.
   2. Limits personal choice of physician.

B. Cost considerations should not override decisions to provide the best care (Donovan & Matson, 1994, p. 44).

C. Utilization review staff (nurses) do not see the complete picture as much as does the care provider at the member's bedside. Often, providers feel that it is a very time-consuming task to share information with the MCO or the plan.

D. Concern that MCOs engage in antiselection or "cherry picking" of members. Recent legislation, called Health Insurance Portability and Accountability Act of 1996 (HIPPA), makes this no longer possible.

■ LEGAL ISSUES FACING MANAGED CARE

A. Government and Legislative Issues
1. Employment Retirement Income Security Act (ERISA) of 1974
   a. Two (of many) provisions
      (i) Does not require people with self-funded plans to pay premium taxes, complying with state mandates or other state regulations for health insurance
      (ii) Requires plans to provide an explanation of benefits statement to a member in the event of a claim denial, explaining the reason for the denial and the appeal process
2. Consolidated Omnibus Budget Reconciliation Act (COBRA) of 1986
   a. Law requiring certain employers to allow qualified employees, spouses, and dependents to continue health insurance coverage when it would otherwise stop, for example, when one quits a job
3. Taft-Hartley Trusts of 1948
   a. Allows unions to form trusts to administer their health benefits (Siefker et al., 1998, p. 36)
   b. Union management trusts, administered by both union management and union representatives.
4. Omnibus Budget Reconciliation Act (OBRA)
   a. Annual tax and budget acts that generally relate to the managed care market and Medicare
5. HIPAA
   a. Main objective is to make health insurance more portable from job to job and to eliminate or decrease waiting periods
   b. Applies to all companies that offer health insurance (Humo, 1998)
   c. Has many parts and provisions, addressing everything from fraud and abuse to minimum maternity stays to medical spending accounts
   d. Prevents "cherry picking" by MCOs

■ OTHER ISSUES IN MANAGED CARE

A. Credentialing and Recredentialing
1. Can be costly to maintain
B. Medical Management (Utilization Management, Case Management, Quality Management, and Disease Management)

   1. All components are needed in a health plan.
C. Claims Processing and Information Systems
   1. Need to be able to produce data, report cards, and monitor performance of providers.
   2. Efficient and accurate claims processing is a necessity.
   3. Systems and software are expensive.
D. Marketing
   1. Stiff competition
E. Profitability of MCOs
   1. Financial viability necessary for both nonprofit and for-profit organizations (Siefker et al., 1998, p. 26)
   2. Increased risk sharing between providers of care and MCOs
F. Provider Reimbursement
   1. Financial viability important for both physicians and hospitals versus the need to keep medical costs under control
   2. Some concern that reimbursement to providers is not adequate to compensate for costs

■ **TYPES OF INSURANCE**

A. Liability
   1. Benefits are paid for bodily injury or property damage, or both
B. No-fault
   1. Auto—for injuries or property damage, or both, incurred involving a vehicle
   2. Workers Compensation—for injuries incurred while on the job
C. Accident and Health
   1. Health—pays benefits for medically related costs. Generally has a lifetime maximum benefit.
      a. Third Party Administrator (TPA)
         (i) Also known as Administrative Services Only (ASO)
         (ii) Performs administrative functions only (i.e., claims processing and medical management) for self-funded employer groups
      b. Indemnity or Traditional Insurance
         (i) Member selects provider of his or her choice; there is no network
         (ii) Provider sets fees.
         (iii) Mechanisms in place to help control cost
            (a) Increased deductibles
            (b) Copays for office visits, emergency room visits
            (c) Coinsurance
            (d) Precertification and preauthorization
            (e) Medical appropriateness and necessity language

(f) Exclusions

(g) Waiting periods (Siefker et al., 1998, p. 21)

2. Long-term or short-term disability (LTD or STD)—insurance to provide replacement of salary when the member is unable to work owing to illness or injury. STD lasts up until 6 months, and LTD usually has a maximum benefit amount.

REFERENCES

Academy for Health Care Management (1997). *Managed health care: An introduction.* Alpharetta, GA: Professional Book Distributors.

Borfitz, D. (1999). Living with the limits of managed care. *Infusion, 5*(6), 37–42.

Chan, F., Leahy, M. J., McMahon, B. T., Mirch, M., & DeVinney, D. (1999). Foundation knowledge and major practice domains of case management. *The Journal of Case Management, 5*(1).

Cohen, E. L., & Cesta, T. G. (1993). *Nursing case management from concept to evaluation.* St. Louis: Mosby.

Donovan, M. R., & Matson, T. A. (Eds.). (1994). *Outpatient case management: Strategies for a new reality.* Chicago: American Hospital Publishing, Inc.

Huggins, K., & Laud, R. D. (1992). *Operations of life and health insurance companies* (2nd ed.). Atlanta: LOMA

Humo, T. (1998). Introduction to health insurance portability and accountability act. In *Employers Guide to HIPAA.* Washington, DC: Thompson Publishing Group.

Kongstvedt, P. R. (1997). *Essentials of managed care* (2nd ed.). Gaithersburg, MD: Aspen.

Kongstvedt, P. R. (1996). *The managed care handbook* (3rd ed.). Gaithersburg, MD: Aspen

Mullahy, C. M. (1995). *The case manager's handbook.* Gaithersburg, MD: Aspen.

Mullahy, C. M. (1998). *The case manager's handbook* (2nd ed.). Gaithersburg, MD: Aspen

Mullent, J. K. (1995). *Introduction to managed care: Fundamentals of managed care coverage and providers.* Atlanta: LOMA.

Powell, S. K., & Dalton, M. E. (1996). Shifting roles. *Continuing Care, 15*(2), 20–30.

Siefker, J. M., Garrett, M. B., Van Genderen, A., & Weis, M. J. (1998). *Fundamentals of case management.* St. Louis: Mosby.

CHAPTER 5

. . . .

Utilization Management/ Resource Management

CAROL CANADA
RUFUS HOWE
CHERI LATTIMER
PAT STRICKER

LEARNING OBJECTIVES

Upon completion of this chapter, the reader will be able to:

1. Identify terms associated with utilization management (UM).
2. List goals common to UM.
3. Discuss the history and impact of managed care.
4. Gain an understanding of the importance of managing resources to maintain cost-effective outcomes.
5. Discuss the basic concepts of reimbursement.
6. Define the criteria used to assess medical necessity and appropriateness.
7. Understand the principles used in the UM in the health care environment.
8. Discuss the review, referral, and adverse-outcome processes.
9. Identify regulatory and accreditation bodies associated with the process of UM.

GLOSSARY OF TERMS

American Accreditation Healthcare Commission/Utilization Review Accreditation Commission (URAC)
Clinical Pathways
Concurrent Review
Denials
Diagnostic Related Groups (DRGs)
Code of Federal Regulations (HCFA)
InterQual, Inc.
Hospital Issued Notice of Non-Coverage (HINN)
Joint Commission On Accreditation of Healthcare Organizations (JCAHO)
Lag Days—Aberrant Days
Level of Care (LOC)
Length of Stay (LOS)
Milliman and Robertson, Inc.
National Committee for Quality Assurance (NCQA)
Notice of Discharge and Medicare Appeal Rights (NODMAR)
Notice of Non-Coverage (NONC)
Precertification—Prior Authorization—Preadmission Review
Peer Review Organization (PRO)
Prospective Payment System (PPS)
Retrospective Review
Resource Management/Service Delivery
Standing Orders
Utilization Management (UM)

■ UM GOALS

  A. Determine medical necessity.

  B. Eliminate or minimize unnecessary care.

  C. Determine appropriateness of care.

  D. Ensure appropriate utilization of resources.

  E. Promote quality patient care.

  F. Evaluate efficient use of financial resources.

  G. Evaluate efficient use of personnel resources.

■ HISTORY OF MANAGED MEDICAL CARE

  A. 1965: Medicare
    1. Health Care Finance Administration (HCFA)
    2. Payment based on costs/charges
    3. Diagnosis related groups—1980 (DRGs)
    4. Quality Screening Program—1986–1987
    5. Medicare health maintenance organizations (HMOs)—1990 (fee-for-service)
    6. Ambulatory patient groups (APG)
    7. Overseen by a peer review organization (PRO). PRO directed scope of work

  B. 1966: Medicaid
    1. Operated by individual states

2. HCFA dictates basic regulations
3. Uses state and federal funds
4. Market characteristics vary widely
5. Regulations, eligible categories, benefits, and access
6. Originally was fee for service
7. Reimbursement DRGs and per diem
8. Managed care enrollment—1970s

C. 1970s: HMO
1. Predetermined payment/per member per month (PMPM) basis
2. Responsible for financials, delivery and quality of care
3. Controls access (PCP/network) through UM
4. Risk agreements
5. HMO Models:
   a. Staff—Employs salaried physicians
   b. Group—Contracts with physician groups
   c. Network—Contracts with two or more physician groups
   d. IPA—Contracts with individual physicians

D. 1975–1980: Preferred Provider Organization (PPO)
1. "Evolving HMOs"
2. Contracted providers and facilities
3. Discounted rates/fees
4. Increased patient out-of-pocket payments for out-of-network care
5. Broad networks
6. Selective contracting with providers
7. UM programs

E. 1987: Point of Service (POS)
1. Strategy for benefit flexibility and cost control
2. Different levels of benefits linked to network use
3. Might require PCP directed in network care
4. UM programs
5. Risk sharing
6. Increased employer involvement

F. 1985–1990: Capitation
1. Prepayment to providers for care
2. Based on membership, not services delivered
3. Payment PMPM varies by age/gender and case mix
4. Risk pools/withholds

■ IMPACT OF MANAGED CARE

A. Three main areas: physicians, facilities, and the consumer
B. Introduced creative reimbursement models, encouraged hospital

partnering and physician hospital organizations (PHO), and created internal UM and quality processes.

C. Impact on physicians

D. Managed care led to less autonomy

E. Adversarial interactions between physicians and patients

F. Perceived quality issues

G. Increased liability

H. Less cost shifting

I. Organized Independent Physician Associations (IPAs) and Managed Care Organizations (MCOs)

J. Increased labor costs in the office

K. Micro management

L. Poor feedback and information

M. Threatened income and changed personal goals

N. Resulted in less autonomy, restricted care, decreased physicians/hospital choices, perceived decrease in quality and increased responsibility

O. Quality of health care caused accountability to shift to the customers and increased emphasis on development of quality processes. Some of these processes are:
   1. National standards for consistency, efficiency, measurement, and comparison
   2. Provider quality concerns
   3. State regulatory processes
   4. Accreditation by national organizations

P. Managed care produced several types of benefit plans.
   1. Transitioned from "loose" to "tight" to "loose" plan management
   2. Forced employer role to evolve
   3. Forced increased responsibility for the provider and member

■ **BASIC CONCEPTS OF REIMBURSEMENT** (Note: For more reimbursement issues and concepts, see Chapter 4: Health Care Delivery and Managed Care.)

A. Medicare Part A
   1. Hospital or inpatient care—These services are covered by Medicare Part A and are under the prospective payment system (PPS). This system has been in place since 1983 and replaced the systems in which vendors were paid on a reasonable cost basis.
   2. Under PPS, hospitals are paid a fixed amount based on operating costs of the patient's diagnosis. The diagnosis fits into one of nearly 500 diagnosis related groups or DRGs.
   3. The assignment of DRG is made according to diagnosis, patient age

and sex, treatment needed, and discharge destination. In some cases, the cost of caring for the individual is higher than the reimbursement. However, payments sometimes are adjusted for expensive or longer lengths of stay.

B. Medicare Part B

1. Physician payments are based on reasonable charges. These charges are defined as the lesser of submitted charges or an amount from a uniform fee schedule. The fee schedule is based on national uniform relative values for all physician services. These values are adjusted for locations by a geographic factor.

2. Skilled nursing payments were paid on a reasonable cost basis with limitations and restrictions. Skilled nursing is now transitioning into a prospective payment reimbursement structure.

3. Home health care and hospice care are paid on a reasonable cost basis. Durable medical equipment and laboratory services are based on a fee schedule.

4. Medicare managed care plans—The insurer receives a monthly payment from Medicare for each enrollee. These "risk" plans assume full financial risk for all care provided. Beginning in 1999, managed care plans will be paid according to the new Medicare + Choice Program. Payments will be based on a blended rate.

5. Services not covered by Medicare (but that may be covered by managed care with copayments) include long-term care or custodial care; dentures or dental care; eyeglasses, except for medical correction; hearing aids; and most prescription drugs.

■ UM CONCEPTS AND DEFINITIONS

A. Defined as, "evaluation of medical necessity, appropriateness, and efficiency of the use of health care services, procedures, and facilities under the auspices of the applicable health benefit plan."

B. Goals

1. Eliminate or minimize unnecessary care and promote the use of appropriate care. This includes hospital admissions, outpatient diagnostic procedures, and imaging studies and visits with specialists. It focuses on real-time management of process.

C. Resource management encompasses processes that monitor appropriateness of resource utilization and delivery.

■ KEY DEFINITIONS

A. Level of Care—Appropriate setting that enhances appropriate resource delivery.

1. UM—Involves determining the appropriate setting and resources for the care to be delivered in order to maintain cost effectiveness and quality.

2. Resource management—Resources are monitored to be appropriate

for the condition presented and the opportunity to maintain or improve care through the use of alternative solutions.

B. Insurance terms

1. Tax Equity & Fiscal Responsibility Act (TEFRA)

C. Cost per discharge, reimbursement targets, and limits

1. Consolidated Omnibus Budget Reconciliation Act (COBRA)

D. Employers must offer continued health insurance.

1. Employee Retirement Income Security Act (ERISA)
2. Regulates corporate pension funds and exempts self-insured plans from including "mandatory" state insurance benefits.

■ TOOLS AND STRATEGIES

A. UM Modalities and Tools

1. Programs, processes, criteria, and screens used to assist the provider in managing the quality delivery and cost of health care services.
2. These avenues vary from health care settings and may be governed by specific rules and regulations for practice and payment.
3. Examples of these tools include practice guidelines, clinical pathways, benchmarks for care, and outcomes management.
4. Length of Stay (LOS). Average LOSs have been established by federal criteria and also private sector organizations to offer the provider of care a guideline for average hospital stays for specific disease or conditional states.

■ UTILIZATION STRATEGIES AND MODALITIES IN THE ACUTE CARE ENVIRONMENT

A. InterQual

1. InterQual, founded in 1976, provides clinical decision support criteria and credentialing systems. Their first set of criteria, the ISD for managing hospitalized patients, was developed in 1978.
2. The ISD criteria allow utilization reviewers to evaluate appropriate use of hospitals by applying clinically specific criteria to patient findings. InterQual is the industry standard and is used internationally.
3. In the 1980s, InterQual developed credentialing and privileging programs, UM program, quality and risk management programs, and the Surgical Indications Monitoring (SIM) criteria.
4. In the 1990s, three more criteria sets were developed:
   a. Surgery, Invasive Procedures and Imaging Appropriateness (ISPR and ISXR)
   b. Primary Care Physician/Specialist Divisions of care (IPSR)
   c. Clinical Management of Workers' Compensation Cases (IWCR)

B. Criteria Sets

1. The sets cover a spectrum of care:

a. Inpatient and outpatient surgery
b. Procedures and imaging
c. Primary care physician/specialist
d. Division of care
e. Work-related injuries and illnesses

C. Criteria Development
1. It is necessary to know how the criteria are developed to understand their validity and why they are the standard in the industry.
    a. The prototype is created with key physician consultants after extensive medical literature review.
    b. Independent physician consultants then review it.
    c. There are over 250 community-based and academic specialists and subspecialists.
    d. Recommendations are reviewed and compiled, taking local medical policy and clinical nonagreement into consideration.
    e. Amended criteria sets are drafted. Second- and third-tier field reviews are then submitted.
    f. The final criteria set is released after consensus, common sense, and evidence-based best practices are acknowledged.
    g. Feedback is obtained from patients, criteria conferences, employer groups, payers, providers, seminar participants, surveys, UM consulting, and user groups.
2. The criteria assist with accreditation standards for HCFA, URAC, NCQA, and JCAHO.
3. This standard is supported with ISP and ISX, which clearly indicate emergent procedures, and as with ISD, review can be conducted retrospectively to validate emergent need without obstructing medical decision making.
4. The criteria is shared with providers because
    a. Mutual review goals are more easily attained.
    b. Collaboration is always good business.
    c. Disclosure is mandated in some states.
    d. It is a requirement of URAC/NCQA.

D. InterQual is used to determine whether proposed services are clinically indicated and provided at the appropriate level or setting. The criteria are applied to all types of reviews and have many advantages:
1. Objective and rule-based
2. Focused on the specific condition of the patient and not the diagnosis
3. Channeled care to the appropriate level of care
4. Based on research and referenced studies, practice guidelines, and pathways that prompt "best practices"
5. Open—no "black box." Providers have access to criteria through proper channels.
6. Based on clinical information/input from external physician panel

7. Reviewed and updated annually

8. Monitoring the delivery of services across the acute stay for fragmentation, duplication, and appropriateness

9. Clinical pathways, algorithms, practice guidelines, and preprinted or standing orders are developed for specific disease states.

  a. Consideration given to best demonstrated practice, along with review of clinical and financial outcome data.

10. Concurrent and retrospective review processes used to monitor patient status for changes.

E. Milliman and Robertson, Inc.

  1. Used by many health care providers for assessing, managing, and improving the quality and cost of health care services. Healthcare Management Guidelines (HMGs) for acute care include inpatient and surgical care guidelines.

  2. Hospital efficiency index

    a. On the basis of Milliman and Robertson's Hospital Efficiency Index, over 53% of all Medicare inpatient hospital days were potentially avoidable in 1997.

    b. The indices measure how efficient an individual hospital is relative to the actual LOS and admission experience of the most efficient hospitals.

    c. At 1997 levels, the U.S. Medicare average LOS could be reduced from 6.6 days to 4.1 days if all care were provided at the most efficient levels, and admissions could be reduced by nearly 38%.

    d. The 53% figure is based on potentially avoidable days due to longer than necessary inpatient LOSs, the LOS Efficiency Index, treatments that could have been provided outside the acute hospital environment, and the ADM (Admission) Appropriateness Index.

  3. Healthcare Management Guidelines (HMGs)

    a. Provide a look at procedure, timing, and sequence of care for typical patient diagnoses and circumstances. Organizations can compare their own practices with these nationally developed best practices and adjust their procedures accordingly. This series of volumes is updated annually.

  4. Health Status Improvement and Management (HSIM)

    a. This proprietary concept was developed to extend the value of the Healthcare Management Guidelines and facilitate healthcare reform.

    b. It presents a construct of how delivery management should evolve and includes the integration of care, the new patient/physician relationship, and the responsibility shift.

  5. Actuarial Health Cost Model

    a. Claims that cost projections incorporating utilization, service intensity, and unit cost information are used to establish realistic premium rates for prospective or existing managed care plans.

6. Selection Model
   a. Actuarial consultants use this model to evaluate provider risk-sharing arrangements for point-of-service care.
7. Hospital Reimbursement Methodology
   a. Using a combination of case rates and per diems, this technique integrates the Healthcare Management Guidelines with contracting strategies to determine realistic reimbursement.
8. Impact Analysis
   a. This analysis of cash flow, risk, and daily operations allows providers to determine the impact of the risk level assumed, or about to be assumed, with a particular managed care contract.
   b. Detailed treatment plans and procedures.
   c. Custom treatment plans and procedures are useful for provider organizations interested in direct contracting.
9. Resource Planning Models
   a. Specific planning models show health care organizations which resources (staff and equipment) are required to provide care to specific closed-group populations. These models, which can either use American Medical Association (AMA) productivity data or be based on patient-specific assumptions, also weigh the cost versus the benefits of contract versus salaried compensation.
10. MEASUR Index
    a. This pricing and planning information is used by developers of ambulatory surgery centers. It is included in Volume 3 of the Healthcare Management Guidelines.
11. M&R Claims Analysis System
    a. Financial analysis of insured-but-not-paid claims liabilities is critical for sound management and financial decisions.
12. M&R Risk Analyzer Program (RAP)
    a. Data and analysis of potential variations in costs, rates of return, and number of expected claims allow organizations to evaluate specific risks.
13. HMO Financial Projection System
    a. Detailed reserve and expense assumptions and payment lag assumptions enable organizations to examine cash flow, incurred profits and losses, capital requirements, and other key financial data. This is valuable for start-up organizations, establishing a new line of business, or developing projections for regulatory filings.
14. M&R Health Cost Guidelines
    a. This proprietary data base of more than 20 million member months of geographically consistent information about costs and utilization is used by M&R actuaries to identify and manage health insurance risks of individual providers.
15. Health Care Operations Benchmarks

a. A collection of operations benchmarks for an insurance plan to assess administration costs. These benchmarks form Best Practice measurements of operational efficiency and quality for specific functions.

16. Workers' Compensation Treatment and Pricing Protocols
    a. These protocols can be customized to specify the most appropriate treatment and related cost for common workers' compensation—related injuries, by body part and type of injury.

17. Scenario Testing Analysis
    a. This analysis of associated costs and resources allows patients to select one of the most advantageous outcomes for their prospective plan or service contract before implementation.

18. Health Care Software Vendor Profiles
    a. This set of health care software vendor profiles is categorized by function and can be used to select the vendor with the best capability for accomplishing a patient's needs.

19. Inpatient/Outpatient Chart Review Models
    a. These software programs are used by consultants (or licensed patients) to evaluate efficiency and identify high-cost areas and significant variations in a hospital or primary care setting.

■ HCIA STANDARDS

A. Collect, manage, and distribute comparative health care information. Customers deliver, purchase, and manufacture health care products and services. By combining industry leading data bases, methodologies, and analytic services, HCIA creates information assets that help customers manage health care costs and improve patient care.

B. Based on all-payer data gathered from nearly 11 million actual inpatient records, representing 1 out of every 3 discharges from U.S. hospitals annually.

C. Based on data from a detail-rich data base—not "goal" scenarios. Unlike panel-derived goals, which are subjective opinion, HCIA LOS uses statistical facts drawn from vast quantities of patients who experienced a hospital stay in the prior year.

D. Provide the exact number of patients contributing to the published LOS value.

E. Address the patient's illness complexity. The standards provide norms for both simple and more complex patients. HCIA LOS provides figures for multiple-diagnosis patients who have had a significant procedure performed and those who have not.

F. Address the issue of patient age with five age group breakouts for every ICD-9-CM code. Panel-based goals have one generic LOS for any patient, regardless of age.

G. Document the statistical range of stays for each patient group. These ranges are represented as percentiles that can allow a more aggressive (benchmark) or less aggressive (norm) LOS for the patient, depending on individual variables, and all backed by actual patient data.

H. Cover all ICD-9-CM codes and incorporate LOS figures for any type of case.

■ PROCESSES WITHIN THE UM WORKFLOW

A. Information Gathering—Information might be obtained from several sources. The provider can fax or call a request for review of an episode of precertification, inpatient admission, continued stay, retrospective review, or specialist referral. Part of information gathering is to determine whether this service is being provided in network or out of network.

B. Documenting—Information is documented in a standard UM application or logbook. If additional clinical information is needed to determine the indication or medical necessity, the nurse will call the provider for additional information.

C. Apply InterQual Criteria—Review clinical information with the use of the approved criteria for the patient.

D. Document Nurse Outcome—If the criteria are met, the nurse will approve the request and inform the provider. If a subsequent review is necessary, the nurse will inform the provider of the next date for that review. There might be specific events that require a case management referral or reporting back to the plan. These would be patient-specific requirements. If no criteria exist to assess a specific diagnosis, procedure, or referral, or if the criteria are not met even after obtaining additional information, the nurse will inform the provider that the request cannot be approved and a physician referral is required. The nurse forwards that request to a supervisor, who will review the case and send it on for a second-level review by a medical reviewer. The medical reviewer might send it on for further (third-level) review by a specialist.

E. Document Medical Review Outcome—The medical reviewer will review the case using personal medical judgment and expertise and make a determination based on the patient's needs. The reviewer will document the findings or send the determination to the UM nurse to enter. If the case is approved, there is no further action unless subsequent reviews are necessary. If the case is not approved, the medical advisor will contact the requesting provider to obtain more information or to explain why the case is being denied and provide an appeal mechanism. If the case is denied, the provider or member can initiate the appeal process.

F. Identification and External Reporting of Sentinel Events—Sentinel events are diagnoses on admission to the hospital. Tracked events are identified by management and are based on patient specifics. This type of quality review is based on the outcomes of services or care. Traditionally, sentinel event tracking is done in all aspects of the managed care industry. Sentinel events are typically identified during the review process.

G. Case Management Referrals—Patients can provide lists of case management services on which they might want the case manager to report. This process can include such things as high-risk pregnancies and catastrophic illness.

■ UM IN THE ACUTE CARE ENVIRONMENT

A. UM in the hospital environment revolves around monitoring the appropriateness of admission, the appropriate level of care, and planning for the discharge of the patient. It also includes the monitoring of services furnished.

B. The above-mentioned processes are further required for hospitals to participate in the Medicare/Medicaid program.

C. The HCFA administers standards or criteria for participation.

D. Qualified hospitals are required by HCFA to have a plan that provides for review of the medical necessity of admission, LOS, and professional services furnished. The plan must also review and provide for meeting the needs of patients after hospitalization.

■ UM IN THE MANAGED CARE ENVIRONMENT

A. Generally speaking, the process of UM in the managed care environment parallels that in the acute care environment.

B. In most settings, it contains criteria for hospitalization, ensuring appropriateness of setting and effectively monitoring resources for cost-effective alternatives. Constituencies affected by managed care include employers, consumers, health care providers, and the workers' compensation arena.

■ PROGRAM AND PROCESS MODALITIES

A. Precertification or preadmission review
   1. Performed before service is rendered. This does not apply in an emergency situation. This process may occur before admission to a hospital or skilled nursing facility or before a surgical event. This may also occur for outpatient services such as radiologic procedures or delivery of home health.

B. Concurrent review
   1. Performed while the patient is in a facility. Most often, the reviewer visits the facility, but the review may be done via telephone. The review is often collaborative in nature, including the facility case manager or UM personnel. Again, appropriateness of setting and resource utilization is considered. The review process is generally performed within 24 to 48 hours and every 2 to 3 days.

C. Retrospective review
   1. Occurs after discharge. The reviewer may deny the admission or parts of the inpatient stay.

2. The reviewer may be a representative of Medicare or other payor source.
3. This process also is used as a tool for quality improvement.

■ UTILIZATION STRATEGIES AND MODALITIES IN THE MANAGED CARE ENVIRONMENT

A. InterQual criteria
   1. Useful and frequently used tool in the managed care environment, in acute and post-acute settings
B. Clinical pathways, practice guidelines, and benchmarks
   1. Developed to obtain best demonstrated practice along with review of clinical and financial outcome data.
C. Milliman and Robertson, Inc. Healthcare Management Guidelines (HMGs)
   1. Used by many health care providers for assessing, managing, and improving the quality and cost of health care services in acute and post-acute settings.

■ APPEAL PROCESS

A. The appeal process is the formal mechanism by which a service provider or a member, or both, can request reconsideration of a decision, with the goal being to find a mutually acceptable solution. The appeal process consists of the following four levels:
   1. Reconsideration (first-level appeal)—A request by telephone for additional review of a UM determination not to certify. It is performed by the peer reviewer who reviewed the original decision and is based on additional information or peer-to-peer discussion. For example, a provider can discuss denial with the AHG medical director for possible reversal of a decision based on additional verbal clinical information.
   2. Expedited (second-level appeal)—A request by telephone for additional review of a decision not to certify imminent or ongoing services requiring a review conducted by a clinical peer who was not involved in the original decision not to certify. The member or provider can request an expedited decision (no longer than 72 hours). AHG provides the decision within 24 hours of having all pertinent medical information. At present, AHG contracts with a national physician peer review group, but is working on setting up our own network of physicians for review.
   3. Standard (third-level appeal)—A request to review a denial of an admission, extension of stay, or other health care service. It is conducted by a peer reviewer who was not involved in any of the previous determinations pertaining to the same episode of care. This is a formal written appeal process defined and handled by the payor.
   4. Arbitration (final level)—Mediation usually handled by objective outside parties. The patient also handles this level.

■ DENIALS OF ADMISSION OR SERVICES

A. A denial notice may be issued when admission to, or continued stay in, the facility cannot be justified as medically necessary.

B. There are different types of denials and specific regulations that govern their use for Medicare and Medicaid patients.

C. Private review agencies may have specific policies and procedures for denials according to their specific payor groups.

■ APPEALS

A. An appeals process is generally in place for reconsideration of the denial. Poor communication and/or documentation are often factors that contribute to a denial.

B. Peer Review Organizations (PRO). PROs contract with HCFA to review the quality and appropriateness of care being rendered to hospitalized patients receiving Medicare benefits. Processes are developed for review and referral when a denial is issued.

C. NONC (Notice of Non-coverage): a generic term for a notification of non-coverage

D. HINN (Hospital-Issued Notice of Non-coverage): notice of noncoverage for fee-for-service Medicare beneficiaries

E. NODMAR (Notice of Discharge and Medicare Appeal Rights): notice of noncoverage for Medicare beneficiaries in managed care plans (Powell, 2000)

F. Expedited Appeals—The expedited appeal is for imminent or ongoing services that must be attended to quickly (within 1 business day) for patient safety (Powell, 2000).

G. Standard Appeals—A standard appeal is usually for retrospective services that do not require immediate attention (within 30 days of receiving the documentation) (Powell, 2000).

■ ADVERSE REVIEW DETERMINATION

A. Adverse review determination is defined as the non-authorization (denial) of payment for a request for care or services.

B. NCQA considers nonauthorization decisions that are based on either medical appropriateness or benefit coverage or experimental treatments to be denials.

C. Partial approvals and care terminations are also considered denials.

D. The UM service might deny authorization based on medical necessity, but denials based on benefits or experimental treatments are handled by the patient.

E. If the review does not meet the InterQual criteria or there are no criteria for that diagnosis, procedure, or imaging procedure, then

1. There could be a supervisor review, then the nurse outcome would refer to a second-level medical review.
2. The medical review might also refer to a third-level review.
3. Nonphysician reviewers at the first level cannot deny payment for any care or procedure.

■ MEDICAL REVIEW OUTCOMES

A. Medical review outcomes are based on the medical reviewer's judgment and expertise after reviewing the case for medical appropriateness. The health plan might also deny a service because it is not covered in the plan benefit coverage or is considered to be experimental. Types of medical review outcomes include:
1. Closed for lack of information
2. Approval or partial approval
3. Awaiting more information
4. Denial (adverse determination)

■ KEY REGULATORY AND ACCREDITATION BODIES ASSOCIATED WITH THE PROCESS OF UM

A. HCFA
1. A federal regulatory agency that oversees Medicare and Medicaid dollars

B. JCAHO
1. A private not-for-profit organization developed to improve the quality of care provided to the public. It provides standards and evaluates for a variety of settings, e.g., hospitals, LTC long-term care, home health.

C. The American Accreditation Healthcare Commission/URAC
1. A nonprofit organization founded to establish standards for the managed care environment

D. NCQA
1. A private not-for-profit organization dedicated to assessing and reporting on the quality of managed care plans

■ UM REGULATORY AND ACCREDITATION PROCESSES

A. It is desirable for UM service companies to obtain accreditation for services. Accreditation demonstrates:

B. Accountability to external customers
1. Compliance with regulations, including state regulatory processes
2. Attentiveness to provider quality concerns
3. Process consistency
4. Process efficiencies

REFERENCES

American Accreditation Healthcare Commission/URAC. (February 2000). World Wide Website. *www.urac.org/sumum.htm. www.urac.org/ur_survey_press_release.htm.*

Cohen, E. L., & Cesta, T. (1997). *Nursing case management* (2nd ed.). St. Louis: Mosby.

Conditions of participation hospitals/managed care. (October, 1998). HCIA—Code of Federal Regulation.

HCIA Inc. and Ernst & Young. (1998). *Comparative clinical and financial benchmarks. The DRG handbook.* (some material adapted from the Website *www.hcia.com*)

InterQual—ISD—AC. (1997). *Adult user guide.* Website: *igeinterqual.com.*

Joint Commission on Accreditation of Healthcare Organizations (1998). *Hospital accreditation standards.* Washington, DC: NCQA.

Milliman & Robertson, Inc. (1999). *Client Notes,* vol. 4, N.1, first quarter.

Milliman & Robertson, Inc. (February 2000). *World Wide Website. http://www.milliman-hmg.com.*

Powell, S. K. (2000). *Case management: A practical guide to success in managed care.* Philadelphia: Lippincott Williams & Wilkins.

CHAPTER 6

· · · · · · · · · · · · · ·

Legal Issues in Case Management

LYNN S. MULLER

This chapter is a survey of legal issues and could not possibly contain all relevant law. Please refer to the Federal or State programs, or both, under which you practice for laws and regulations governing professional licensing, workers' compensation, automobile liability, available benefits, and so on. Public and university libraries are a good source for such information. You may also contact the local offices of elected officials to request copies of state and federal legislation.

LEARNING OBJECTIVES

Upon completion of this chapter, the reader will be able to:

1. Understand a wide range of legal terms and identify sources for additional legal research.
2. Gain an appreciation for the interaction of conflicting areas of law and ethical practice.
3. Discuss the role of the case manager in relation to the legal community.
4. Understand the patient's rights and case managers' responsibility.

IMPORTANT TERMS AND CONCEPTS (GARNER, 1996)

Advocate: A person who assists, defends or pleads . . . for another.
Agent: One who is authorized to act for or in place of another.
Battery: In tort law (civil law), an intentional and offensive touching of another.
Breach: Violation or infraction of a law

or obligation. A failure on one's part to conform to the standard required.
Breach of Contract: Violation (failure to perform) a contract obligation.
Case Law: The collection of reported cases that form the body of jurisprudence within a given jurisdiction.

Causal Connection: The relationship between cause and effect.

Civil Law: The law of civil or private rights.

Codify: Codification. The process of compiling, arranging, and systematizing the laws of a given jurisdiction into an ordered code.

Common Law: The body of law derived from judicial decisions and opinions, rather than from statutes or constitutions. Also known as case law.

Conflict of Interest: A real or seeming incompatibility between one's private interests and one's fiduciary duties.

Contract: A set of promises, for breach of which the law gives a remedy, or the performance of which the law in some way recognizes as a duty.

Contribution: The right to demand that another, who is jointly responsible for a third party's injury, supply part of what one is required to compensate a third party.

Damages: Monetary compensation for loss or injury to person or property.

Decision: A court's (judge's) ruling in a case.

Defendant: The party being sued in a civil lawsuit.

Deposition: A witness' out-of-court testimony that is reduced to a writing, usually by a court reporter, for later use in court or for discovery purposes.

Discovery: The act or process of finding and learning something that was previously unknown. (Each state's court rules govern the discovery process.)

Duty: An obligation recognized by the law, requiring a person to conform to a certain standard of conduct, for the protection of others against reasonable risks.

Expert Witness: A witness qualified by knowledge, skill, experience, training, or education to provide scientific, technical, or other specialized opinions about the evidence or a fact issue.

Fundamental Right: (1) A right derived from natural or fundamental law. (2) Fundamental rights as enumerated by the Supreme Court including the right to vote and interstate travel, along with various rights of privacy.

Harm: Actual loss or damage resulting from the actions or inactions of another.

Informed Consent: (1) A person's agreement to allow something to happen, made with full knowledge of the risks involved and the alternatives. (2) A patient's intelligent choice about treatment, made after a physician discloses whatever information a reasonably prudent physician in the medical community would provide to a patient regarding the risks involved in the proposed treatment.

Intentional Tort: A tort committed by someone acting with general or specific intent; examples: battery, false imprisonment, and trespass. May also be termed a willful tort and is distinguished from negligence.

Interrogatories: A numbered list of written questions submitted in a legal context, usually to an opposing party in a lawsuit as part of discovery.

Joint Liability: Liability shared by two or more parties.

Law: (1) A set of rules that orders human activities and relations. (2) The collection of legislation and accepted legal principles; the body of authoritative grounds of judicial action.

Lawyer: One who is designated to transact business for another; a legal agent.

Liable: (1) Legally obligated or responsible. (2) To have a duty or burden.

Liability: The quality or state of being legally obligated or responsible.

Malpractice: Negligence or incompetence on the part of a professional. Professional negligence.

Medical Malpractice: A tort that arises when a doctor (or other health professional, including registered nurses, dentists, or social workers) violates the standard of care owed to a patient and the patient is injured as a result. (Often shortened to "Med Mal".)

Negligence: (1) The failure to exercise that standard of care that a reasonably prudent person would have exercised in the same situation. (2) A tort (civil wrong) grounded in this failure.

Opinion: The court's (a judge's) written statement explaining its decision in a given case, including statements of fact, points of law, rationale, and dicta.

Plaintiff: The party who brings a lawsuit in a civil action.

Proximate Cause: A cause that directly produces an event and without which the event would not have occurred.

Remedy: The enforcement of a right or the redress of an injury, usually in the form of monetary damages, that a party asks of a court.

Res Judicata (Latin term meaning "a thing [already] adjudicated"): An issue that had been definitively settled by judicial decision.

Several Liability: Liability that is separate and distinct from another's liability, so that the plaintiff may bring a separate action against one defendant without joining the other liable parties.

Standard of Care: In the law of negligence, the degree of care that a reasonable person would exercise.

Statutory Law: The body of law derived from statutes rather than from constitutions or judicial decisions.

Subpoena: A court order commanding the appearance of a witness, subject to penalty for noncompliance.

Tort: (1) A civil wrong for which a remedy may be obtained, usually in the form of damages. (2) Breach of a duty that the law imposes.

Verdict: A jury's findings or decision on the factual issues of a case.

Waiver: (1) To voluntarily relinquish or abandon. Waiver may be expressed or implied (by one's actions). A person who is alleged to have waived a right must have had both knowledge of the existing right and intention to relinquish it. (2) Waiver may also refer to the document by which a person relinquishes a right.

Witness: (1) One who sees, knows, or vouches for something. (2) One who testifies under oath or affirmation, either orally or by affidavit or deposition.

■ INTRODUCTION

In our litigious society, case managers are concerned with an ethical-legal conflict in which they want to provide quality case management services, obey the law, meet licensing requirements and regulations, please their employers or contractors, and still act as an advocate for their patients. The good news is that it is possible. Legal issues affecting case management are interwoven in the complex matrix that is case management practice. Just as each patient is an individual who presents with uniquely different life experiences, expectations, and outcome potential, so the interplay of the law is unique and will affect decision-making. Case managers have recognized the need for greater understanding in this area, but must always be mindful of the parameters of practice. It is knowing those parameters of practice or "knowing your sandbox" that reduces liability (Garner, 1996) exposure for the case manager.

■ BACKGROUND

A. Legal Basics: Understanding the law is much like learning a new language. It is especially important to learn legal terms, because some legal terms are words that have other meanings in common usage.

  The legal system is divided into two major categories, criminal and civil law. Civil law is also the law that applies to private rights especially, as opposed to the law that applies to criminal matters. Civil law is the body of law that permits an individual who believes that he has been wronged to sue another and recover damages (dollars). The purpose of tort law is to adjust losses, to compensate one person because of the actions of another. Criminal Law is public law that deals with crimes and their prosecution. Substantive criminal law defines crimes, and procedural criminal law sets down criminal procedure. A tort is a civil or personal wrong, as compared with a crime, which is a public wrong.

B. Intentional Torts: There are intentional torts, including assault, battery, false imprisonment, and trespass. These terms are often confused because they also exist in criminal law. When they are used in criminal law, they are defined by statute and can vary from state to state. Each intentional tort represents a direct interference with a person's physical integrity or right to property. Personal freedom is a fundamental right. One does not waive a fundamental right, such as personal integrity, automatically, but a person must be aware that he or she possesses the right and can intentionally relinquish it.

  Informed consent is a good example of a knowing and voluntary waiver in the medical setting. In the absence of such a waiver of rights, a person touching or keeping another in a clinic, hospital, or any place he or she chooses not to be may be liable for assault, battery, or false imprisonment. Informed consent is a statutorily created right, given to potential recipients of medical treatment. Many states have enacted a "Patient's Bill of Rights" (Box 6–1). When a law exists, such as a Patient's Bill of Rights in one setting (e.g., the hospital setting), the health practitioner can reasonably assume that the policy established in that law may apply to a setting not articulated specifically. In other words, if a case manager finds himself or herself in the field setting or on the telephone and in a decision-making dilemma and, to complicate the matter, the patient is very argumentative and difficult, the case manager must be cognizant of the statutory language that states, " [A patient (client) has a right] to considerate and respectful care consistent with sound . . . practices, which shall include being informed of the name and licensure status of a . . . staff member who . . . observes or treats the patient" (see Box 6–1). There is no doubt that a case manager is making observations about a patient, whether on the telephone or at arm's length. Even if there is no statute di-

BOX 6–1
Bill of Rights for Hospital Patients
• •

Every person admitted to a general hospital as licensed by the State Department of Health and Senior Services pursuant to P.L. 1971, c. 136 (C. 26:2H-1 et al.) shall have the right:

a. To considerate and respectful care consistent with sound nursing and medical practices, which shall include being informed of the name and licensure status of a student nurse or facility staff member who examines, observes or treats the patient.;

b. To be informed of the name of the physician responsible for coordinating his diagnosis, treatment, and prognosis in terms he can reasonably be expected to understand. When it is not medically advisable to give this information to the patient; it shall be made available to another person designated by the patient on his behalf;

d. To receive from the physician information necessary to give informed consent prior to the start of any procedure or treatment and which, except for those emergency situations not requiring an informed consent, shall include as a minimum the specific procedure or treatment, the medically significant risks involved, and the possible duration of incapacitation, if any, as well as an explanation of the significance of the patient's informed consent. The patient shall be advised of any medically significant alternatives for care or treatment, however, this does not include experimental treatments that are not yet accepted by the medical establishment;

e. To refuse treatment to the extent permitted by law and to be informed of the medical consequences of this act;

f. To privacy to the extent consistent with providing adequate medical care to the patient. This shall not preclude discussion of a patient's case or examination of a patient by appropriate health care personnel;

g. To privacy and confidentially of all records pertaining to his treatment, except as otherwise provided by law or third party payment contract, and to access to those records, including receipt of a copy thereof at reasonable cost, upon request, unless his physician states in writing that access by the patient is not medically advisable; to give this information to the patient, it shall be made available to another person designated by the patient on his behalf;

h. To expect that within its capacity, the hospital will make reasonable response to his request for services, including the services of an interpreter in a language other than English if 10% or more of the population in the hospital's service area speaks that language;

i. To be informed by his physician of any continuing health care require-

(continued)

BOX 6–1
Bill of Rights for Hospital Patients (*Continued*)

- -

ments which may follow discharge and to receive assistance from the physician and appropriate hospital staff in arranging for required follow-up care after discharge;

j. To be informed by the hospital of the necessity of transfer to another facility prior to the transfer and of any alternatives to it which may exist, which transfer shall not be effected unless it is determined by the physician to be medically necessary;

k. To be informed, upon request, of other health care and educational institutions that the hospital has authorized to participate in his treatment;

l. To be advised if the hospital proposes to engage in or perform human research or experimentation and to refuse to participate in these projects. For the purposes of this subsection "human research" does not include the mere collecting of statistical data;

m. To examine and receive an explanation of his bill, regardless of source of payment, and to receive information or be advised on the availability of sources of financial assistance to help pay for the patient's care, as necessary;

n. To expect reasonable continuity of care;

o. To be advised of the hospital rules and regulations that apply to his conduct as a patient;

p. To treatment without discrimination as to race, age, religion, sex, national origin, or source of payment; and

q. To contract directly with a New Jersey licensed registered professional nurse of the patient's choosing for private professional nursing care during his hospitalization. A registered professional nurse so contracted shall adhere to hospital policies and procedures in regard to treatment protocols and policies and procedures so long as those policies and procedures are the same for private duty and regularly employed nurses. The registered professional nurse shall not be considered an agent or employee of the hospital for purposes of any financial liabilities, including, but not limited to, State or federal employee taxes, worker's compensation payments or coverage for professional liability.

N.J.S.A. 26:2H-12.8

rectly on point regarding case management practice, you can assume that a court will use existing law as a basis for an alternative practice setting for as much as is practical. This is how new laws are developed.

C. Negligence: For a lawsuit to be successful in negligence, it requires four elements. These elements are commonly referred to as duty, breach, cause, and harm. All of the elements must be present. Lots of duty and an obvious breach are not sufficient without establishing the causal connection to the harm claimed (Prosser, 1984). Proof of damages (harm) is an essential element to a negligence case. Negligence is sometimes referred to as simple negligence as compared with malpractice or professional negligence. The standard of proof for a simple negligence case is that of a reasonably prudent person.

The concept of negligence is based on the idea that there can be a generally uniform standard of human behavior. The simplest example of this is that when one drives a car, there is a generally accepted expectation that each person will operate the vehicle in a reasonably prudent and careful manner. Each time that there is a motor vehicle accident, it is likely that one or more persons deviated from the reasonably prudent person's standard and liability may attach. However, state statutes may limit or expand one's ability to bring a cause of action. No-fault insurance is an example of such a limitation, particularly when there is an express limitation on one's ability to sue for certain personal injuries (N.J.S.A 39:6B, *et seq*).

D. How Cases Are Decided: What we refer to as "the law" is a combination of legislated rules—statutory law and case law. Case law is the compilation of common law. Common law, with its historical roots dating back to 12th-century England, provides the foundation for the collection of decisions. Such decisions are outcomes of particular cases and are either jury verdicts or judges' decisions. Judges' decisions may be verbal, on the record, or in the form of a written opinion. *Res judicata* is the legal term explaining that today's law is based on decisions that came before. Once an issue on a particular set of facts has been decided, there is no reason to relitigate the issue. For example, it has already been decided that if a surgeon excises the left limb when the informed consent clearly states the right limb, the surgeon is liable and has committed a battery. Whether a new case relates to ears, legs, arms, or breasts, the court will rely on the existing law relating to battery and professional negligence, also known as malpractice. Therefore, most cases are not reported. A reported case is one that can be found in an official reporter. There are state as well as federal reporters. When entered into a reporter, the case is printed and becomes part of the ever-growing body of case law.

E. Professional Negligence and Malpractice: Each of us comes to case management with education and experience from a profession. We are often licensed in that underlying profession. In fact, this is one of the qualifications for a person seeking to become a case manager. It is critical that the case managers maintain current licensing requirements and update his or her knowledge each year in both the field of case management and the underlying profession. The standard by which any case manager will be judged remains one derived from an external authority, such a governmental standard. If you are a nurse, this would be derived from the Nurse Practice Act. (Each state has a Nurse Practice Act of one variety or another [N.J.S.A. 45:11–23, *et seq*]). When these laws were drafted, the concept of managed care had not been thought of by the legislatures.

Each profession develops a standard for itself through a complicated process of interaction with other professions, professional journals, meetings, and networking with colleagues. In the developing world of new names and new roles, the law has not caught up with these rapid changes. Over time, hundreds of separate standards and comments become the "standard practice" (Eddy, 1982). Each profession has an obligation to monitor itself.

F. Burden of Proof: In the case of professional liability, (malpractice), the law requires that an expert witness be employed to establish the accepted standards of practice. Such experts base their opinions and their testimony on their knowledge, education and experience. State and federal rules of evidence require that a patient claiming that a professional is responsible for his or her injuries and damages use a "like-kind" expert witness to prove his or her case (Fed. R. Evid. 703, 704, N.J.S.A. 2A:84A2, *et seq*). In other words, if the case manager who is being sued is a nurse, then it will be necessary for another nurse to act as the expert witness. The plaintiff cannot proceed or be successful in a lawsuit unless a causal relationship is established between the harm claimed, the duty of the nurse case manager, and an alleged breach of such duty. It is not enough to have a generally experienced nurse testify against a nurse in a unique role; rather, case managers require a nurse case manager expert, utilization review nurses require a utilization review expert, and social workers require a social worker case manager expert.

G. Affidavit of Merit: In many states, it is now necessary on the filing of a malpractice lawsuit that an Affidavit of Merit is filed (N.J.S.A. 2A:53A-27).[1] This is a safeguard for the defendant, the purpose of which is to eliminate lawsuits filed without a genuine cause of action against a professional (licensed) person. In New Jersey, for example, this was part of major tort reform legislation. A person who wishes to bring a negligence or malpractice action against a licensed person must submit the affidavit

---

1 Affidavit required in certain actions against licensed persons. In any action for damages for personal injuries, wrongful death, or property damage resulting from an alleged act of malpractice or negligence by a licensed person in his profession or occupation, the plaintiff shall, within 60 days following the date of filing of the answer to the complaint by the defendant, provide each defendant with an affidavit of an appropriate licensed person that there exists a reasonable probability that the care, skill, or knowledge exercised or exhibited in the treatment, practice, or work that is the subject of the complaint fell outside of the acceptable professional or occupational standards or treatment practices. The court may grant no more than one additional period, not to exceed 60 days, to file the affidavit pursuant to this section, on a finding of good cause. The person executing the affidavit shall be licensed in this or any other state; have particular expertise in the general area or specialty involved in the action, as evidenced by board certification or by devotion of the person's practice substantially to the general area or specialty involved in the action for a period of at least five years. The person shall have no financial interest in the outcome of the case under review but this prohibition shall not exclude the person from being an expert witness in the case. (N.J.S.A. 2A:53A-27.)

within 60 days from a neutral-licensed person. This independent person must state that the services were not acceptable, and the law requires that the person providing the affidavit be a qualified expert (N.J.S.A 2A:53A-27). The only exception to the affidavit requirement is in those cases in which the defendant (licensed professional) failed to provide necessary records that would reveal malpractice (N.J.S.A. 2A:53A-27). In a recent case, an affidavit prepared by an independent expert was found to be sufficient when the author (expert) submitted his *curriculum vitae*, delineating education, experience specific to the defendant's practice, and scientific presentation and papers he had authored (*Wacht v. Farooqui*, 1998).

H. Liability Exposure for Case Managers: Case managers must be aware of what the law says about case management practice. Because many case managers come from a scientific discipline, with finite rules and measurable answers, it is difficult sometimes to understand the fluid, fact-driven dynamic that is the law. Now case managers have been recognized by some courts as potential defendants.

Until there are more reported cases in which case managers have either been held to be liable or relieved from liability, or states create statutes controlling case management practice, the profession must rely on its own developing standards.

Recently, the New Jersey Supreme Court held that a health maintenance organization (HMO) was liable for the contribution toward the malpractice of a physician they hired as an independent contractor (*Dunn v. Praiss*, 1995). Logically it would follow that a case manager performing telephonic or field case management services for an HMO, who deviates from the "accepted standards of practice," could be held liable for his or her actions. In addition, the HMO could share in that liability. This is known as joint liability.

In an Alabama case, the allegation by a plaintiff/employee, "that the nurse [case manager] was more concerned with saving money than with the employee's recovery," was found to be insufficient to support a claim (*Reid v. Aetna Casualty & Surety Co.*, 1997). In this case, the client was offered a variety of choices for the treatment of pain management and the provider chosen was also the least expensive. In addition, there was an allegation of fraud on the part of the defendant or insurance carrier, in that they had suppressed the following material information (among other things): "that the nurse [case manager] was not acting as a registered nurse with the normal professional obligations toward the worker [client]" (*Reid v. Aetna Casualty & Surety Co.*, 1997). The court held that even if that were true (and made no finding that it was true), there was no evidence that the actions of the case manager caused any harm to the patient. "It is undisputed that Aetna hired [a case management company] to perform medical case management, that the [case manager] was employed as a registered nurse . . . and that she worked on the client's case." Although the patient claimed that the case manager "prevented her from undergoing beneficial treatments," she failed to offer proof of such alternative beneficial treatments, and the case was dismissed (*Reid v. Aetna Casualty & Surety Co.*, 1997).

It is very important to note that in the concurring opinion, another judge is this case stated the following: "My objection to this practice is not so much that the insurance carriers are employing these nurses [case managers] but that the [case managers] are usually not forthcoming in revealing the existence, nature, and purpose of their employment. Thus, injured employees are presented with [case managers] who appear to be assisting them, when in actuality the [case manager] might be testifying in court using information gained through the employee's trust in them" (*Reid v. Aetna Casualty & Surety Co.*, 1997).

Case managers should view this case as a "red flag." It is one example of a court that had a bad experience with case management. The majority of case managers are forthcoming about who they are, whom they are employed by, and why they are meeting with the patient. This case supports the need for case managers to clarify these issues at the first and subsequent meetings with the patient. Once the case manager has disclosed this information to the patient, any information obtained by the case manager about the patient's illness, injury, prior history, work history, present income, and source of income can be freely shared with the relevant parties. These may include the physician (as is needed for proper treatment), the payor source, and, in some limited circumstances, the employer.

■ CONTRACTS

A. Contract Basics: In the discussion of torts and negligence, you learned that a duty is a legally recognized obligation for which a remedy may be sought in the event of breach of that duty. Contract is another example of a source of duty. When a contract is formed, it creates one or many legal obligations for which damages may be available, in the event of a breach of contract. A lawsuit based on contract is a separate and distinct cause of action.

B. Elements of Contract: There are three elements to a valid or binding contract—offer, acceptance, and consideration.

1. Offer: A promise to do or refrain from doing something in exchange for a promise, an action, or refraining from action. An offer is a demonstrative of one's (*offeror—the one who makes the offer*) willingness to enter into a contract. The offer must be made known to the *offeree* (*one to whom the offer is made*) at the time of contract formation.

2. Acceptance: Once the offer has been made, acceptance is a voluntary act of the one who is given a contract offer. That person, by his or her action or promise, exercises his or her consent and willingness to enter into agreement and a legal relationship, known as a contract.

3. Consideration: Something of value. A contract must be supported by a benefit for believed benefit to the parties.

C. The Case Manager and Contract: A simple example of contract creation is the following: You are an independent case manager. You receive a telephone call from XYZ Insurance, asking you to provide case management services for Mr. Smith. In addition, XYZ offers you a fee if you visit Mr. Smith and submit a report. There are several ways to bind you to this contract. The first is to simply say, "Thank you, I'll do it." The second is to do what is requested and submit the report. The problem arises when you make a telephonic contact with Mr. Smith, submit the report anyway, and later XYZ discovers your "breach." This the foundation for contract litigation. Questions would be asked, such as "Was there a meeting of the minds at the time of contract formation?" "When was the contract formed?" "Was the information contained in the report so complete that the contract was substantially performed, and what is the value of the report and services rendered?" (Williston Contracts, 1957).

There are entire courses on this subject. What is important for the case manager to know is that your words and your actions are very important as you perform your day-to-day work. You have entered a phase of your professional life in which your words are central to the creation of obligations. You may be an agent of your employer or the purchaser of case management services, or both. Your actions and your words may effectively bind (obligate) the payer (insurance company, employer, or health benefits provider) to provide disability benefits, medical expenses, and services or any other service or benefit that you include in your verbal or written report. This concept should not intimidate you but rather aid you in your assessment and recommendations.

■ THE CASE MANAGER AND THE LEGAL COMMUNITY

Throughout your career, you have used a variety of resources to increase your knowledge. Attorneys are another source of valuable information. A case manager is an advocate for the client.[2] When you share a client with his or her lawyer, many of your goals should be the same. In a personal injury case, the attorney wants his or her client to receive any and all necessary services to improve their medical and physical condition. So do you. The difference is that the case manager has an obligation to accomplish the delivery of medically necessary services in a cost-effective and efficient manner. In general, the attorney does not become concerned with the expense to the payer but simply wants the client's needs to be met. These goals are not inconsistent; in fact, there are times when the attorney can be of assistance to the case manager. If you share a client with a lawyer, and that client is uncooperative in some way, a telephone call or short note to his or her attorney may go a long way.

When the case manager learns that a client is represented by a lawyer, the case manager has an obligation to contact that attorney, identify himself or herself and for whom he or she is working, the purpose in wanting to meet or communicate with the client, and generally what the case manager's goals are.[3] If you present yourself by saying, "I represent your client's automobile policy carrier and I'm here to save money," that will be the last conversation you have with the client or the attorney. However, if you say or write, "I am a case manager working for XYZ Insurance, your client's automobile carrier. I have been asked to meet with your client to assess present and future needs

---

2 Client: The individual who is ill or disabled who collaborates with the case manager to receive services (Case Management Society of America, 1995).

3 Note: In some states, particularly in the case of workers' compensation, an attorney cannot keep the case manager from meeting with the patient. Please refer to your practice state for this information.

and to facilitate the delivery of those services. I plan on meeting with your client on Tuesday. I look forward to communicating with you," the result should be far more to your liking. Both statements are true, and both statements have the same ultimate goal—cost-effective case management. Remember, there are times when presentation counts. When the case manager communicates with a lawyer, the telephone call should be outlined in advance (a simple note to yourself will do) and written notes or faxes should be presented in a professional manner. Attorneys practice the art of persuasion. Case managers are capable of being persuasive without being combative. If you can cultivate the lawyer as an ally, it can do much to accelerate the progress of your case.

A. The Case Manager and Litigation: There are times when the case manager is called as a witness in a patient's case. If the case manager receives a subpoena, it will be asking for one of two things—either an appearance by the case manager at a deposition or court, or the submission of records kept by the case manager relating to a client—or both. In most jurisdictions (states), interrogatories, which are written questions and answers under oath, are served only on parties to an action. Therefore, the only time the case manager may receive them is in the event of a lawsuit against the case manager as an individual. Even if the case manager is an expert witness, most states' discovery rules would not include interrogatories.

B. The Case Manager as Witness: More and more, the legal community is recognizing the case manager as a valuable source of information. There are two general categories of witnesses.
   1. The first is the *fact* witness. In that case, you would simply be asked to speak about things that you had seen or heard yourself. In other words, you might be asked to describe the condition of the patient as you observed her on a particular date, the treatment that you observed and documented, and to identify records previously made by you. Most likely, you would be appearing on behalf of the patient, as plaintiff, in a civil lawsuit. It is also possible that the defendant insurance carrier in a civil case may also use the case manager as a fact witness. This is nothing to fear. Most attorneys will invest time and prepare you before you testify. All you have to do is to tell the truth, which you would do without preparation.

      In Louisiana, a case manager's determination was used to ascertain whether a claimant's injury was work related. The claimant alleged that the case manager's assessment was not sufficient "investigation of the claim." The case was decided in favor of the employer, who retained the services of the case manager and held that the case manager's visit, assessment, and recommendations did constitute "reasonable effort" to ascertain an employee's exact medical condition [668 So.2d I161 (La. App. 5 Cir)].
   2. The expert witness is used when specialized information is required. Case managers are well qualified to provide such information to the court. In a liability lawsuit, the expert witness does not speak to the specific facts of a case because he or she would not be one of the persons involved in direct care. An expert witness is expected to be im-

partial. He or she may discuss items such as standards of practice, trends in an industry, educational background, and criteria for entry to a profession. Case managers have been used to clarify procedure and define case management process and practice.

In an unreported New York case, an insurance carrier was joined in a lawsuit initiated by a home care provider. After providing more than $65,000 of home care to a cancer patient, the carrier rejected the claim on the death of the patient. When the home care provider received the case, they immediately and repeatedly contacted the representative of the insurance company. The initial claim was sent to a "nurse approver," a nonmedical person, then on to a "nurse reviewer" who was a registered nurse. The reviewer forwarded the claim to the "medical management center," where a nurse would review the claim again, with additional documentation. When the claim was denied at this level, it was sent to a "medical director," a physician, for final determination. Initially, the case was dismissed by the court. However, a case manager with particular expertise in health benefit contract analysis (Krul, 1998) reviewed the contract under which the patient had received home care services. She discovered that the contract required case management and found that the insurance carrier had breached the contract by failing to provide the requisite case management services. The case returned to the New York Superior Court. With the sworn testimony of the case manager, the court found in favor of the home care company, thereby relieving the grieving family of the $66,000 burden. At any step of the approval process, it would have been simple for a case manager to assess the case and discuss the possibility of giving the patient a hospice classification with the physician. This would have triggered another contract obligation, and 100% of the home care would have been covered without the expense and aggravation of litigation.

■ FREQUENTLY ASKED QUESTIONS

A. *I am a new case manager. My boss gave me a case load immediately. I've been in the clinical setting for years. How can I be a case manager overnight?* There once was a day when you were a new nurse, social worker, or other health professional. The difference is that as a new case manager, you have been developing the necessary skills from the first day of clinical practice in your primary profession. Unless and until your state has enacted a statute or regulation under your licensing structure, there is no legal restriction regarding representing yourself as a case manager.

It is critical that you never forget your professional roots, because the law is slow in developing. In the event that you are sued for malpractice, the basis of that allegation would go first to your primary profession. For example, if you are a nurse, any action brought against you for work as a case manager would be a suit for nursing malpractice.

B. *The insurance carrier who assigned my latest patient wants me to ask the patient questions about "how the accident happened and who might be at fault." Can I do this?* Difficult questions call for complex answers, and this question is actually several questions. When your employer (whether it is an insurance carrier or intermediary) asks you to collect liability information, you are going outside the scope of practice. Your obligation is to collect information relevant to a patient's injuries or illness. A patient is "the individual who is ill or disabled who collaborates with the Case Manager to receive services." There is nothing contained in the definition of a patient that would indicate that your role, as you collaborate with that individual, is to collect facts or evidence pertaining to liability.

Note: Having been fully informed of your role, including your duty to report relevant information to the carrier, should the patient volunteer information about the accident or onset of the illness, you can and should deliver that information to the appropriate party. It is important that you relate such information accurately and factually, without editorial or judgmental overtones. Using an example of a soccer injury, when that information is reported, it should simply be written, "Client reports playing soccer on the Sunday immediately preceding the reported accident date." This gives the carrier the information it needs to investigate the report further. (See the discussion of the Alabama case in the Section on Liability Exposure for Case Manager.)

Insurance investigators are in the business of delving into the history and details of an injury or illness. They have various resources available to them, such as surveillance, photographs, and telephone and personal canvassing. None of those investigative tools falls within the role of the case manager.

C. *How can I honestly advise the patient, upon initial contact, whom I represent and why we are meeting (whether in person or by telephone)?* Honesty is always the best policy. If you are an "in-house" case manager, you should tell the patient that you are a case manager from XYZ Insurance, the company handling his or her claim. If you are employed by a case management company, simply modify the answer, "I am a case manager working for ABC Case Management Services, and in your case, we are working for XYZ Insurance, the company handling their claim."

The reason why this is so important is seen in the potential conflict between confidential information and the duty of the case manager to disclose information to the insurance company. Both of these obligations can exist simultaneously but require the case manager to be clear, particularly on the first patient contact.

D. *What if a patient tells me things that may affect his or her coverage under the insurance program through which I was hired?* This is not a new dilemma, merely an old one in a new environment. In your clinical experience, you were required to take patient histories on a regular basis, no matter what your underlying professional background. It is not unusual for a patient in the clinical setting to say, "I'm going to tell you something, but it's just between us." In the clinical setting, the response would be, "I appreciate your feeling comfortable enough to share that information, but I must report it to your physician, because it may affect his diagnosis. Would you prefer telling him yourself?"

In the role of case manager, the scenario is much the same. Typically a patient will say, "I told my boss I fell at work, but I'm telling you that I was injured playing soccer on Sunday. It will be our little secret." The response is similar to that in the clinical setting. "Remember at our first visit I explained that I was hired by the Workers' Compensation carrier. I also told you then that I have an obligation to report relevant information to them, and I will be passing this along." Do not apologize. It is your job.

E. *What if the patient asks me to keep something "off the record?"* Same answer as in D.

F. *What if I observe something that indicates that the patient is working?* Same answer as in D. Once you have fully informed the patient of who you are, who you are employed by, and the purpose of your visit, you can and will report all relevant information that you observe.

G. *What if I see or smell illegal drugs in a patient's home?* Case managers must be very careful not to be judgmental in their observations and assessments. The case manager is not a law enforcement person; however, such substances may impact on the potential recovery of the patient. The case manager should remove himself from the situation as quickly as possible and report only accurate facts to the supervision. You would not want to accuse someone of something as serious as drug use and learn later that your olfactory sense had misled you. Do not guess.

H. *What if I see my patient abuse a child or parent in my presence?* Most states now require medical and educational professionals to report actual acts of child or elder abuse that take place in their presence. Know your state's law on the subject. Contact your state board of medicine, nursing, social work, or other professional body to obtain such information. Again, do not guess. When it is necessary to report such information, the result will be an intrusive investigation by the appropriate state agency.

I. *What if my patient asks me to change a dressing?* As a case manager, it is not appropriate to perform "hands-on" care, even if you have the education and training to do so. The case manager's role is to coordinate and facilitate medically necessary treatment; therefore, it would be appropriate to contact the home care provider, physician, or family, depending on the circumstances of the particular case.

J. *What do I do if I walk into a medical emergency in a patient's home?* You should be familiar with the "Good Samaritan Act" where you practice.[4] When you enter someone's home as a case manager, you are not there to act as a "hands-on" nurse or other practitioner. It would be appropriate to respond to the best of your ability, based on your education and experience.

---

4 N.J.S.A. 2A:62A-1. Emergency care (commonly known as the Good Samaritan Act). Any individual, including a person licensed to practice any method of treatment of human ailments, disease, pain, injury, deformity, mental or physical condition, or licensed to render services ancillary thereto, or any person who is a volunteer member of a duly incorporated first aid and emergency or volunteer ambulance or rescue squad association, who in good faith renders emergency care at the scene of an accident or emergency to the victim or victims thereof, or while transporting the victim or victims thereof to a hospital or other facility where treatment or care is to be rendered, shall not be liable for any civil damages as a result of any acts or omissions by such person in rendering the emergency care.

A recent revision of one state's law provides that "any one [including RNs, LPNs, MDs, etc] who in good faith renders emergency care at the scene of an accident or emergency to the victim . . . shall not be liable for any civil damages as a result of any acts or omissions by such person in rendering the emergency care" (N.J.S.A. 2A:62A1). The purpose of such legislation is to encourage knowledgeable licensed persons to act, rather than shy away in fear of being sued.

K. *My supervisor edits all my reports. I feel like I'm back in high school. Is that OK?* It is important that the product, your report, be presented in a clear, concise, and professional manner. Stylistic and grammatical changes are simply a matter of taste and not a problem. The problem occurs when the substance of your report is changed by another, particularly if this change is without your knowledge.

Example: You make an observation about a patient and report that he or she has improved significantly since your last contact. You recommend a reduction of services to telephonic case management, with an anticipated closure in 30 to 45 days. The reviewer changes that information to read, "minimal improvement noted" and changes your recommendation from closing the file to "two to three more visits required to monitor progress."

Several things have happened here. First, the report is no longer your professional opinion, based in observation and assessment, but rather is a misrepresentation. It may go so far as to be considered fraud and places you, as well as the employer, in the position of having committed fraud on an insurance company. States vary on the consequences of this kind of action, but certainly the reviewer is risking the company and your presumably good reputation. If the problem is discovered, the company would not hire you again. Not all legal consequences are settled in court. Because litigation is costly, the cost-effective response would be to change case management service providers. Depending on the severity of the fraud, it could result in a lawsuit in which the company would be a named defendant.

L. *What is the significance, if any, of signing my reports?* If reports are signed, they should be signed by the writer. It is common practice for the report to be submitted in either a rough form, on a floppy disk, or in some instances entered directly into a company computer network. All of these methods still permit editing, revision, and the temptation for the editor to fall to the temptation described above in K. If you are the last person to review a report before submission to the carrier or another person who has purchased the case management services, then it certainly can be signed by you. On the other hand, if you are in a situation in which you do not get to see the final product before mailing, that, too, should be indicated on the report. Such methods as, "dictated but not read," alert the reader that the author of the report might not have seen the final product.

There is no magic in the signature itself. It is merely another indication that the author is submitting a completed project. In the ideal situation, the report should be submitted, edited, and returned to the author for review and signature.

M. *My employer does not pay for continuing education (CE) or make it available in-house. Do I still have to attend CE programs?* As the field of case management grows and is better recognized by the law, practitioners will be expected to have up-to-date information. To reduce your liability exposure, it is important to read, discuss, and earn continuing education credits. It is anticipated that as states codify case management practice and as other professions are regulated by state law, CE will be required. If you are to become a certified case manager (CCM) or other certified professional, CE credits are required.

If you were ever called as a fact or expert witness in a case relating to your case management practice, one of the first questions you would be asked is, "Do you have any special training or certification, and do you have any continuing education in the field of case management?"

N. *Is there any value in belonging to a professional organization?* The benefits of belonging to a professional organization, such as Case Management Society of America (CMSA), are immeasurable. The reason that this becomes a legal issue is that your source of case management practice information and guidelines should come from a reliable source. CMSA is a leader in the case management industry and works constantly to improve and standardize the practice. As a member, you will receive educational opportunities, practice updates, and opportunities to interact with other members of the profession, and be part of the development of the Standards of Practice.

O. *Can I refuse to see a patient?* Of course. The real question is "why?" Patient assignments and services can never have a discriminatory basis. If you sense a potential conflict of interest, this should be reported to your supervision and a decision should be made as to whether another case manager would be more appropriate for the assignment. The difficulty occurs when there are personality conflicts. This is best dealt with through consistent professional contacts with the patient and does not become a legal issue.

P. *Do I have to go back to that patient's home?* Your duty to provide services should never place you in personal or professional danger. If you have been exposed to a danger in a patient's home, the neighborhood, or work environment, there are alternative ways of obtaining necessary information. Such genuine fears should be reported to your supervisor and documented, if appropriate.

Remember, do not be judgmental in your report writing. A smart attorney will use this information to demonstrate that you had some prejudice in your decision-making in areas in which the patient is concerned. Describe what you see but do not characterize the information. For example, "The patient was dressed in pajamas when I arrived at his home at 1:30 PM. I asked him three times to turn off the television before I could begin the interview." This description simply tells the reader what you saw and what happened. "The patient appeared lazy. It was early afternoon, he was still in his pajamas and appeared more interested in the soap opera he was watching than in anything having to do with his recovery." This description is your opinion of why the patient presented in a particular way, which may be based on your life experience and not that of the patient. Be cautious.

Q. *What if I refer a patient to a provider and that provider commits malpractice? Could I be liable?* Each health (and other) professional is responsible for his or her own actions. Cost-effective medical care is an essential part of case management. Identifying the highest-quality service or product for the lowest price is consistent with one's professional obligations and ethical duty. When price alone dictates your professional decision-making, liability may follow. When you are placed in a position to make a referral, you should not do so blindly. What is the source of your referral? Is it a provider that your coworkers have been very pleased with, or is it simply the lowest price you can find? Are you able to procure an identical product or one that performs as well or simply a lesser product?

Make a reasonable inquiry to determine what will be provided for the dollars spent. Sometimes, a dollar saved in the short term can represent long-term expense. It may also expose the decision-maker to unnecessary risk. Potential liability rests with whether you acted within the scope of your profession and accepted standards of practice (CMSA, 1995).

REFERENCES

Black's law dictionary. (1966). St. Paul: West Publishing Co.

Case Management Society of America (CMSA) (1995). *Standards of practice for case management.* Little Rock, AR: CMSA.

Dunn v. Praiss, 139 N.J. 561 (1995).

Eddy, J. (1982). Clinical policies and the quality of clinical practice. *New England Journal of Medicine,* 343.

Fed. R. Evid. 703, 704, N.J.S.A. 2A:84A-2, et seq.

Keeton, W. P. (1984). *Prosser and Keaton, the law of torts* (5th ed.). St. Paul: West Publishing.

Krul, R., personal communication.

N.J.S.A. 39:6B, *et seq.*

N.J.S.A. 45:11–23, *et seq.*

Reid v. Aetna Casualty & Surety Co., et al., 692 So.2d 863 (Alabama App. 1997).

Wacht v. Farooqui, 312 N.J. Super. 184, 711 A.2d 405 (App. Div. 1998).

Williston Contracts §1(3d ed. 1957), Restatement 2d, Contracts §2, See Muller, L. (1998) Provider contracts: What case managers need to know. *The Journal of Care Management, The Official Journal of The Case Management Society of America, 4,* 5.

668 So.2d 1161 (La. App. 5 Cir.)

CHAPTER 7

. . . .

Ethical Issues in Case Management

PATRICIA M. PECQUEUX

LEARNING OBJECTIVES

Upon completion of this chapter, the reader will be able to:

1. Define ethical principles of case management practice and cite patient examples for each principle.

2. Describe several ethical decision making tools and when to use them.

3. Explain the importance of codes of ethics for professional case management practice.

4. Explain the Patient Self Determination Act of 1990 and its importance in the case management process.

5. Discuss several patient management scenarios that have significant ethical dimensions and how you would manage them as a case manager.

IMPORTANT TERMS AND CONCEPTS

Advance Directives
American Nurses Association's Code of Ethics
Assisted Suicide
Case Manager as Gatekeeper
Code of Professional Conduct for Case Managers
Commission on Rehabilitation Counselor Certification's Code of Professional Ethics

Ethical Dilemma
Ethics
Ethics Committee
"Gag Rules"
Guide for the Uncertain in Decision Making Ethics (GUIDE)
Medical Necessity
Patient Advocate
Patient Self Determination Act of 1990

Rationing of Health Care	Statement of Ethical Case
Standards of Professional Performance	Management Practice
	"Unnecessary" Treatment

■ INTRODUCTION

A. Ethics is the study of values and human conduct with the study of right conduct.

B. Ethical conduct means doing the right thing for the right reason at the right time.

C. Ethical decision-making is an attempt to identify and analyze ethical dilemmas in order to resolve them.

D. There are several ethical principles that are particularly important to the practice of case management: autonomy, beneficence, nonmaleficence, justice, and veracity.

E. A relationship exists between the law and ethics. Both the law and ethics are social sanctions and functions and both serve as action guides. "Law is created for the purpose of maintaining order and continuity in society; it generally sets a minimum standard for social behavior. The force behind the law is some form of enforceable punishment (e.g., imprisonment, fines). Ethics is often regarded as higher than the law and a source of judgment of the law itself. Disobedience to ethical norms does not carry the same force of punishment as the law does. Violation of an ethical rule may elicit moral disapproval from others, such as anger or ostracism" (Fowler & Ariff, 1987).

■ KEY DEFINITIONS

A. Advance Directives—Legally executed documents that are drawn up while the individual is still competent and used only if that individual becomes incapacitated or incompetent (Powell, 2000)

B. Advocacy—In the legal context, advocacy refers to defending basic human rights on behalf of those who cannot speak for themselves (Fowler & Ariff, 1987)

C. Autonomy—A form of personal liberty of action when the individual determines his or her own course of action in accordance with a plan chosen by himself or herself (Case Management Society of America [CMSA], 1996)

D. Beneficence—The obligation or duty to promote good, to further a person's legitimate interests, and to prevent or remove harm actively (CMSA, 1996)

E. Distributive justice—Deals with the moral basis for dissemination of goods and evils, and burdens and benefits (CMSA, 1996)

F. "Gag Rules"—Provisions in managed care contracts that prevent physicians and other health care employees from being fully open with their patients (Powell, 2000)

G. Justice—Maintenance of what is right and fair (CMSA, 1996)

H. Medical Necessity—Comparison of the state of illness with the treatment rendered. Medical necessity asks if the treatment or level of care is appropriate for this set of medical conditions (Powell, 2000).

I. Nonmaleficence—Refraining from doing harm to others (CMSA, 1996)

J. Veracity—Truth telling (CMSA, 1996)

■ ETHICAL PRINCIPLES

A. Ethical principles guide behavior in the clinical setting.

B. Ethical principles may conflict with one another (i.e., patient advocacy versus control of resources).

C. Autonomy can refer to self-determined choice, freedom of action, individual liberty, or self-governance. These different uses of autonomy reflect two origins of the concept: respect for the unconditional worth of the person and respect for individual thought and action.
  1. Respect for the unconditional worth of the person was the philosophical view of autonomy proposed by Immanuel Kant.
  2. Respect for individual thought and action was the philosophical view of autonomy proposed by John Stuart Mill.
  3. The principle of autonomy does not apply to a young child, comatose patient, or person who is severely mentally ill or incapable of making decisions for himself or herself.
  4. Autonomy is often compromised due to illness or the ability of the person to make his or her own decisions, or both.
  5. Examples of health care situations that apply to this principle are "gag rules" and the "right to die" issue.

D. Advocacy is defending basic human rights on behalf of those who cannot speak for themselves. There are three models of advocacy:
  1. Rights Protection Model—The case manager is viewed as the defender of patient rights against an impersonal health care system that violates patient rights (Fowler & Ariff, 1987).
  2. Values-Based Decision Model—The case manager helps a patient discuss his or her needs and assists the patient to make choices that are consistent with his or her values by informing and supporting the patient (Fowler & Ariff, 1987).
  3. Respect for the Person Model—The patient is viewed as possessing certain human characteristics that require our respect. The patient is respected whether he or she is autonomous or not. As an advocate, the case manager respects the basic human values of the patient by protecting his or her human dignity, privacy, and honoring his or her choices, if the patient is competent (Fowler & Ariff, 1987).

E. Beneficence in health care requires a case manager to behave in a way such that important and legitimate outcomes for the patient are focused on, while avoiding harm to the patient. This principle focuses on "doing good and causing no harm." Professional codes of ethics and a patient's bill of rights are based on this principle.

1. Professional codes of conduct
   a. American Nurses Association "Code of Ethics and the Standards of Professional Performance" (1985)
   b. Commission on Rehabilitation Counselor Certification's Code of Professional Ethics
   c. Commission for Case Management Certification "Scope of Practice for Case Managers and the Code of Professional Conduct for Case Managers"
2. The Consumer Bill of Rights and Responsibilities is a document that was developed by a Presidential Advisory Committee and released in November, 1997. The bill makes recommendations in seven areas of health care:
   a. Information disclosure
      (i) Health plan information
      (ii) Health professional information
      (iii) Health care facility information
      (iv) Information about consumer assistance programs
   b. Choice of plan and provider
      (i) Provider network adequacy
      (ii) Women's health services
      (iii) Access to specialists
      (iv) Transitional care
      (v) Choice of health plans
   c. Participation in treatment decisions
   d. Respect and nondiscrimination
   e. Confidentiality of health information
   f. Complaints and appeals
   g. Consumer responsibilities
3. Situations relating to the withholding or withdrawing of a patient treatment would pertain to this principle (Quinlan case, 1975).

F. **Nonmaleficence** means that a case manager must not knowingly inflict harm on a patient. It requires that a case manager act carefully and thoughtfully toward the patients and others.

G. **Justice** means that like cases should be treated alike and different cases should be treated differently. The challenge for the case manager is to know when differences exist in patient situations.
1. Distributive justice is the most important application of the principle of justice relating to case management. It is the allocation of goods and services, usually in times of scarcity.
2. Examples of health care situations that apply to this principle include organ donation, allocation of services, and the use of expensive technology in patient care.

H. **Veracity** means to tell the truth. This principle is applicable to patient situations involving informed consent and the "patient's right to know" about his or her diagnosis and treatment options.

I. Ethical Decision-Making Processes

1. Ethics committees are composed of a multidisciplinary group of health care professionals who collect and carefully analyze all aspects of an ethical patient situation with the intent of rendering an opinion on the appropriate course of action. Ethics committees are usually institutionally based.

2. Ethical tools that can be used in the decision-making process include the following (Powell, 2000):

   a. Schools and theories of ethical thought

   b. Humor

   c. Contemporary thought on a particular issue

   d. Effective communication skills

   e. Honesty

   f. Balancing your own values with those of the patient and the family, the institution, and existing laws

3. A problem-solving process, which includes the following steps, can be used in the decision-making process:

   a. Assessment

   b. Planning

   c. Implementation

   d. Evaluation

4. The guide for the uncertain in decision-making ethics (GUIDE) (Levenson & Pettrey, 1994) takes into consideration advance directives, proxy decision-makers, and health care teams' preferences in the ethical decision-making process.

REFERENCES

American Nurses Association. (1985). *Code for nurses with interpretive statements*. Kansas City, MO: ANA.

Banja, J. (1999). Ethical decision-making: Origins, process, and applications to case management. *The Case Manager, 10*(5), 41–47.

Blancett, S. S., & Flarey, D. L. (1996). *Handbook of nursing case management*. Gaithersburg, MD: Aspen Publishers.

Case Management Society of America (CMSA). (1996). *Code of professional conduct for case managers*. Rolling Meadows, IL: Commission for Care Management Certification.

Fowler, M. D., & Levine-Ariff, J. (1987). *Ethics at the bedside*. Philadelphia: J. B. Lippincott Company.

Kohnke, M. E. (1980). The nurse as advocate. *American Journal of Nursing, 80*, 2038–2040.

Levenson, J. & Pettrey, L. (1994). Controversial decisions regarding treatment and DNR: An algorithmic guide for the uncertain in decision making ethics (GUIDE). *American Journal of Critical Care, 3*(2), 87–91.

Meaney, M. E. (1999). Building a professional ethical culture in case management. *The Case Manager, 10*(5), 63–67.

Mullahy, C. M. (1999). Case management: An ethically responsible solution. *The Case Manager, 10*(5), 59–62.

Powell, S. K. (2000). *Nursing case management: A practical guide to success in managed care*. Philadelphia: Lippincott-Raven.

Saulo, M., & Wagener, R. J. (1996a). How good case managers make tough choices: Ethics and mediation. *The Journal of Care Management, 2*(1), 8–14, 51–55.

Saulo, M., & Wagener, R. J. (1996b). How good case managers make tough choices: Ethics and mediation, Part 2. *The Journal of Care Management, 2*(2), 10–16, 35–42.

CHAPTER 8

• • • • • • • • • • • •

Quality Reviews and Risk Management

NANCY CLAFLIN

PATRICIA M. PECQUEUX

LEARNING OBJECTIVES

Upon completion of this chapter, the reader will be able to:

1. Describe the similarities between quality improvement and risk management.
2. Describe important components of a risk management program.
3. List elements of quality reviews.
4. Describe how quality reviews can enhance a risk management program.
5. Explain the case manager's role in quality and risk management.
4. List several key concepts related to documentation about which a case manager should be knowledgeable.
5. Explain the case manager's role in quality and risk management.
6. List several key concepts related to documentation about which a case manager should be knowledgeable.

IMPORTANT TERMS AND CONCEPTS

Adverse Patient Outcome
Continuous Quality Improvement/Total Quality Management
Important Aspects of Care

Incident
Incident Report
Indicators
Occurrence Report

<table>
<tr><td>Outcomes</td><td>Quality Reviews</td></tr>
<tr><td>Potentially Compensable Event</td><td>Risk Management (RM)</td></tr>
<tr><td>Quality Assurance (QA)</td><td>Variances</td></tr>
<tr><td>Quality Improvement (QI)</td><td></td></tr>
</table>

■ INTRODUCTION

A. Quality health care has evolved from a quality assurance (QA) approach to a focus on continuous quality improvement (CQI)/total quality management (TQM) and, ultimately, to doing procedures right the first time.

B. QA traditionally has focused on monitoring, preventing, and correcting quality deficiencies (Powell, 2000).

C. QI incorporates a proactive, CQI approach to patient care.

D. Risk management (RM) focuses on identifying potential risk areas and on interventions that will enhance patient safety and prevent losses before they occur (Powell, 2000).

■ KEY DEFINITIONS

A. Adverse Patient Occurrences (APO)—An APO is defined as any adverse patient occurrence, which, under most conditions, is not a natural consequence of the patient's disease process or the end result of a procedure (Powell, 2000).

B. CQI/TQM—A management philosophy for continually improving quality and satisfying customers that is directed from the top levels of the organization and involves all of its members in the improvement of processes, products, and services (Claflin, 1998).

C. Important Aspects of Care—These are the aspects of care that occur frequently, affect large numbers of patients, or place patients at risk for serious consequences if not provided for optimally. These aspects are often the target of performance improvement activities and, therefore, must be measurable (Powell, 2000).

D. Incident—An incident is an accident or a discovery of a hazardous condition that is inconsistent with standards of care (Powell, 2000).

E. Incident Report—An incident report is a communication tool to record adverse events or unusual occurrences. Incident reports assess potential liabilities, are used for discovering existing problems, and assess the need for revising current policies or procedures (Powell, 2000).

F. Indicators—Tools used to measure the performance of functions, processes, and outcomes of important aspects of patient care or services (Claflin, 1998).

G. Occurrence Report—A report of a concurrent review of patient records to determine whether an adverse event has occurred that is the result of health care management and not of the disease process (Claflin, 1998).

H. Outcomes—Outcomes describe the results and consequences of the care received; outcomes also result from care not received (Powell, 2000).

I. Potentially Compensable Event—A potentially compensable event is one in which the end result could be litigation (Powell, 2000).

J. QA—Activities designed to monitor, prevent, and correct quality deficiencies (Powell, 2000).

K. Quality Management (QM)/QI—A process that determines whether the care provided meets medical standards (Powell, 2000).

L. Quality Reviews—The process of screening the clinical content of the patient's medical record and treatment plan to determine if professionally recognized standards of care were met (Powell, 2000).

M. RM—The science of the identification, evaluation, and treatment of perils and hazards that represent the threat of financial loss; a program that attempts to provide positive avoidance of negative results (Claflin, 1998).

N. Variance—A measure of the differences in a set of observations (Claflin, 1998); deviations from expected care (Powell, 2000).

■ QUALITY IMPROVEMENT ACTIVITIES

A. Quality care includes five major components:
  1. Good professional performance by all health care practitioners
  2. Efficient use of resources
  3. Minimal risk to the patient of injury or illness associated with care
  4. Patient satisfaction
  5. Compassionate care

B. CQI/TQI are based on the assumptions that organizations that deliver health care can improve patient care quality or increase the probability of desired patient outcomes, including patient satisfaction.
  1. QI builds on the strengths of QA by broadening its scope, refining its approach to assessing and improving care, and diminishing the negative connotations sometimes associated with QA.
  2. The role of leaders in improving quality is emphasized.
  3. The scope of assessment and improvement activities is expanded beyond the clinical to the interrelated governance, managerial, support, and clinical processes that affect patient care outcomes.
  4. Ongoing monitoring continues, but other sources of feedback are also used to trigger evaluation and improvement of the care and services provided.
  5. The health care organization's customers are defined as everyone affected by its services.
  6. QI seeks to improve patient care outcomes by focusing on the processes of care and structures that support those processes in producing patient outcomes (Claflin, 1993).
  7. Quality reviews provide data for QI activities.

■ RISK MANAGEMENT

A. RM is the process of making and carrying out decisions that will minimize the adverse effects of accidental losses. Risks and their prudent management are viewed as matters of patient safety.

B. RM is usually an administrative undertaking intended to protect the financial assets of a health care provider in four ways:
   1. By ensuring adequate, appropriate insurance coverage against potential liability.
   2. By reducing liability when potentially compensable events or adverse patient outcomes occur.
   3. By preventing those events that are most likely to lead to liability.
   4. The case manager can help reach the goals of RM, which include identifying actual or potential causes of patient incidents and recommending strategies to eliminate or reduce those incidents.

■ SIMILARITIES BETWEEN QUALITY IMPROVEMENT AND RISK MANAGEMENT

A. Poor quality care that creates risk of injury to patients also creates potential financial risks both to the health care practitioner and to health care organizations and facilities.

B. Both QI and RM emphasize identification and resolution of problems in patient care, which require coordinated QI, RM activities, and information systems.

C. Both depend on establishing relevant screening criteria (quality reviews), collecting and analyzing data related to those criteria, and correcting problems through improvements in systems and in individual practices.
   1. A timely flow of information between QI and RM will assist with the identification of problems and the evaluation of the success of corrective actions.

■ RISK MANAGEMENT PROGRAM

A. RM includes risk identification and risk reduction.
   1. Risk identification is the first step in meeting the goals of reducing liability when untoward events occur and preventing those events that are most likely to lead to liability. Risk identification includes identifying loss exposures and loss prevention.
   2. Risk reduction aims to lower the severity of a particular loss either before the loss occurred or after. This is accomplished through programs such as claims management and resource preservation.

B. The case manager can assist in the risk management processes by providing input into the review of areas of risk, including performing quality reviews of medical record documentation, and information obtained from occurrence screens and incident reports involving patients and families in all health care settings.

C. The case manager is responsible for sharing this information as appropriate with members of the health care team and the RM department.

D. The case manager can also assist in identifying areas of risks, such as those related to admission and discharge, safety, equipment and supplies, clinical activities, emergency situations, informed consent, confidentiality, and documentation requirements.

E. The case manager can assist in performing quality reviews of medical record documentation to identify potential problem areas. Whether in the hospital, skilled nursing facility, rehabilitation facility, or home care, there are some common requirements for medical records that can be identified through quality reviews. They include

1. Identification data
2. Medical history, including chief complaint, details of the present illness, relevant past, social and family histories appropriate to age, and an inventory by body system
3. A summary of the patient's psychosocial needs, as appropriate to age
4. A report of relevant physical examination
5. A statement on the conclusions or impressions drawn from the admission history and physical examination
6. A statement on the course of action planned for the patient for an episode of care and of its periodic review, as appropriate
7. Diagnostic and therapeutic orders
8. Evidence of appropriate informed consent
9. Clinical observations, including the results of therapy
10. Progress notes made by the medical staff and other authorized staff
11. Consultation reports
12. Reports of operative and other procedures, such as pathology and clinical laboratory examinations and radiology and nuclear medicine examinations or treatments
13. Records of donations and receipt of transplants
14. Final diagnoses
15. Conclusions at termination of hospitalization
16. Clinical resumes and discharge summaries
17. Discharge instructions to the patient and family as appropriate
18. Results of autopsy (Claflin, 1998)

F. The case manager can assist in collecting RM data through quality reviews, which include incident reporting, event reporting, and occurrence screening.

1. The case manager should be involved in the incident reporting system. Data from incident report forms include information about the person involved in an incident, the type of incident, the time and location of the incident, any hazards associated with the incident, treatment provided, and the outcome of the incident. Incidents that should be reported include
   a. Disruptions of facility functions

    b. Adverse public relations occurrences

    c. Undesirable events inconsistent with routine client care

    d. Violations of established policy and procedure

    e. Events that may or do result in injury

    f. Security breaches

    g. Sudden, unexpected adverse results of treatment

    h. Biomedical equipment and mechanical failures or problems

    i. Defective premises conditions

    j. Incidents involving voiced hostility by a client, visitor, or family member

    k. Other adverse events (Claflin, 1998)

2. All staff members fill out incident reports when warranted; the case manager is included.

3. The case manager can also assist in identifying immediate corrective actions that include immediate care of the patient and instructions to any health care providers involved.

4. The case manager may also participate in an objective assessment of the problem's cause and scope. This problem assessment is followed by comprehensive corrective actions to reduce the possibility of similar incidents in the future.

    a. For example, the case manager may assist in developing guidelines and revising policies, procedures, and equipment.

    b. Areas of risk most often identified through a review of incident reports involve patient falls and injury to patients' skin. Most organizations have fall-risk and skin integrity–risk assessment programs as part of risk identification activities. The case manager can participate in this program, which involves developing policies and procedures for classifying each patient on admission according to the risk of falls or skin integrity risk. The case manager can also participate in the development of a protocol to guide classification of patients into levels of risk. Each level of risk is associated with mandatory safety precautions. As part of the quality review, the case manager can help determine whether patients are appropriately classified and are receiving appropriate safety precautions.

G. One of the most common methods of loss prevention is the use of informed consent. The requirement of informed consent in health care is based on the tort law of assault and battery.

1. A battery consists of the touching of a first person by a second person or by any substance put in motion by the second person.

2. The health care professional who performs any procedure that involves touching a patient should first obtain permission.

3. The patient's understanding of informed consent is based on adequate information about his or her disease or condition, recommended therapy, available alternatives, and collateral risks.

4. A signed consent form is evidence that the patient's informed consent has been obtained.

5. The case manager can assist in identifying proper informed consent through quality reviews of the patient's medical records.

H. Staff education is a critical component of a RM program.

1. The case manager can assist in ensuring that staff, patients, and families are educated about risks by providing education programs.

2. Education programs for staff related to RM should contain information about legal aspects of nursing, medication errors, patient confidentiality, and liability. Other information to be provided includes policies and procedures regarding RM and informed consent and guidelines on reporting and resolving incidents and claims.

3. Education programs for patients should include information on the benefits and risks associated with clinical services and programs.

I. Successful RM depends on early intervention, prevention, and use of available resources. The case manager can assist in all of these areas. RM should be an interdisciplinary team effort that increases awareness of the importance of prevention (Claflin, 1993).

■ IMPLICATIONS OF AGE AND CULTURE FOR RISK MANAGEMENT

A. Every patient has unique care needs. Age and culture are part of what makes each person unique. The case manager plays an important role by helping identify age and cultural factors that could impede successful patient outcomes. The case manager can help educate staff regarding age and cultural differences. Every person grows and develops in his or her own unique way. Not every member of a cultural group may share all of its values, beliefs, or practices. A patient may appear similar to the caregiver but still be different in certain ways.

B. Factors that may differ from patient to patient include ethnic, religious, and occupational factors. These factors may jeopardize the patient's health or place the patient at risk if they are not taken into account. The case manager can help implement cultural protocols that take into account the following factors:

1. Some people belong to more than one ethnic group, as well as cultural groups. Other people have fewer group identities.

2. The importance of religion can vary from person to person. For example, some people keep many daily traditions, such as eating certain foods, whereas others keep traditions only on special occasions or not at all.

3. For many different reasons—for example, religious, ethnic, health, or personal preference—a person may eat or avoid certain foods at certain times or not eat some foods at all. The case manager needs to be aware that this practice may jeopardize the patient's recovery or place the patient at risk if nutritional needs are not met.

4. Different cultures have different ideas about how to express and respond to pain. Some cultures value bearing pain silently, whereas others expect expressiveness.

5. Different cultures have different views about when to seek profes-

sional medical help, treat oneself, or be treated by a family member or traditional healer.

C. Patients who do not speak English may be at greater risk. The degree to which a patient or family member is fluent in English may affect his or her care. Those whose English is limited often say that they speak their native language when possible because both their explanations and their understanding can be more accurate, and because it is more comfortable. The case manager can help implement language protocols to assist staff and non-English—speaking patients.

1. Language can be likened to a song that has both lyrics and melody. The lyrics—the vocabulary, grammar, and syntax—are easier to learn, especially for adults, than the melody—the pitch, inflections, and tone of the adopted language. Staff can help overcome this barrier by paying attention to the sound of the patients' accents they deal with most frequently and by learning the most common substitutions people make. Examples are the interchanging of "sh" and "ch" by Spanish speakers and the use of "p" and "f" and "s" for "sh" sounds by Filipinos. Remember, too, that even when someone has an extensive vocabulary in an acquired language, word order and the use of articles (the, a, and an), pronouns, and prepositions may be confusing and difficult.

2. Another frequent confusion occurs when native speakers of Tagalog, a Filipino dialect, which does not have separate masculine and feminine pronouns, use "he" for "she" and vice versa.

D. Cultural influences are complex and multifaceted. It is impossible to know all of the rules about each specific group. Cultural generalizations categorize areas of similarity in preferences, norms, and values, which should not be applied with certainty to each individual. Therefore, when treating a patient who is from a different background, the case manager should know that it is more effective to investigate and check out one's assumptions than to operate on incorrect predictions. The case manager can share the following information to educate caregivers in treating patients from other cultures:

1. Avoid making judgments about the patient's beliefs and practices.
2. Consider analogous beliefs or practices in which you are engaged.
3. Ask questions that help you learn about the patient's view of his or her condition.
4. Find out what other treatments the patient may be using.
5. Ask the patient to bring all medications that he or she is using.
6. Explain procedures carefully before an examination, especially when they may be embarrassing or uncomfortable for the patient. Assure the patient that all attempts will be made to preserve modesty.
7. Avoid touching the patient's head unless necessary and then explain the reasons before touching.
8. Ask the patient who he or she wants to be involved in discussions about diagnoses, treatment, and prognosis.
9. Ask patients how much they want to be informed and who should re-

ceive information if they do not want full disclosure themselves (Gardenswarz & Row, 1998).

■ THE CASE MANAGER'S ROLE IN QUALITY AND RISK MANAGEMENT

A. The case manager identifies and anticipates potential problems.
   1. Identifies patient care situations that are high risk, problem prone, or frequently occurring
   2. Assesses the patient's physical, psychosocial, emotional, and spiritual condition to determine whether they are at risk to develop problems
   3. Functions as a patient advocate, assessing concerns and complaints from the patient or the family early in order to deal with them before they become problems
   4. Acts as a liaison between the patient, the family, the health care facility, and the insurance company, anticipating needs and developing discharge plans that address these needs
   5. Conducts quality reviews of the patient's medical record to identify any quality concerns, to determine whether a quality problem exists, and if a quality problem is confirmed, conducts the necessary follow-up
   6. Develops quality indicators that identify potential quality of care issues, such as readmission to the hospital within 30 days of discharge

The case manager's role in RM includes
   1. Consulting a risk manager when questionable patient situations arise
   2. Communicating with the RM department when an incident has occurred
   3. Listening willingly and responsively to all patient and family issues, even when they are angry and upset
   4. Notifying the RM department of potential suits
   5. Including the patient and family in as much of the decision-making process about the patient's care options as is possible
   6. Carefully evaluating all readmission to a facility or unit
   7. Placing special emphasis on high-risk neonates and their care needs, as well as the informational needs of the family
   8. Practicing quality documentation
      a. Documenting all communications between the case manager and physician
      b. Dating and timing all entries
      c. Stating information clearly, factually, objectively, and completely
      d. Avoiding ambiguous statements and words with multiple meanings
      e. Documenting follow through and follow-up
      f. Documenting incidents factually and not placing blame
      g. Documenting any threats or complaints, using quotes if necessary
      h. Documenting patient and family concerns
      i. Documenting patient noncompliance

    j. Documenting informed consent

    k. Documenting the discharge plan and transfers to other facilities

REFERENCES

Blancett, S. S., & Flarey, D. L. (1996). *Handbook of nursing case management*. Gaithersburg, MD: Aspen.

Claflin, N. T. (Ed.) (1998). *Guide to quality management* (8th ed.). Glenview, IL: National Association for Healthcare Quality.

Claflin, N. T. (1993). Safety, risk management, and infection. In G. S. Wlody (Ed.), *Managing clinical practice in critical care nursing*. St. Louis: C. V. Mosby.

Gardenswartz, L., & Rowe, A. (1998). *Managing diversity in health care*. San Francisco: Jossey-Bass.

Powell, S. K. (2000). *Case management: A practical guide to success in managed care*. Philadelphia: Lippincott Williams & Wilkins.

CHAPTER 9

. . . .

Credentialing, Accreditation, Standards, and Pathways in Case Management

GARY WOLFE

LEARNING OBJECTIVES

Upon completion of this chapter, the reader will be able to:

1. Define credentialing.
2. List six components of credentialing.
3. Define certification.
4. List eight criteria for any certification.
5. List four certifications and criteria for case managers.
6. Define accreditation.
7. List the nine categories of accreditation standards for case management organizations.
8. Define Standards of Practice.
9. List three components of the Standards of Practice.
10. List the five uses of the Standards of Practice.
11. Define clinical pathway.
12. List eight benefits of clinical pathways.

IMPORTANT TERMS AND CONCEPTS

Accreditation
Accreditation of Case Management
  Organizations
Accreditation Standards
Benefits of Clinical Pathways
Certification for Case Managers
Clinical Pathways
Components of Standards of
  Practice
Content of Clinical Pathways

Credentialing
Definition of Case Management
Definition of Certification
Developing Clinical Pathways
Philosophy of Case Management
Specific Certifications in Case
  Management
Standards of Care
Standards of Performance
Standards of Practice

■ INTRODUCTION

A. Credentialing is an essential activity to case management in order to ensure that individuals hired to practice case management are providing quality case management services and to protect the consumer.

B. There are many certifications in case management. Certification is but one aspect of credentialing.

C. American Accreditation Healthcare Commission/Utilization Review Accreditation Commission (URAC) has developed accreditation standards for case management organizations.

D. Standards of Practice for Case Management, adopted by the Case Management Society of American in 1995, are authoritative statements defining the behavior of case managers.

E. Clinical pathways may be part of the case management process and help guide care, treatment, and processes and measure desired outcomes.

■ CREDENTIALING CASE MANAGERS

A. Credentialing is the process of evaluating a person's education and experience against a standard to determine whether he or she is qualified to perform the job, taking into consideration community standards, national standards, and state practice acts and liability.

B. Components of Credentialing
   1. Definition of Case Management: "A collaborative process that accesses, plans, implements, coordinates, monitors, and evaluates the options and services required to meet an individual's health needs, using communication and available resources to promote quality, cost-effective outcomes" (Certified Case Manager [CCM] Certification Guide).
   2. Philosophy of Case Management
      a. A philosophy is a statement of belief, setting forth principles, that guides the case manager.

  b. Philosophy of Case Management developed by the Commission for Case Manager Certification:

  (i) "Case management is not a profession in itself, but an area of practice within one's profession. Its underlying premise is that when an individual reaches the optimum level of wellness and functional capability, everyone benefits: the individuals being served; their support systems; the health care delivery systems; and the various reimbursement sources.

  (ii) "Case management serves as a means for achieving client wellness and autonomy through advocacy, communication, education, identification of service resources, and service facilitation. The case manager helps identify appropriate providers and facilities throughout the continuum of services, while ensuring that available resources are being used in a timely and cost-effective manner in order to obtain optimum value for both the client and the reimbursement source. Case management services are best offered in a climate that allows direct communication between the case manager, the client and appropriate service personnel, in order to optimize the outcome for all concerned." (CCM Certification Guide)

3. Job Description—This is an important part of credentialing because the job description is used as the day-to-day working document delineating the role, responsibilities, and work of the case manager.

  a. Components of job description

  (i) Job title

  (ii) Reports to

  (iii) Summary of position

  (iv) Duties and responsibilities

  (v) Required knowledge

  (vi) Functions

  (vii) Qualifications, including education, experience, licenses, and certifications

4. Employment application or contract, which sets forth in writing the education, work experience, and skills of the individual.

5. Applicant interview

  a. By supervisor

  b. By peers

  c. By subordinates

6. Verification of licenses or certifications, or both.

C. Credentialing is a dynamic process in determining the qualifications of a person compared with standards to perform a given responsibility safely and legally.

D. Credentialing is a recurring process that occurs usually annually and includes a competency-based performance appraisal. Re-credentialing ensures the continued meeting of standards.

■ CERTIFICATION FOR CASE MANAGERS

A. Certification is a process of validation of knowledge, skills, and abilities of individual practitioners.

B. Certification is based on predetermined standards, including education, acceptable experience, and a test, as well as building on an existing, defined health license such as registered nurse (RN), medical doctor (MD), or licensed clinical social worker (LCSW).

C. It is governed by independent bodies created to define and set standards for certification and administer the certification process and the recertification process.

D. Certification governing bodies are composed of individuals certified by that body and a variety of other individuals who represent the broad spectrum of individuals served, including consumers.

E. Certification is for an initial period, which is typically 5 years, at which time recertification is required to maintain certification.

F. Recertification is based on continued acceptable employment in the field and a predetermined number of continuing education requirements or by retaking the examination.

G. Individuals who are certified have a specific designation they are allowed to use after their name, such as CCM, for as long as they are certified.

H. Certification is voluntary.

I. Certifying bodies have a code of professional conduct for the individuals they certify.
   1. A code of professional conduct protects the public interest.
   2. Codes of professional conduct contain
      a. Principles
      b. Rules of conduct
      c. Guidelines for professional conduct. Individuals may have more than one code of professional conduct if they are licensed or a member of a profession

J. Certification examinations should be free of bias and nondiscriminatory.

K. There should be validity of the examination established through a job analysis survey.

L. There are many certifications, but the above general criteria are useful in evaluating any certification.

M. Benefits of certification
   1. Provides a standard of knowledge for employers of case managers
   2. Provides a standard and assurance to the consumer and public that the case manager has a sufficient level of knowledge
   3. Provides a recognized benchmark for health care workers and consumers of case management services

4. Is an indication that the person certified is knowledgeable, informed, and current in area of certification

N. A case manager should choose a specific certification depending on his or her job function and responsibilities matched to the certifying requirements.

■ SPECIFIC CERTIFICATIONS IN CASE MANAGEMENT

A. CCM by the Commission for Case Manager Certification.

1. This was the first certification developed specifically for case managers.
2. In 1992, The National Case Management Task Force organized a meeting with representatives of various national organizations with interest in case management. This meeting was organized because of the growing concern that there were no standards or qualifications for people calling themselves case managers.
3. In the early 1990s, case management was a "loose cannon" with no protection for the case manager or the consumer.
4. Consensus was reached in the 1992 meeting to appoint the Commission of Insurance Rehabilitation Specialists (now known as the Commission for Disability Management Specialists) to develop a certification for individual case managers, based on the work of the National Task Force.
5. This work culminated in the creation of the Commission for Case Manager Certification and certification for individual case managers.
6. Certification requirements for CCM
   a. Good moral character, reputation, and fitness for the practice of case management
   b. Licensure and certification requirements:
      (i) License or certification must be based on a minimum educational requirement of a post-secondary degree program in a field that promotes the physical, psychosocial, or vocational well-being of the persons being served.
      (ii) The license or certification awarded on completion of the educational program must have been obtained by passing an examination in the areas of specialization.
      (iii) The license or certification process must grant the holder the ability to legally and independently practice without the supervision of another licensed professional and to perform the following six essential activities of case management:
         (a) Assessment
         (b) Planning
         (c) Implementation
         (d) Coordination
         (e) Monitoring
         (f) Evaluation
      (iv) All licenses and certifications must be current.

   c. Employment experience categories

     (i) One of the following experiences must be met:

       (a) Twelve months of acceptable full-time case management employment or equivalent under the supervision of a CCM for the 12 months.

       (b) Twenty-four months of acceptable full-time case management employment or equivalent. Supervision by a CCM is not required under this category.

       (c) Twelve months of acceptable full-time case management employment or its equivalent as a supervisor, supervising the activities of individuals who provide direct case management services.

     (ii) All experience must be verifiable by a manager, supervisor, or employer. Self-employment is acceptable but also must be verified.

     (iii) To qualify as acceptable employment, the applicant must demonstrate as part of his or her employment the six essential activities of case management (listed earlier) applied to each of the following five core components:

       (a) Coordination and service delivery

       (b) Physical and psychological factors

       (c) Benefit systems and cost–benefit analysis

       (d) Case management concepts

       (e) Community resources

     (iv) The core components must

       (a) Be applied across a continuum of care

       (b) Be applied in multiple environments

       (c) Involve interactions with the client's health care system

       (d) Deal with the client's broad spectrum of needs without providing direct patient care

   d. The CCM examination is administered twice a year.

   e. The CCM certification is the most widely held certification by case managers.

   f. Applicants who successfully pass the examination use the designation CCM.

   g. The first examination for CCM was offered in 1993.

   h. The person must be recertified every 5 years.

B. Nursing Case Management (Cm) by the American Nurse Credentialing Center.

   1. Eligibility requirements to sit for the examination:

     a. Hold an active RN license in the United States.

     b. Currently hold a baccalaureate or higher degree in nursing.

     c. Have functioned within the scope of a registered nurse case manager for a minimum of 2000 hours within the past 2 years.

     d. Show proof of a current, core nursing specialty certification from the American Nurse Credentialing Center.

e. If the applicant does not hold a core nursing specialty certification from the American Nurses Credentialing Center, the applicant is still eligible to sit for the examination, but candidates must complete an additional 50 questions related to the American Nurses Association Standards of Clinical Nursing Practice.

2. The nurse case manager examination is administered twice a year by the American Nurse Credentialing Center.

3. The first examination for nurse case manager certification was offered in 1997.

4. Applicants who successfully pass the examination use the designation RN, Cm.

5. The person must be recertified every 5 years.

C. Care Manager Certified (CMC) by the National Academy of Certified Care Managers.

1. Eligibility requirements to sit for examination:

a. Hold a master's degree in social work, nursing, gerontology, counseling, or psychology

b. Must have 2 years of supervised, paid, full-time care management experience

c. Experience must include personal, face-to-face interviewing, assessment, care planning, problem solving, and follow-up, or

d. Applicants with a bachelor's degree in social work, nursing, gerontology, counseling, or care management and

e. Four years of paid, full-time work experience with clients in practice settings of social work, nursing, mental health, counseling, or care management. Two of those years must be supervised, paid, full-time care management experience, or

f. Applicants with a high school diploma or any degree in an area not related to care management and

g. Six years of paid, full-time, direct experience with clients in social work, mental health, nursing, counseling or care management; 2 of those years must be supervised.

2. The first examination for care manager certified was administered in 1996.

3. The person must be recertified every 3 years.

D. Certified Case Management Administrator (CCMA) by the Center for Case Management.

1. Case management administrators supervise employees who perform the following role functions or, if applying as an experienced case manager, perform at least eight of the following functions on a daily basis:

a. Case finding

b. Comprehensive assessment of client situation

c. Evaluation and coordination of the plan of care

d. Matching client resources to client needs

e. Monitoring delivery of services

f. Critical thinking, appropriate prioritization, and time management

    g. Measurement and evaluation of financial, clinical, functional, and satisfaction outcomes

    h. Accountability for financial, clinical, functional, and satisfaction outcomes

    i. Effective leadership displayed in the performance of current role

    j. Effective communication

    k. Evaluation of and response to learning needs of clients, clinicians, and community

2. Eligibility requirements to sit for the examination:

    a. Master's degree and 1 year experience in case management administration, or

    b. Master's degree and 3 years of experience as a case manager, or

    c. Bachelor's degree and 5 years of experience as a case manager

3. Recertification is required every 5 years.

4. The certification examination is a written examination composed of a maximum of 200 multiple-choice, objective questions.

5. The content is approximately the following:

    a. Identification of at-risk population: 20%

    b. Assessment of clinical system components: 10%

    c. Development of strategies to manage at-risk populations: 10%

    d. Assessment of organizational culture: 15%

    e. Market assessment and strategic planning: 15%

    f. Human resource management: 10%

    g. Outcomes measurement, monitoring, and management: 20%

6. The examination for case management administrators was first administered in 1998.

7. Individuals who successfully pass the examination use the designation CMAC (Case Management Administrator Certified).

■ OTHER CERTIFICATIONS

A. There are many certifications for individuals working in health care.

B. To determine credibility of certification, refer to Certification for Case Managers II (earlier).

C. Case managers relate to individuals who perform some tasks of case management but not all or not across the continuum. See Table 9–1 for a listing of certifications and contact information.

■ ACCREDITATION OF ORGANIZATIONS PERFORMING CASE MANAGEMENT

A. Accreditation is a process of reviewing all aspects of an organization against published standards to see if the organization meets all the standards of providing services. Accreditation is a voluntary process.

B. Accreditation organizations and standards

(text continues on page 110)

TABLE 9–1
Case Certifications and Contact Information

Certification	Acronyn	Specialization	Sponsoring Organization	Contact Information
American Board of Disability Analysts	ABDA	Rehabilitation medicine, case management	American Board of Disability Analysts	ABDA Central Office, Park Place Medical Building, 345 24th Ave. N, Suite 200, Nashville, TN 37203, 615-327-2984
American Board of Quality Assurance and Utilization Review Physicians	ABQUA URP	Utilization management for physician and allied health	American Board of Quality Assurance and Utilization Review Physicians	American Board of Quality Assurance and Utilization Review Physicians, 2120 Range Rd., Clearwater, FL 33765, 900-998-6030
Advanced Certification Continuity of Care	A-CCC	Multidisciplinary discharge planners, case managers	National Board for Continuity of Care Certification	National Board for Continuity of Care Certification, 638 Prospect Ave., Hartford, CT 06105, 203-586-7525
Certified Case Manager	CCM	Multidisciplinary case managers	Commission for Case Management Certification	Commission for Case Manager Certification, 1835 Rohlwing Road, Suite D, Rolling Meadows, IL 60008, 847-818-0292
Certified Disability Management Specialist	CDMS	Disability managers Insurance-based insurance rehabilitation specialists Vocational counselors	Certified Disability Management Specialist Commission	Certified Disability Management Specialist Commission, 1835 Rohlwing Road, Suite E, Rolling Meadows, IL 60008, 847-394-2106
Case Management Administration Certified	CMAC	Case management administration	The Center for Case Management	Professional Testing Corporation, 1350 Broadway, 17th Floor, New York, NY 10018, 212-356-0660
Care Manager Certified	CMC	Gerontology, counseling, social work, mental health	National Academy of Certified Care Managers	National Academy of Certified Care Managers, 3389 Sheridan St., Suite 170, Hollywood, FL 33021

continued

TABLE 9–1

Case Certifications and Contact Information

Certification	Acronyn	Specialization	Sponsoring Organization	Contact Information
Certified Managed Care Nurse	CMCN	Nurses in managed care	American Board of Managed Care Nursing	American Board of Managed Care Nursing, 4435 Waterfront Drive, Suite 101, Glen Allen, VA 23060, 804-747-9698
Certified Occupational Health Nurse–Case Manager	COHN-CM	Occupational health nursing case management	American Board of Occupational Health Nursing	American Board for Occupational Health Nurses, 201 E. Ogden Ave., Suite 114, Hinsdale, IL 60521, 630-789-5799
Certified Professional Disability Management	CPDM	Disability managers	Insurance Educational Association	Insurance Educational Association, 1201 Dove Street, Newport Beach, CA 92660, 800-655-4432
Certified Professional in Healthcare Quality	CPHQ	Quality managers, utilization managers, risk managers	Healthcare Quality Certification Board of the National Association for Healthcare Quality	Healthcare Quality Certification Board of the National Association for Healthcare Quality, PO Box 1880, San Gabriel, CA 91778, 818-286-8074
Certified Professional Utilization Review	CPUR	Utilization managers, case managers	InterQual	InterQual, 44 Lafayette Road, PO Box 988, North Hampton, NH 03862

Certified Rehabilitation Registered Nurse, Certified Rehabilitation Nurse–Advanced	CRRN, CRRN-A	Rehabilitation nurses	Rehabilitation Nursing Certification Board	Rehabilitation Nursing Certification Board, 4700 W. Lake Avenue, Glenview, IL 60025, 800-229-7530
Certified Nursing Case Manager	RN, Cm	Nurse case manager	American Nurse Credentialing Center	American Nurse Credentialing Center, 600 Maryland Ave. SW, Suite 100 West, Washington, DC 20024, 800-284-2378
Certified Rehabilitation Counselor	CRC	Rehabilitation counseling, case managers	Commission on Rehabilitation Counselor Certification	Commission on Rehabilitation Counselor Certification, 1835 Rohlwing Road, Suite E, Rolling Meadows, IL 60008, 847-394-2104
Professional, Academy for Healthcare Management	PAHM, FAHM	Managed care	Academy for Healthcare Management	Academy for Healthcare Management, 2300 Windy Ridge Parkway, Suite 600, Atlanta, GA 30339, 800-667-3133
Fellow, Academy for Healthcare Management				

1. In June 1999 the American Accreditation HealthCare Commission/ URAC (Commission/URAC) adopted accreditation standards for organizations performing case management.
2. Commission/URAC used an expert panel, advisory committee with representatives from all case management stakeholders to develop the standards.
3. Organizations represented included the Case Management Society of American, the American Medical Association, the American Nurses Association, American Association of Health Plans, Commission/ URAC accredited companies, Association of Managed Healthcare Organizations, business representatives, Washington Business Group on Health, American Health Quality Association, American Hospital Association, Blue Cross Blue Shield Association, Health Care Financing Administration (HCFA)/Medicare, representatives from the Department of Defense, and the Commission for Case Manger Certification.
4. These are the first standards that specifically address case management organizations and set standards as to what constitutes a quality case management organization.
5. There are 33 standards addressing the following:
   a. Structure and organization
   b. Staff structure and organization
   c. Staff management and development
   d. Information management
   e. Quality improvement
   f. Oversight of delegated functions
   g. The case management process
   h. Organizational ethics
   i. Complaints
6. The standards were tested in three case management organizations.
7. Commission/URAC defines a case management organization as an organization or program that provides telephonic or on-site case management services in conjunction with a private or publicly funded benefits program. All such organizations are eligible to apply for accreditation.
8. The accreditation process consists of
   a. An application
   b. An internal Commission/URAC review of the application, commonly referred to as a Desk Top Review
   c. An on-site review
   d. After the review team completes their review and recommendations, a review by the Commission/URAC Accreditation Committee with a recommendation concerning accreditation status is forwarded to the Commission/URAC Executive Committee.
   e. Final approval is granted by the Commission/URAC Executive Committee.
9. Full accreditation by Commission/URAC lasts for 2 years. The accredited organization must remain in compliance with the standards throughout the accreditation period.

10. Because there are no other generic case management organization standards, the standards developed by Commission/URAC are the standards all organizations—both accredited and nonaccredited organizations—will be evaluated against and held to.

■ STANDARDS OF PRACTICE FOR CASE MANAGEMENT

A. Standards of Practice are authoritative statements that describe the responsibilities for which case managers are accountable.

B. Standards of Practice define accountability to the consumer and delineate client outcomes.

C. The Case Management Society of America (CMSA) developed and published Standards of Practice for Case Management in 1995.

D. Until 1995, there was no defining document that was accepted nationally. Many organizations and individuals were trying to incorporate standards of practice but did not have a reference tool that would define and set the standards.

E. The CMSA Standards of Practice were developed by a committee of case managers who, using a modified consensus Delphi model, gathered, considered, and evaluated input from case managers from across the United States.

F. The CMSA Standards of Practice has become the standard of the case management field. It is recognized as an important and milestone document in case management.

G. By de facto, these standards of practice define acceptable behavior of case managers and liability for negligence.

H. The standards define
1. Who case managers are
2. Where they practice
3. Benefits to clients and society
4. Accountability
5. The future directions of case management

I. Components of the standards of practice
1. Case management functions
   a. Assessor
   b. Planner
   c. Facilitator
   d. Advocate
2. Standards of care delineate a competent level of case management services.
   a. Assessment and case identification and selection
   b. Problem identification
   c. Planning
   d. Monitoring

  e. Evaluating
  f. Outcomes
  3. Standards of performance
      a. Quality of care
      b. Education, preparation, certification, and qualifications
      c. Collaboration
      d. Legal
      e. Ethical
      f. Advocacy
      g. Resource Utilization
      h. Research
J. Not all standards are achieved by all case managers, but the standards are a guide toward achieving excellence.
K. Use of Standards of Practice for case management
  1. Reference tool to guide the behavior of case managers on a daily basis
  2. A tool for the development of a job description
  3. A reference for organizing or evaluating a case management program
  4. When interviewing for a position
  5. When determining potential liability and performance of a case manager

■ PATHWAYS

A. A pathway is a predetermined written guide for a plan of care for a specific health situation and is usually used as a medical management or utilization guide.
B. A pathway may also be referred to as a guideline, algorithm, care map, progress map, practice parameter, critical path, or clinical path.
C. Pathways can be developed for a specific condition, disease, symptom, event or process, diagnosis-related group (DRG) diagnosis, chronic condition, and timeline of care.
D. Benefits of clinical pathways:
  1. Improve communication
  2. Delineate process and expected outcome
  3. Focus on the patient
  4. Identify performance expectations
  5. Ensure quality
  6. Define accountability
  7. Improve documentation
  8. Define a consistent standard of care for a specific condition, event, or process
E. Developing clinical pathways

1. Coordinate across the continuum of care using staff from all providers in the continuum.
2. Use state-of-practice, evidence-based research when available.
3. Select a target population, diagnosis, condition, or event.
4. Use a central, core working group with all stakeholders represented.
5. Review existing data, programs, and services.
6. Complete a needs assessment of the target population, diagnosis, condition, or event.
7. Develop the clinical pathway in a graphic process flow.
8. Establish benchmarks.
9. The greater the input and consensus in development, the greater the acceptance, use, and application.
10. Clinical pathways are dynamic, so they need a constant process of monitoring and re-evaluation and a continuous quality improvement focus.
11. Initially test the clinical pathway on a small sample before it is finalized.

F. Content of clinical pathways
   1. Assessment
   2. Plan
      a. Diagnosis
      b. Care
      c. Teaching
      d. Discharge
   3. Intervention
   4. Resource utilization
   5. Patient and caregiver teaching
   6. Discharge planning
   7. Work and disability issues
   8. Psychosocial issues
   9. Special considerations
   10. Anticipated outcomes
   11. Variance
   12. Each of the above-mentioned issues is delineated over specified time intervals and frequencies.

G. Clinical pathways are only used as a guide but must always consider the individual's response to care and treatment.

H. The pathways are a process of providing care with consistent interventions.

I. Clinical pathways are useful to share with patients and all providers so they can also understand the care and treatment.

J. Chronic conditions and conditions, symptoms, and care processes that have a fairly predictable outcome and course lend themselves to clinical pathways.

REFERENCES

Birdsall, C., & Sperry, S. (1997). *Clinical paths in medical-surgical practice.* St Louis: Mosby.

Case Management Society of America (1995). *Standards of practice for case management.* Little Rock, AR: CMSA.

Case management standards. (1999). Washington, DC: American Accreditation HealthCare Commission/ URAC.

CDMC certification guide, certified disability management specialist. (1999). Rolling Meadows, IL: Certification of Disability Management Specialists Commission.

CCM certification guide, certified case manager. (1999). Rolling Meadows, IL: Commission for Case Management Certification.

CRC certification guide, certified rehabilitation counselor. (1999). Rolling Meadows, IL: Commission for Rehabilitation Counselor Certification.

Gardner, S. (1999). Academy for Healthcare Management offers managed care programs. *Inside Case Management, 6*(2), 12–21.

Handbook for candidates, certification examination for case management administrators. New York: The Center for Case Management/Professional Testing Corporation.

Smith, D., et al. (1998). *Case management 101—A training guide.* Los Angeles: AMS Press.

St. Coeur, M. (1967). *Case management practice guidelines.* St Louis: Mosby.

CHAPTER 10

• • • • • • • • • • • • • •

Case Management Tools and Technology

NANCY NASUTI WHIPPLE

LEARNING OBJECTIVES

Upon completion of this chapter, the reader will be able to:

1. Understand the subtle differences between case management strategies, clinical pathways, extended care pathways, protocols, and guidelines.

2. Identify tools that are available to support the case management process.

3. Describe the goals and benefits of an automated case management information system and how case management informatics can support standards of care.

4. Define the features and functions that are necessary in the case management system.

5. Identify key, meaningful data elements and required data format that will support reporting.

6. Understand how data collected and processed can be used to measure outcomes and the effectiveness of case management activities.

7. Describe the steps involved in choosing and implementing a case management system.

8. Identify the critical steps in developing clinical content to be used in a case management system.

IMPORTANT TERMS AND CONCEPTS

Algorithm
Batch Processing
Case Management (CM)
Critical or Clinical Pathways
Decision Support System
Disease Management (DM)
Extended Care Pathway (ECP)
Guidelines
Integration
Interface

Knowledge Base (KB)
Management Information System
  (MIS)
Outcomes Analysis
Protocols
Remote Access
Return-on-Investment (ROI)
Telemedicine
Variance

■ INTRODUCTION

A. Many tools are available to the case manager and the medical management team. These tools include guidelines, practice standards, pathways, critical pathways, and "tickler" or reminder systems. Some of the tools are computer-based information systems, and some are traditional paper-based systems. Many case managers have long been using guidelines to simplify and standardize their interactions with the patient.

B. This chapter focuses on automated case management information systems (CMISs), which are designed to streamline the case manager's workflow and eliminate much of the "busy work" that comes with managing patients, such as duplicate documentation, photocopying files to share with associates, placing "yellow stickies" everywhere to remember interventions, and filling out numerous forms to authorize services. The power of a CMIS comes from its ability not only to support data collection but also to provide efficient data storage, data sharing, data retrieval, and decision-making functions.

C. Information systems are becoming key elements of case management and disease management (Fig. 10–1).

D. Other tools for case management include telephonics and Internet-based communication to the patient and providers, as well as Internet exploration. However, most of these tools are simply used for data collection or information gathering. With the exception of computer-based demand management, these tools do not support decision-making based on the information gathered. Case managers independently determine which actions to take.

E. An organization's primary goal when using any tool is to produce results that are valued by the customers. Customers include not only the patients but the users of the tools, the providers of services, and the organization's management.

F. Medical informatics is becoming pervasive in all areas of health care. Case managers must become knowledgeable in all aspects of medical in-

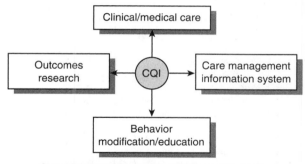

Organizational Structure, Skills, and Culture

FIGURE 10–1 Continuous quality improvement (CQI) is key in a successful case management program. Accomplishing CQI requires a coordinated effort to manage clinical care and affect patient behavior. A CMIS is an integral component that allows the care manager to focus on these goals and measure the outcomes of his or her efforts.

formatics to maximize the benefits of these systems. They must be open to whatever the technology is available to them, and be consistent and persistent in using them to their maximum potential.

G. In today's era of cost containment, case management organizations of all sizes and structures cannot afford not to automate, and today's case managers must be computer literate (Dause, 1997). Health care value can be calculated by factoring the overall financial, time, resource, and problem costs into improved clinical, economic, service, and humanistic outcomes.

H. Case managers are experiencing heavier caseloads, both in the quantity and the complexity of their cases, and they are increasingly required to justify their value. Tools are needed to be able to provide proof of effectiveness.

I. Case managers who use computerized case management systems estimate that they can complete a comprehensive plan in one third to one half the time previously required (Smith, 1998).

J. Career opportunities are available for case managers and other health care providers to work as consultants to developers of information systems and organizations who wish to use this technology.

■ KEY DEFINITIONS

A. Rule-Based Systems: Systems that generate patient-specific recommendations based on all of the information gathered up to that point

B. Clinical or Critical Pathway: Provides an overview of care, and tracks patient movement and flow through the health care system. Essentially, a clinical pathway is a traditional nursing care plan mapped to standardized protocols on a specified time-line. Critical pathways, being somewhat more limited, are usually implemented in acute care inpatient settings (Fig. 10–2).

C. Practice Guideline: A decision support tool that specifies whether a pa-

ID No.	Activity name	Duration (hours)	Precedent Activities
1	Thoracic Surgery Clinic Visit	3	None
2	Anesthesia Clinic Visit	3	1
3	Physical Therapy Visit	1	1
4	Preop Assessment	1	2,3
5	Preop Identification of Postdischarge Caregiver	1	4
6	Pre- and Postop Patient and Family Teaching	1	5
7	Operative Procedure CABG	6	6
8	Pharmaceutical Support	16	7
9	Hemodynamic Monitoring	16	7
10	Cardiac Monitor	16	7
11	Maintain Ventilator Support	16	7
12	Stabilize Hemodynamics	1	8,9,10
13	Discontinue Hardwire Monitor	1	12
14	Discontinue Hemodynamic Monitoring	1	12
15	Adequate Blood Gases, with Reduced Oxygenation	1	11
16	Extubate	2	15
17	Transfer to Step-Down Unit	1	13,14,16
18	Cardiac Monitoring via Telemetry	48	17
19	Discontinue Telemetry	24	18
20	Normal or Preop Cardiac Rhythm	0	19
21	Monitor Intake and Output, Vitals, etc. (ongoing)	0	17
22	Diuretic Protocol	36	21
23	Monitor Weight	1	22
24	Weight Approaching Preop Weight	0	23
25	Increasing Activity (plus other related activities)	85	17,27,28
26	Bowel Movement	1	25
27	Wean to Nasal Cannula	3	16
28	Discontinue Nasal Cannula	34	27
29	Room Air x 24 Hours	24	28
30	Tolerates Activity on Room Air	0	29
31	Discharge	4	20,24,26,30
32	Positive Life Style Activities		31
33	Postop Appointments Kept		31
34	Weight at Preop Level		31
35	Cardiac Rhythm Stable		31
36	Activity at Least at Preop Level		31

FIGURE 10–2. Excerpt from a sample activity/precedent table for uncomplicated CABG patients. (Reprinted from Coffey, R.J., Othman, J. E., & Walters, J. I. [1995]. Extending the application of critical path methods. *Quality Management In Health Care, 3*[2],24. © 1995, Aspen Publishers, Inc.)

tient should receive a specific treatment or prescription. It contains criteria used to determine the appropriate treatment for specific clinical circumstances. It assists in key decision-making for a select group of patients. Practice guidelines are based on scientific evidence, accrediting and regulatory agencies, and quality outcomes. Their goal is to enhance patient, provider, and case management knowledge; decrease variation in care; define proper use of medical technology; eliminate inappropriate care; and control health care costs (Casanova, 1997). Practice guidelines are primarily used by providers of care. However, the case manager can refer to them to assess the appropriateness of delivered care and identify any treatment that is not consistent with the selected guideline.

D. Practice Standards: Define a treatment protocol that is applied to all patients, not just a select group. Also referred to as "best practice." Usually a minimum set of standards that is not intended to cover all aspects of the patient's care (Table 10–1).

E. Extended Care Pathway (ECP): A set of policies and procedures that providers use to address a specific disabling chronic condition over time and across various service settings. It is a standardized approach to the multidisplinary care of an individual with a particular diagnosis. An ECP is designed to increase the continuity of care between settings, and thereby improve both the quality and cost-effectiveness of care. ECPs indicate what key events are necessary for patients to meet expected outcomes. They are tools to be used for managing, monitoring, and evaluating care (National Health Care Consortium [NHCC], 1995).

1. Information systems were important forerunners to the formulation of ECPs, because they standardized information and guided case managers toward similar practices.

2. The challenge to link acute care with the community and long-term care systems is now being addressed. Case management, using such tools as information systems with integrated ECPs, is helping to meet the challenge of supplying this missing link.

F. Protocol: A tool for deciding which care to provide under which circumstances. To assist in decision-making, it may contain a decision tree or flow chart. It frequently covers a smaller segment of care rather than the whole illness. It can describe the particular order of events, but in most cases it does not suggest a time-line.

G. Demand Management: Provides risk appraisals, telephone health information services, and prevention and wellness initiatives. Frequently, demand management involves patients calling either an independent call center, a center set up by their health plan, or a special number available to them by their provider. The call can be initiated because the client is experiencing symptoms and is looking for guidance in determining necessary treatment, or the client may be requesting general information about preventive health care or access to and information about a provider of health care.

H. Algorithm: Flow diagrams that consist of branching logic pathways that permit the application of defined criteria to the task of identifying a terminus (Fig. 10–3). The terminus can be an identification, a classification,

TABLE 10–1

Practice Standards for Inpatient Day by Day Care for an Uncomplicated CABG Patient

	Postop Period of Operative Day	Postop Day 1	Postop Day 2
Treatment	Maintain ventilator support until extubation Wean to nasal cannula Hardwire monitoring Vital signs monitored Hemodynamic monitoring Cardiac output every 4 hours Pharmaceutical support Initiate diuretic protocol	Oxygen by nasal cannula Telemetry Vitals every 4 hours Pharmaceutical support Continue diuretic protocol	Room air Monitor intake and output tid Vitals every 4 hours Telemetry Pharmaceutical support Continue diuretic protocol
Patient activity	Bed rest until extubated Up in chair at bedside	Ambulate to tolerance qid	Increase ambulation to tolerance qid
Diet	NPO Advance to clear liquids	No added salt, low-cholesterol solid diet	No added salt, low-cholesterol solid diet
Discharge planning		Assess additional home care needs Transfer to step-down unit	
Teaching	Explain ICU procedures Explain transfer to step-down unit	Reinforce incentive spirometer use Reinforce increasing activity	Reinforce increasing activity
Medications	Potassium as needed Magnesium as needed Diltiazem 30 mg tid Nitroglycerine 1 ug/kg	Diltiazem CD once a day	Potassium as needed Diltiazem CD once a day
Tests	Electrolytes (potassium × 2) CBC Arterial blood gases Chest x-ray Pulse oximetry	Electrolytes Pulse oximetry	

(Courtesy of University of Michigan Hospitals, Ann Arbor, MI.)

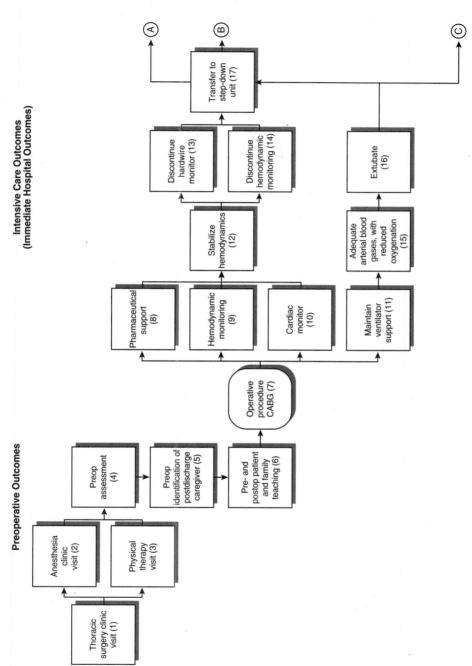

FIGURE 10-3. An excerpt from a sample flowchart of activities and desired outcomes for an uncomplicated CABG patient.

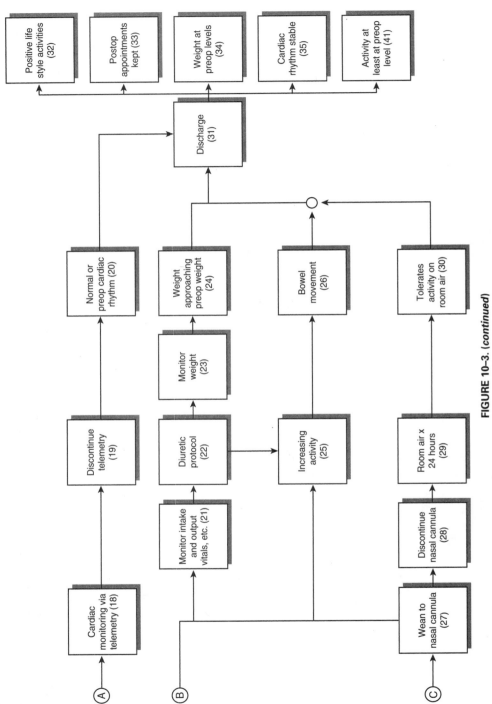

FIGURE 10–3. (*continued*)

or an activity (Horan, 1994). Algorithms, both formally and informally defined, have been used in health care for many years—for example, the algorithm for approaching an unconscious heart attack victim.

1. Algorithms have been criticized as being too rigid. Opponents say that patients are too variable to fit into any one box. Another criticism is that algorithms impose too many restrictions, preventing the health care professional from using his or her own expertise. However, any reasonable system that incorporates algorithms provides the ability to override decisions made by the algorithm or to customize any embedded algorithm.

I. Decision Support System: A decision support system (DSS) enriches a case manager's professional judgment by quickly verifying or invalidating business decisions. The user has at his or her fingertips all of the pertinent elements needed for evaluation.

1. The heart of a DSS system is a medical information warehouse containing all of the information about the patient, as well as data and outcomes of patients identified as having similar medical conditions (Dietzen, 1997).

2. Data come from a variety of sources (e.g., laboratories, pharmacy, authorizations), although the majority of information comes from claims. Data must be organized in a way that facilitates easy retrieval for meeting the identified business needs.

J. Telemedicine: Accessing health care services using any medium besides hands-on, direct patient contact. Although it can include simple telephonic contact like telephonic triage, the more accepted definition includes the use of computers, video equipment, and remote medical monitoring (Wrinn, 1998b), for example, electrocardiogram (EKG) hook-ups, blood pressure monitoring, quality-of-life assessments, and self-risk assessments. Case managers should be aware of the uses, benefits, and limitations of telemedicine so that they can use the technology in the appropriate way. In addition, case managers can perform long-term monitoring of patients using the same telemedicine tools.

■ GOALS OF A CASE MANAGEMENT INFORMATION SYSTEM (CMIS)

A. Eliminates double data entry by same user. Data can be viewed in several places within the system and in several formats.

B. Eliminates double data entry by multiple users. Data-sharing capabilities for all users with appropriate access security in place.

C. Provides the ability to run in parallel with other systems and communicate with other systems either real-time (data are accessible as soon as they are entered anywhere in the system or in a legacy system to which the CMIS is integrated) or in batch mode (data are updated on a preset timed periodic schedule). Data that are used in decision making must be available in real-time.

D. Acts as central repository for all the information about a patient. In other words, it must be patient centered. However, users should have the ability to access quickly the information that is most important to them and to filter out messages, reminders, and other prompts that are not directed to them.

E. Views comprehensive patient data over the entire continuum of his or her illness. A patient's information is not fragmented as he or she moves from one setting to another or from one provider to another.

F. Patient census, medical history, psychosocial history, financial status, goals and problems, plan of treatment, and intervention target dates can be quickly identified and accessed. Supports the key elements of case management, including assessment, problem and goal definition, planning, monitoring and evaluation.

G. Stores relevant clinical information indefinitely to provide for long-term population trending and analysis. Provides cost details as well as the clinical causes of patient variances (Favor, 1996).

H. Simplifies accreditation updates by tracking the minute details required by the regulatory agency.

I. Standardizes terminology, documentation, and data management practices.

J. Provides the ability to document and retrieve case manager interventions and cost of care information, and directly relate the activities to patient outcomes and cost savings realized as a direct result of the case manager coordinating the appropriate level of care at the appropriate site in the appropriate time frame. In other words, it links the financial aspects of care with clinical data, giving organizations the advantage of knowing what the cost of care is and where specifically dollars are spent.

   1. Although cost savings reports are still important to an organization's operation, more organizations are making patient outcomes the critical indicator of how well they are doing. As Intergrated Delivery Systems (IDSs) become more popular, the opportunities for direct cost savings and cost avoidance decrease.

   2. In the past, each case manager could measure outcomes differently. A CMIS should allow objective, standardized reporting over the entire managed population by all case managers.

   3. Case managers are accountable for facilitating solutions that match cost–benefit to case outcomes (Dietzen, 1997).

     a. In the past, fee schedules and capitation agreements were helpful in controlling costs.

     b. Later, case managers had criteria-driven utilization management and clinical pathway tools to use.

     c. Now, decision support systems turn data into actionable information, leading to additional cost savings. Data must be timely to be effective as a tool for intervention.

■ LIMITATIONS OF A CMIS

A. The system cannot take the place of what is sometimes called the "gut factor." Any decisions made by the system must still be reviewed by a health care professional (McGarvey, 1998).

B. Health care lags behind other industries in information management. Standardization of data across the health continuum at different locations is not yet a reality, although much progress has been made within the last few years with several different initiatives. In IDSs, data sharing is less of a challenge because there are no issues of ownership and security.

1. Health Level Seven, Inc. (HL7): HL7 is a nonprofit standards-developing organization accredited by the American National Standards Institute (ANSI). HL7 is a standard vocabulary for clinical and health care administrative data.

2. Systemized Nomenclature of Medicine (SNOMED): SNOMED is a complete dictionary of medical terms containing the relationships between the SNOMED terms and other coding systems such as billing codes and diagnostic codes. Requiring care providers to use the same dictionary of medical terminology to capture data allows analyses to be done comparing "apples to apples."

3. Read Code is sponsored by the Department of Health and National Health Service in Great Britain. There is an initiative under way to merge SNOMED with Read Code to become the English language standard.

4. Logical Observation Identifiers, Names, and Codes (LOINC): LOINC is a terminology developed to focus on standardized nomenclature for laboratory observations.

5. NANDA, NIC, NOC: The American Nurses Association–recognized nursing classifications vocabulary for assessment, intervention, and outcomes. The systems are being merged with SNOMED.

6. The recently enacted Kennedy-Kassebaum Bill (Health Insurance Portability and Accountability Act [HIPAA]) mandates development of standards to facilitate exchange of patient information.

C. There is no centralized data base for patient data as the patient moves from one management organization to another, one facility to another, or one provider to another.

■ BENEFITS OF A CMIS

A. The benefits of using a CMIS can be divided into three categories: workflow, patient care, and organizational.

1. Workflow benefits include support of the case management process, allowing the case manager to focus on the patient and patient outcomes and not be overwhelmed by clerical tasks; reduction of duplication of documentation; elimination of "double-data" entry; generation of reminders or "ticklers" when a case manager intervention is required; improving data entry and storage; improving data access for sharing and reporting; and simplifying and streamlining of mundane tasks.

2. Patient care benefits include keeping patients from "falling through the cracks"; monitoring and recording the progress of the patient throughout the health continuum; promoting a consistent, best-practice approach to managing patients with similar medical conditions;

and incorporating national standards and reducing the variability of case management practices. For example, when a patient with congestive heart failure is discharged from the hospital, scheduling a follow-up visit within 2 weeks seems like a routine task. However, keeping that appointment has implications both clinically and financially. Some studies have shown that if patients wait even 1 month after discharge to follow up with their provider, readmission rates are significantly higher (Barr, 1998).

3. Organizational benefits include improving the efficiency in the case management process; improving case manager job satisfaction; increasing staff accountability and empowerment; improving patient satisfaction; improving relationships with providers; increasing consistency in providing care; and providing the ability to document and report outcomes. Documentation is integrated, streamlined, simplified, standardized, and reportable.

■ CMIS SUPPORTING STANDARDS OF CARE

A. Case identification and selection defines why a patient is being cared for by a case manager. Many criteria can be used to identify suitable candidates for case management, including the primary disease or illness, medical complications, exacerbations and comorbidities, the cost of care, psychosocial status, the prevalence of the disease, and the amount of treatment variation. The system can automatically identify patients for case management based on user-defined triggers, or the case manager can review the patient against the criteria to determine the suitability for case management.

B. Patient assessment: Provides the case manager with a method of conducting a thorough and objective analysis of the patient's current status (Case Management Society of America [CMSA], 1995). The case manager can perform a baseline assessment, ongoing assessments, psychosocial assessments, quality-of-life assessments, patient satisfaction surveys, and clinical status reviews. In addition, the system can track changes in responses over time. An integral part of the assessment is to move patients with a particular disease or condition into homogeneous subgroups, called stratification groups. The system guides the user through the stratification process, applying criteria as appropriate and available, to reduce subjectivity and variability. Patients will naturally move from one stratification group to another as the illness progresses. For example, the population identified as having asthma can be broken down further into the following stratification groups: severe persistent, moderate persistent, mild persistent, and mild intermittent. The system automatically tracks the stratification history and supports a restratification process.

C. Identification of problems: Problems can be defined as issues that may affect the health and functioning of the patient or barriers to effectiveness of their care. Default problems can be automatically assigned to a patient by the system based on the patient's illness and the subgroup to which he or she belongs.

D. Planning: Planning involves the identification of immediate, short-term, and long-term goals, as well as coordination of treatment based on identified problems and needs of the patient. Goals can appear in many forms such as patient centered (e.g., return to previous level of function), case management (e.g., patient's endurance will improve with physical therapy), or clinical (e.g., stabilization of diabetic status with proper use of insulin). The system can keep track of the status of goals. In addition, default goals can be defined by the system based on the patient's diagnosis and the subgroup to which they have been assigned.

E. Monitoring: Throughout the course of the patient's continuum of care, the case manager must monitor and assess the patient's status as well as collect information regarding the delivery of services. Many times, patients "fall through the cracks" owing to lack of follow-up by their provider. The case manager has a vital role in proactively monitoring the patient as he or she progresses through critical junctures in the course of the disease. The system can define and schedule time-critical interventions.

F. Evaluation: The case management process requires continuous evaluation. The patient's status and response to treatment is evaluated; the provider's plan of care is evaluated and refined for effectiveness and consistency with established standards; the status of goals is evaluated to determine the progress made; and the case manager must evaluate himself or herself against adopted guidelines and protocols. Evaluation is more meaningful and effective when status and outcomes can be measured consistently and objectively. After each evaluation, the case manager modifies the intervention strategy or plan as necessary.

G. Outcomes: Outcomes can be defined in a variety of ways depending on what elements of the patient's health status the case manager has an interest in or can affect. The same bits of data can provide different information to different users based on the way the data are reported (Steinhauser, 1999). For example, the CMIS reports how many patients met their goal of "Understanding their disease process" by the target date.
   1. The case manager looks at the data to determine if his or her intervention strategy with the patient was appropriate.
   2. The medical director looks at the results of assessments. For example, based on the fact that the patient was unable to recite the basic aspects and goals of his or her treatment, it is determined that the providers were not explaining the disease adequately to the patient or involving him or her in the treatment plan.
   3. The case management director identifies that the target date of the goal was too aggressive, based on the target population.
   4. The health plan uses the data to support the development of a disease management program for the specific disease to promote patient education and improve outcomes.
   5. There are many different ways a CMIS system can be used to measure outcomes.
      a. Medical: Readmission rates, emergency department visits signifying

treatment failure, exacerbations, complications, too frequent or too infrequent office visits, reduced lengths of stay (LOSs).

    b. Case management: Defined processes followed, goals met and variances reported, time-dependent interventions completed, compliance improved (patient and provider), patient knowledge increased.

    c. Patient: Improved quality of life, satisfaction with provider and the care he or she is receiving, and empowerment.

    d. Organizational: Cost savings, population profiling, improved working relationships, improved community image.

■ FEATURES OF A CASE MANAGEMENT INFORMATION SYSTEM (CMIS) (BOX 10–1)

A. Storage of clinical knowledge, divided into three major categories:

    1. Reference: This aspect of clinical knowledge pertains to the underlying medical knowledge, facts, or treatment standards that are used as rationale within the software. It can remain strictly in the background as the clinical justification for the software-driven clinical outputs and may not be visible to the user, or references and facts are visible within the application and serve as resource and support in the form of lookup tables, lists, indices, or glossaries.

    2. Informational knowledge: The informational knowledge base conveys data and information about patients and providers. Also included in this category are the various types of patient and user education material, including audio, text, or scripts formatted and accessible through the software as well as clinical data.

    3. Software-driven clinical outputs: The last type of clinical knowledge base relates to the actions or recommended actions that stem from software logic. Often, this takes the form of alerts, reminders, or recommendation prompts. To a large extent, this knowledge base is subjective and is based on an extrapolation of clinical facts or a consensus agreement among clinical experts. Risk assessment criteria are also in this category. Based on input prompted for by the system, the system makes a decision regarding the intervention strategy or the approach the case manager should take. For example, an algorithm is applied to the treatment, diagnostic, and pharmacy history of a group of patients. The output consists of the following:

        a. A list of patients who are at high risk for developing complications and exacerbations or requiring a hospital admission in the near future. These patients should be actively managed.

        b. A list of patients who are relatively stable or at moderate risk. These patients may be enrolled in a disease management program or have a case management contact scheduled for every month for follow-up and assessment.

        c. A list of patients who are stable and at low risk for complications. These patients may still benefit from intervention by a case manager in the form of educational material being mailed directly to their homes.

BOX 10–1

• •

A case management system is a complex, integrated tool that can include many features, functions, and elements. To have a maximum benefit to the users, all these components must work together. Because they are primarily used by clinicians, clinical components make up the major part of the systems. However, without the inclusion of the nonclinical, business-based components and data items, the system would have limited value.

Clinical Components

Assessments
Baseline
QOL
Disease specific

Disease Stratification
Sub-populations
Criteria
Problem identification

Goals
Identification
Target date
Tracking
Variances

Clinical Variables
Lab values
Vital signs
Medication dosing

Look-Up Tables
ICD-9
CPT-4
DSM-IV

Lists
Drug formularies

Documentation of Medical Treatment Plan

Documentation of Care Management Plan

Patient Milestone Identification

Intervention Strategies

ID of Care Management Candidates

Nonclinical Components

Member Data:
Demographics
Admission status
Benefits/coverage

CM's Active Patient List

Tickler System/To-Do List

Documentation (Notes)

Provider Data

Utilization Management

Cost Calculation

B. Promote awareness of guidelines, pathways, and protocols (Casanova, 1997).
   1. Prompting case managers with reminders (e.g., follow-up with patient regarding compliance with medication regimen).
   2. Providing treatment recommendations tailored to the individual patient (e.g., patient enrollment in a weight reduction program).
   3. Generating appropriate alerts for immediate issues (e.g., contact physician regarding possible treatment failure).
   4. Allowing access to guideline specifics (e.g., schedule for laboratory tests, office visits, and eye exams).

C. Provide exception tracking when the patient varies from the guideline.

D. Facilitate accurate and simplified data entry and collection.

E. Support data retrieval for reporting and outcomes measurement.

■ CMIS FUNCTIONAL REQUIREMENTS

A. Integration of clinical and nonclinical components
   1. Assessments: The responses to any individual question can be tracked over time. Responses can trigger entries on the to-do list (tickler feature) or generate a goal or problem. For example, if the case manager asks the patient whether he or she is able to tolerate mild activity and the patient responds negatively, the CMIS can generate a problem on the patient's problem list that states "patient has poor stamina" and a goal may appear that states "patient's stamina will improve." The system can also generate a reminder when the time is appropriate to perform an assessment. In addition, notes can be automatically generated that contain the responses to key questions.
   2. Goals: The system can automatically remind the case manager when the target date for a goal is approaching and track the progress toward the goal.
   3. Problems: The system can link problems and goals with plans to resolve each problem.
   4. Milestones: Again, the system can track the status of patient milestones. Is the patient reaching the milestones by the target dates? If not, what are the primary reasons? Is the case manager performing the appropriate interventions at the designated time once the patient meets a milestone?

B. Customization of system parameters: The system must be flexible enough to support a wide range of environments and unique business processes while reducing variance and subjective reporting. For example, two employer groups subscribe to the same HMO. One group has opted for an aggressive disease management program for diabetes, whereas the other has not identified diabetes as a major issue for its employee population.

C. Security: Confidentiality of patient data to unauthorized individuals and organizations as well as encryption capabilities and secure electronic data transfer must be guaranteed by the system.

D. Instantaneous key stroke, screen update, and query response times: Encounters with patients and with the system can be as short as a minute, so the amount of time documenting the encounter or accessing information relevant to the encounter is extremely limited. The system should perform at "think speed" (Casanova, 1997).

E. Portability and remote access with synchronization to host system: The data must be able to go with the user. Case managers are no longer spending all their time behind a desk; on-site visits are an essential part of the assessment process. For case managers, this means visits and meetings in places such as hospitals, patient homes, provider facilities, and home offices. Access to key data should be available at all times. Synchronization of data between remote and on-site systems can occur as needed and should be easy, reliable, and quick.

F. Intuitive user navigation: The information must be arranged and accessed in a way that makes sense to the user. "Jumping" from one area to another must be quick, without requiring specific paths.

G. Rule-based alerts, messages, and reminders based on information gathered or clinical recommendations. Structured data entry with discrete data elements must be in place to meet this requirement. Reminder rules used in the system assess patient states, determine what issues need attention, and then generate the system reminders.

  1. Rules can be related to overlooked treatments, preventive care (reducing complications and exacerbations), proper follow-up, or monitoring current treatment and interventions (McDonald et al., 1994).

  2. Reminder rules consist of two parts. The first part, specified by one or more criteria, defines a particular patient state, for example, "The patient is not using inhaler properly." The second part specifies the required response to that state, for example, "Send written instructions on the proper use of inhaler."

  3. The suggested response can be based on empirical data but more likely is based on anecdotal evidence with its intrinsic uncertainty–that is what worked "best" in the past. Responses must be re-evaluated based on outcome studies. For example, 1 month after receiving educational material about using inhalers properly, 70% of identified patients still use them incorrectly. A new response may be indicated, such as "Patient receives home visit by asthma specialist to give live demonstration about how to use inhaler, evaluate patient feedback, and reinforce importance of compliance."

  4. The success of reminder rules depends on an organization's ability to identify, analyze, and select a set of simple principles for building them, for example, "Simplicity is a required attribute." If a developer recommends a more complex rule, there must be proof to support the complexity.

H. Patient education material can be accessed on-line as well as sent directly to the patient or provider.

I. Tracking of services, admissions, procedures, and equipment approved for the patient.

J. Access to real-time updates with other systems within the organization.

K. Ability to send messages, referrals, and review requests to other users of the system.

L. Ability to scan documents into the system. These may include documents from providers' offices or illustrations.

M. Communication tools to support meaningful dialogues.

■ **CMIS DATA REQUIREMENTS**

A. *Data* do not equal *information*. Data are specific, relevant, comparable, timely, meaningful, and actionable. Information must be provided to the decision makers closest to the "action." Data must be transformed into useful knowledge that shows what works. Edward Deming is attributed as saying, "You can only manage what you measure." This statement is particularly true for today's case managers.

B. Data must have integrity. Data must be consistent and mean the same thing to all users. Data must be valid. Data must be complete; the same type of information must be available for all patients in a group.

C. Data must support the health and disease management initiatives.
   1. By case manager: Change activity of case manager; change behavior of patient or provider, based on responses to interventions and treatment; change guidelines, protocols, or clinical pathways.
   2. By organization: Patient population profiles, cost of treating and managing diseases, outcomes analysis, variance identification, and tracking.

D. Information should be shared among all the members of the health care team. Collaboration with the provider or patient, or both, will improve outcomes.
   1. Once action is taken, assess the impact of that action. Compare this impact against alternative actions to determine the best practice.

E. Any system must support simplified, accurate data entry. If data entry becomes more cumbersome or error prone, the system will not be used as intended. This could lead to inconsistent data collection, which can then lead to misleading and inaccurate reports. Without consistency, all data are suspect and data integrity is lost.

F. Data should be stored in a structured, standardized format that can be aggregated and captured as discreet data for reporting. Queries should be possible that can extract data from multiple files with speed and integrity. The end user cannot wait for days, weeks, or months for information.

G. Data breadth (what) and depth (about whom) as well as completeness (by whom) must be supported consistently for all data collected. Reduce the number of "holes" in the data, making reports more accurate and meaningful.

H. Provide feedback on demand with a user-specified denominator, that is, the subpopulation that will be reviewed.

I. Graphic display of data allows more data to be displayed, making it easier to view and allowing the user to detect trends or track key indicators.

■ CMIS DATA CONTENT REQUIREMENTS

A. Patient demographics, including address, contact information, employment or student status, and date of birth

B. Patient clinical information, including medical directives, primary diagnoses, and allergies

C. Insurance, including providers, plan, eligibility, coverage, benefits, and authorization

D. May include access to most or all of the following tables:
   1. International Classification of Disease (ICD-9) Codes
   2. Current Procedural Terminology (CPT-4) Codes
   3. *Diagnostic and Statistical Manual of Mental Disorders*, 4th Edition (DSM-IV) Codes
   4. Table of drugs
   5. Patient claims
   6. Patient pharmacy (pharmacy benefits manager [PBM]) information
   7. Provider data base
   8. Facility data base
   9. Community resources data base
   10. Medical dictionary and medical spell-check system

■ CMIS CLINICAL CONTENT DEVELOPMENT

A. Many guidelines, protocols, and pathways are available for physician practice, call center triage, hospital care (e.g., Milliman and Robertson, Inc.), and concurrent review. Each of these groups may have quite different guidelines for the same patient populations. However, very few are available for the unique role and environment of a case manager. In addition, most organizations address the process of case management in different ways based on patient population, provider network, case management availability and expertise, and available tools. Therefore, most organizations develop their own guidelines based on the case management process and standards of care as defined by CMSA.
   1. Barriers that exist to the development of clinical content acceptance include:
      a. Users are not involved in development and subsequently do not have sense of ownership
      b. Lack of proper dissemination and training
      c. Weak implementation infrastructure
      d. Controversial content
      e. Poorly designed: based on weak or nonexisting evidence, failure to stratify patients, or the wrong focus

B. The basic elements of a case management guideline development process include the following (Nash & Todd, 1996):

1. Identification of issues
2. Identification of desired outcomes
3. Creation of measuring devices and yardsticks to measure against
4. Determination of cause and effect in relation to outcomes
5. Definition of practice or intervention

C. Clinical process is necessary in the development of a CMIS because
   1. Case managers are usually clinicians with varying clinical experience and varying areas of expertise
   2. Varied approaches among users to perform the basic functions of case management
   3. Identification of best-practice initiatives
   4. Definition of software-driven clinical outputs
   5. Identification of the type and format of clinical information to be gathered
   6. Identification of system functionality and performance requirements to support the steps of case management
   7. Identification of appropriate timing of interventions based on patient needs and the case management process

D. The steps of guideline development are as follows:
   1. Development of disease maps: Before a patient can be effectively case managed, the course of the disease must be fully understood. Disease maps are general "best-practice" algorithms for patient care, including the evaluation and diagnosis of the disease, inpatient and outpatient management, and long-term management of the chronic-stable patient. They illustrate the path patients take within the health care system.
      a. Maps can form the basis for provider process redesign efforts that increase collaboration, enhance communications, and reduce waste by showing where duplication or unnecessary or inappropriate health care processes occur.

      Information is obtained from (in order of value) randomized, control clinical trials with adequate population, randomized control clinical trials with a smaller study group, nonrandomized studies, retrospective studies, and final general consensus and expert opinion. Information sources include journal articles, recently published textbooks, publications from regulatory organizations, and publications from disease-focused organizations (e.g., American Diabetic Association) (Campazzi & Lee, 1997).

   2. Identification of stratification groups: Stratification allows patients to be classified into homogeneous subgroups based on a number of different criteria. The criteria you use will depend on the goal in stratifying your patients. For example:
      a. Stratification based on insurance group (ABC Widge Co.) or product (e.g., Medicare) will support your workflow if, as a case manager, you are assigned to patients based on their coverage and benefits.
      b. Stratification based on severity of illness will allow you to make accurate comparisons when reporting outcomes. For example, an un-

controlled, noncompliant asthmatic will have far different outcome goals than the mild, controlled patient with asthma.

c. Stratification based on patient location supports organizations that assign case managers according to their current location, for example, hospital, nursing home, or in the patient's home with home care services. Each of these situations requires special case management skills.

Once the stratification groups have been determined, it is possible to assign default goals with associated target dates that are appropriate for that stratification group.

3. Determination of critical junctures or milestones in patient management. These critical points are different from what might be identified by the providers. For example, a physician treating a patient may set a milestone as the time the patient is weaned off a ventilator. However, the case manager is more interested in milestones such as "start of chemotherapy" or "stable for 1 month" or "pain free for 1 week."

4. Identifying key areas of concern to the case manager and defining a strategy for managing these patients. These key areas are defined in terms of patient milestones and case manager interventions. As the patient progresses through stratification groups in the continuum of his or her care, these areas of concern will change accordingly, as will short-term and possibly long-term goals.

■ SELECTING AND IMPLEMENTING A CMIS

A. At present, there is an explosion of medical informatics systems and, specifically, software to support case management.

B. However, some organizations choose to develop their own system.

1. The advantages of developing a CMIS from within an organization are

a. Intimate knowledge of existing systems, making interface development less complicated and more streamlined

b. Intimate knowledge of the medical and case management processes that must be automated

c. Ability to make rapid changes to the software based on business decisions and changes in the processes

2. The disadvantages of developing a CMIS from within an organization are

a. It is a huge resource drain of both information system specialists and clinicians, not just for initial design and development but for maintenance and upgrades.

b. Each stakeholder wants a system that will meet all of his or her needs. Design can get bogged down in arbitration among departments regarding system functionality.

c. Lack of standardization. The future of cost-effective health care lies partially in the ability to share vital patient data across the spectrum of health care providers and payers. When each information system develops its own proprietary data coding and storage protocols, the ability of these systems to "talk with each other" becomes complex and costly.

C. Case managers at all levels within an organization can be directly or indirectly involved with choosing and implementing a CMIS. However, many other people from several different areas or departments can also be involved. The system must meet the needs of all the stakeholders.

1. Purchasers (e.g., employer groups): The people who are responsible for managing the overall health costs. They are also vested in improving outcomes and the health, productivity, and satisfaction of their subscribers. Key analysis: Are they getting a favorable return on their investment (ROI)?

2. Payers: This group includes the insurers and managed-care organizations. Their primary interest is in decreasing cost while improving the patients' health status. One of the primary needs of the payer organization is the ability to justify the cost of case management as an effective method for reaching their organizational goals.

3. Providers: This group includes essentially any person, organization, or facility that participates in the care of the patients, including hospitals, long-term or short-term care facilities, skilled nursing facilities, rehabilitation hospitals, clinics, physicians, physical and occupational therapists, speech therapists, group homes, and home care. The primary needs of the provider group are to maximize effective resource utilization, promote timely movement through the system, and improve outcomes. The challenge is to provide a smooth transition between provider settings and to provide access to key clinical data across the continuum.

4. Patients: Patients seek out health care to maintain or improve their health status, quality of life, and functionability. They also are interested in maximizing their health care dollar while decreasing their out-of-pocket costs.

D. Human component of implementing a CMIS

1. Commitment: Not all case managers will commit to go forward at the same time and at the same pace. The case manager must see value in the system directly relevant to his or her investment.

2. Motivation: Implementation takes time. Not all case managers will have the "staying power" to see the technology reach its maximum potential.

3. Training: Depends on the skills of each user, but usually starts with basics, such as using a mouse and learning keyboarding skills, to learning a complex application.

4. Resistance to change: Implementation of any CMIS requires some change in the case management process. Change management must be built into the implementation process.

5. Resistance to the concept of guidelines, protocols, and pathways.

E. The process of selecting and implementing a CMIS is modeled after the case management process itself. The five steps in choosing and implementing a CMIS include the following:

1. Establish teams: preselection team, selection team, implementation team, and postimplementation support team.
   a. Some members may belong to more than one team.
   b. Assign "alternates" to fill in for team members who can no longer participate.
   c. Choose committed people who can stay involved throughout the entire process.
   d. Include representatives from any department that will be impacted by the decision—for example, case managers, medical directors, information system specialists, financial officers, strategic planners, and an arbitrator who will facilitate compromise when conflicts arise.
   e. Identify who will be the final decision makers.
2. Assessment
   a. Assess the requirements, goals, and desired outcomes each department would like to achieve with the system. Be prepared to validate the needs of each stakeholder.
   b. Assess current program and processes. Are they working well? Can they be streamlined? A CMIS will not eliminate problems in your processes; it will simply automate them, which in some instances compounds them.
      (i) Develop a clearly defined workflow that supports the business process.
      (ii) Software that is either designed or purchased is only as good as the process it supports and the people using it.
   c. Assess what resources will be needed to implement the system, including training and backup when users are being trained. You cannot shut down your operation. It is easy to underestimate the time needed to implement a CMIS.
   d. Assess the vendors who have systems that generally meet your needs. Gradually limit the list to two to three vendors. Prioritize your system requirements and submit a request for information (RFI) to each vendor. Assess
      (i) How many of the high-priority requirements does the vendor meet?
      (ii) How well does the system communicate to legacy systems? Is there an open, clearly defined, built-in interface?
      (iii) Is the core data base of the system open and accessible?
      (iv) How does the vendor support implementation and training?
      (v) How flexible is the system (not custom but customizable to fit unique situations)? Remember that there are tradeoffs. The more flexible a system is, the more complex it is. Make sure that common activities are straightforward and easy to perform; rarely performed activities can be more complex and difficult.
      (vi) What is the company's "track record?" Can you talk to other customers? How long has the company been in business? What are the vendor's strategic plans for the CMIS and other related systems?

    e. Assess the cost of building your own CMIS if this is a feasible alternative. Keep in mind that building a system is usually more expensive than purchasing an available system in terms of finances and personnel time.

       (i) The market offers a wide range of systems with a range of costs, features, functions, and integration capabilities.

      (ii) Even if the software is purchased from a vendor, once a relationship is established, the organization may have the opportunity to offer suggestions for future enhancements (Daus, 1997).

3. Planning

    a. Define the role of each team member and the meeting schedule. Each team member must be committed to attending all relevant meetings and to performing action items that are identified in these meetings. More time spent at the beginning of the process will yield time savings after implementation because fewer changes will need to be made.

    b. Create a time-line project plan that identifies resources, which must be used at each phase.

    c. Standardize processes, terms, and data elements such as goal definitions, target dates, measuring tools, and intervention strategies.

    d. Map existing case management processes to system functions.

    e. Define what data you need to collect to obtain the information you need to be successful.

    f. Rewrite any policies, procedures, or job descriptions that are changing as a result of the system.

    g. Assign an administrator who understands the functional and technical sides of the system. The administrator will be responsible for setting up configurable parameters and communicating problems and requests to the vendor.

    h. Hardware is typically the smallest expense in implementing a system. Equipment purchased should support the current data storage needs and processing power and the projected needs for the next 5 years.

4. Implementation

    a. Set realistic expectations with the staff.

    b. Set up training for all users and coverage for the staff while they are involved in training. Assess each user's training needs. Are keyboarding skills weak?

    c. Set up a test environment that mimics the real world. Verify that the system performs as expected.

    d. For the first group to use the system live, choose a pilot group made up of people who are excited about the project, comfortable with technology, and possess good communication skills. Gradually add to small groups and anticipate an initial drop in productivity.

5. Evaluation

    a. Evaluate system performance and user acceptance shortly after implementation and then periodically. Are you seeing a return on your investment?

b. Review processes for optimization and enhancement opportunities as well as creative new ways to use the system.

c. Keep an open path of communication for feedback from users and among users to share ideas.

■ CLINICAL PATHWAYS

A. Development is based on the concerns of health care professionals, purchasers, and consumers regarding quality, utilization, and cost of health care services. Research has identified substantial variations in clinical practice, including overuse, underuse, and inappropriate use of services (Kelly, 1996). Many national, professional, governmental, and private organizations have developed clinical pathways for a wide range of diseases, medical conditions, and procedures.

B. Pathways emphasize coordination of all clinical activities and can be presented in a number of formats:
1. Activity and precedent table format: Lists all the activities and shows their required precedents, duration, and resource requirements. Some may also show start, finish, and slack times as well.
2. Gantt chart format: Shows the beginning and ending times for each activity to be done each day on a bar chart along a time scale. The activities are frequently grouped into consults, tests, patient activities, treatments, medications, diet, and patient and family education. Gantt charts clearly display when activities are to be done in each time period but do not show precedent relationships among activities.
3. Flowchart format: Graphically illustrates the precedent relationship among activities and shows the critical path. In general, flowcharts require more space than tables and can be quite large. This format does not work well in showing which activities have to be done on each day.

C. Although pathways outline best practice for day-to-day management of a patient, they must be tailored to meet the needs of the individual patient by allowing for variance.

D. Uses of clinical paths:
1. Show the overall management of a patient across disciplines, so that activities can be coordinated. Dependencies are identified. For example, a patient who suffered a cerebrovascular accident must be able to stand before being able to ambulate with help.
2. Expectations of actions, timing, and outcomes are established and agreed on by the multidisciplinary team.
3. Reduces variance in care.
4. Effective tool to educate and orient health care staff.
5. Clarifies the recovery process and expectations for the patient.

E. Even though the individual user can tailor pathways, there is still a great amount of resistance from many health care professionals who reject the notion of what they call "cookbook medicine." This can be addressed by involving all clinical practice areas, including physicians, registered nurses, pharmacists, and therapists, in the creation of the pathways.

F. Benefits of using clinical pathways:
1. Source of reliable (defined by the process and resources used to create them) and expert opinion.
2. Foster collaborative goal setting among care providers for specific case types. Expected and desired outcomes are more likely to be achieved because they have been discussed and agreed on by the whole team.
3. Can be used as a basis for a disease management program.
4. Essential for measuring outcomes and modifying treatment based on analysis.
5. Basis for the creation of patient education tools.
6. Can have different focus depending on disease or location:
   a. Inpatient care: Goal to reduce LOS beginning at time before the admission and following the patient through discharge.
   b. Complete episode of care: Begins at time of diagnosis and includes preadmission care, inpatient care, outpatient care at clinic or physician office, and home care.
   c. Specialized: Models of managing patients with special conditions or in a single environment, for example, dialysis patients or patients in an intensive care unit.
   d. Life and health management: Used for managing chronic diseases such as asthma, diabetes, hypertension, and cancer.

G. Disadvantages of using clinical pathways:
1. Difficult to keep up to date with changing practice patterns.
2. Different pathways for the same condition can have conflicting recommendations. For example, hospitals, physician groups, and HMOs have their own clinical pathways to follow. Care must be taken that although the focus may change, the essence and goals of the pathways should be consistent across disciplines.
3. No one pathway for any disease addresses the full continuum of care (i.e., acute care in the hospital to subacute care to home health care to outpatient to patient independence).
4. It is difficult to evaluate the validity of the pathway without extensive outcomes testing.
5. Recommendations may be difficult to implement, mainly due to provider or patient noncompliance.

■ CLINICAL PROTOCOLS

A. Terminology of clinical pathway, clinical guideline, and clinical protocol is blurred and often used interchangeably.

B. Protocols provide the case manager with a list of the minimum standards of care. With few exceptions, they can be applied to all patients assigned to a group because they are independent of individual patient differences. Most protocols are rigidly enforced and guarantee a single standard of care. If patients have multiple problems, protocols can be combined.

C. Goals are not usually included in the definition of a protocol, nor is a time-line or resource allocation recommendation.

D. The success of a protocol depends on organizational processes and governance to develop and deploy them (Drazen, 1999).

E. Protocols are frequently employed in telephonic triage DSSs. These protocols include branching logic based on information obtained.

■ OTHER TECHNOLOGY TOOLS AVAILABLE TO THE CASE MANAGER

A. The Internet. The Internet has been a boon for people searching out information, and its value to case managers is no exception.

1. Stay abreast of the current regulatory requirements, accreditation criteria, and standards of care as set by government and non-government disease-focused agencies (e.g., National Committee for Quality Assurance, American Accreditation Health Care/Commission, Health Plan Employer Data and Information Set, Joint Commission on Accreditation of Healthcare Organizations).

2. Research the latest guidelines. This information can be included in any guidelines you have created in your own organization.

3. Review studies that support best-practice methods of treatment. Again, this information can be included in guidelines you have created or are using.

4. Obtain copies of public domain assessment tools, for example, a quality-of-life assessment tool.

5. Review patient education material.

6. Access health care statistics to help you plan your organization's case management needs for the future.

7. Early stages of allowing access to patient information across the Internet. Case managers can communicate directly with the patient, physician, or hospital to gather information and to manage the services required. The biggest obstacles to this functionality are patient access, technology skills, security, and patient confidentiality and other legal issues.

8. Identification of resources for treatment (i.e., specialists, clinics, equipment, and providers).

B. Claims review systems. Although the case manager may not use these systems directly, they can still have a significant impact on how case managers do their jobs.

1. Identify which providers are outliers.

2. Identify which diagnoses are the biggest consumers of health care dollars and could benefit from case management.

3. Identify which procedures are ordered inappropriately. The results of this investigation may lead to a policy that anytime this procedure is ordered, it must be preapproved.

4. Identify which procedures are not performed when a particular condition or diagnoses warrants it. May lead to a case manager working with a provider to ensure consistency of care.

5. If claims can be reviewed in a timely fashion, they can be used to help in the identification of patients who may benefit from case management interventions.

C. Electronic medical records. Data can be shared among all providers, delivery locations, and case managers in a standardized, fully automated format (Shaffer, 1999).

D. Red flags: Indicators for case management (Kongstvedt, 1996). In the basic system, claims or authorizations are analyzed. User-defined criteria are used to identify patients who would benefit from case management. For example:
1. Patients with admissions lasting longer than "x" number of days
2. Patients with specific diagnoses
3. Patients with a specified procedure ordered or performed
4. Patients whose cost for the current episode exceeds "x" number of dollars
5. Patients receiving "x" number of services during a user-defined period of time

E. More sophisticated systems may look at combinations of events. For example:
1. Patients with a specific diagnoses and on a specific medication
2. Patients with a specific diagnosis and a specific procedure ordered
3. Patient who has not refilled a maintenance prescription at the appropriate time
4. Patient who is refilling a prescription more often than indicated

F. In the future, once electronic medical records have become more widespread, patients will be able to be identified by more clinical criteria. For example:
1. Vital signs out of normal range for a user-defined period of time
2. Laboratory values out of normal range for a user-defined period of time
3. Any combination of vitals signs, laboratory values, diagnoses, procedures, and medications

REFERENCES

Barr, C. E. (1998). The role of information technology in disease management supporting identification of best practices. *Disease Management, 1*(3), 121–132.
Campazzi, E., & Lee, D. (1997). *How to assess clinical guidelines, tools for the task: The role of clinical guidelines.* Tampa, FL: Hillsboro Printing.
Casanova, J. (1997). *Tools for the task: The role of clinical guidelines.* Tampa, FL: Hillsboro Printing.
Case Management Society of America. (1995). *Standards of practice for case management.* Little Rock, AR: CMSA.
Daus, C. (1997). Software solutions: Case management gets automated for success. *Case Review, 3*(2), 54–56.
Dietzen, J. (1997). Decision support systems: Technology enhancing case management. *The Journal of Case Management, 3*(6), 12–17.
Drazen, E., & Metzger, J. (1999). *Strategies for integrated health care.* San Francisco: Jossey-Bass.
Favor, G., & Ricks, R. (1996). Preparing to automate the case management process. *Nursing Case Management, 1*(3), 100–106.

Horan, D. (1994). *Use of algorithms in clinical guideline development. Clinical practice guideline development methodology perspectives.* Washington, D.C.: U.S. Department of Health and Human Services.

Kelly, J., & Bernard, D. (1996). *Disease management: A systems approach to improving patient outcomes.* Chicago: American Hospital Publishing.

Kongstvedt, P. (1996). *The managed health care handbook.* Gaithersburg, MD: Aspen.

McDonald, C., Tierney, W., & Overhage, J. (1994). *Computer based reminder rules, data bases, and guideline development. Clinical practice guideline development methodology persectives.* Washington, D.C.: U.S. Department of Health and Human Services.

McGarvey, L. (1998). Technology's role in case management. *The Case Manager, 9*(2), 69–72.

Nash, D., & Todd, W. (1997). *Disease management, a systems approach to improving patient outcomes* (pp. 52–53). Chicago: American Hospital Association.

National Health Care Consortium. (1995). *Conceptualizing, implementing and evaluating extended care pathways.* Bloomington, MN: NHCC.

Shaffer, C. (1999). Case management law. *Continuing Care, 18*(4), 14–16.

Smith, R. (1998). Simplifying tasks: Computer software programs increase efficiency for case managers. *Case Review, 4*(3), 42.

Steinhauser, K. (1999). Tracking numbers. *Continuing Care, 18*(2), 16–21.

Wrinn, M. (1998a). A new frontier for case management: Outcomes measurement. *Continuing Care, 17*(6), 16.

Wrinn, M. (1998b). The emerging role of telehealth in health care. *Continuing Care, 17*(8), 18–19.

· · · · · · · · · · · · · ·

CHAPTER 11

Workers' Compensation Case Management

SHARON BRIM

Upon completion of chapter, the reader will be able to:

1. Define terms and acronyms specific to health care management in the workers' compensation field.

2. Learn of the role workers' compensation programs play in American business and what case managers need to know.

3. Understand the impact state workers' compensation laws have on case management practices and the need to vary the practices in each state jurisdiction.

4. Describe the market forces in the cost of workers' compensation programs that produced opportunities for skilled case management.

5. List the types of workers' compensation cases typically assigned for medical management and ways to successfully apply case management skills to them.

6. Understand the burden medical, legal, and financial issues place on the practice of ethical, advocacy-based case management.

7. Prepare for trends projected to occur in workers' compensation issues.

IMPORTANT TERMS AND CONCEPTS

Disability Impairment Rating
First Report of Injury
Functional Capabilities Evaluation and
    Functional Capacity Evaluation
Indemnity
Independent Medical Evaluation
Maximum Medical Improvement,
    Maximum Medical Recovery,
    Medical End
Partial Permanent Disability
Partial Temporary Disability

Repetitive Stress Injury and
    Cumulative Trauma Injuries
Reserves
Return to Work
Scheduled Injury
Second Injury Fund
Self-Insured
Third-Party Administrator
Total Permanent Disability
Total Temporary Disability

■ INTRODUCTION

A. Skillful case management in the field of workers' compensation demands a knowledge and understanding of pertinent terms, practices, and parameters not usually taught in health care settings. Because the terms are used throughout the industry, knowing them is essential for the case manager.

B. Review of the history of workers' compensation programs in U.S. business points to an understanding of today's system.

■ DEFINITIONS

A. First Report of Injury: This is a formal document completed by the employer on report of a work-related injury or condition that begins the process of a workers' compensation claim. The report is filed with the appropriate state jurisdiction and sent to the workers' compensation carrier or third-party administrator (claims handlers for self-insured employers). The injured worker or his or her attorney may file the first report of injury.

B. Indemnity: In this context, the term is defined as money paid as a wage replacement when the injured worker is determined to be medically unfit to work. The amount is based on the worker's usual wage, factored by a formula set by the state that has jurisdiction for the claim.

C. Temporary Total Impairment: Status in which indemnity is paid when an injured worker is unable to work in any capacity while treatment continues, with the expectation of recovery and return to employment. In most states, the injured worker receives benefits for the entire time he or she is medically deemed to be unable to work.

D. Temporary Partial Disability: Status in which impairment prevents injured worker from returning to usual job, but the worker can be employed in some capacity. A benefit is paid when the restrictions to work activity result in a decrease of usual wages.

E. Medical End (ME), Maximum Medical Improvement (MMI), Maximum Medical Recovery (MMR): Terms used to indicate that the injured worker has recovered from injuries to a level that a physician states further treatment will not substantively change the medical outcome. If the injured worker has a medically substantiated permanent change to preinjury health and function, an impairment rating may be done.

F. Impairment Rating: The basis for determining the medical outcome of a workers' compensation claim. Many states require an impairment rating to be based on the findings of a licensed physician using an impairment rating system such as the American Medical Association *Guides to the Evaluation of Permanent Impairment*. The final decision on a disability rating rests with an adjudicator in the state workers' compensation system.

G. Permanent Partial Disability: This is the designation used to indicate that there is a presumptive or actual decrease in wage-earning capacity due to injury. A benefit is paid according to the severity of impairment in a formula derived by the state. Most states have "scheduled" injuries (benefit paid by a formula based on loss of or loss of the use of specific body members) and "nonscheduled" injuries (a benefit is based on the percentage of impairment in a formula computed by the state).

H. Permanent Total Disability: This award is based on a medical assertion that the injured worker is precluded by the extent of his or her disability from gainful employment. Each state has guidelines on which this designation and subsequent benefits are paid (United States Chamber of Commerce, 1997).

■ HISTORICAL PERSPECTIVE

A. The industrial evolution in America that began the transformation of the work force from agrarian to industrial in the late 19th and early 20th centuries spawned the workers' compensation system that is taking us to the 21st century.

   1. Common-law practices held that an employer was responsible for injuries or death to his or her workers only if they were caused by a negligent act.

   2. The injured employees or their survivors had to bring suit to establish that there was negligence on the part of employers. This process was difficult and out of the reach of most employees or family members.

   3. Injured workers' financial and health needs were absorbed by their families or the communities around them.

B. As the workplace became larger and more mechanized, the risk to workers increased. Social reformers recognized the need for legislated standards to protect individual workers and the community as a whole.

C. The first laws passed in the various states merely replaced common law with enacted laws, but the burden remained on the injured worker to prove employer responsibility.

D. In 1911, the first state workers' compensation laws were enacted that established a no-fault system to deal with work-related injuries.

E. Today, all 50 states and several U.S. territories have workers' compensation laws. Federal legislation has been enacted to cover federal workers in several different programs (Douglas, 1994; United States Chamber of Commerce, 1997).

■ BASIC AIMS OF ALL WORKERS' COMPENSATION PROGRAMS

A. Provide injured workers prompt medical care and wage replacement for the workers, their dependents, or their survivors regardless of responsibility for the injuries.

B. Establish a single, primary remedy for workplace injuries to decrease the legal costs and relieve the judicial system of heavy caseloads of personal injury cases.

C. Relieve both the public and private sectors from demands on financial and medical services.

D. Promote workplace safety and accident prevention.

■ UNDERSTANDING THE IMPACT OF WORKERS' COMPENSATION COSTS

A. Nearly 100 million workers (85% to 90% of the U.S. workforce) are covered by workers' compensation programs (Stoddard, 1998). The rising costs associated with these programs affect all of society and are driving industry to demand cost-containment strategies. This then sets the stage for medical managers to work throughout the industry (Akabas, Gates, & Galvin, 1992).

B. Workers' compensation program costs are borne by the employer through purchased insurance policies or as a "self-insured" entity meeting requirements imposed by state laws. State and federal employees' programs are publicly supported.

C. There are misconceptions about workers' compensation programs that can result in abuse or overuse of them. Although, as stated above, the employer bears the total cost of workers' compensation programs, two of the most common mistaken ideas about workers' compensation are the following:
   1. Workers' compensation is a tax-supported program that is provided to all employees by state or federal governments.
   2. Worker' compensation insurance is paid for by employees and supplemented by payments from the employer, like health insurance programs.

D. The cost of workers' compensation insurance and all costs associated with workplace injuries are reflected in the price of goods and services sold by the employer. Besides the direct cost of buying insurance premiums, there are several indirect costs (worker replacement, productivity loss) that increase the totals appreciably (Douglas, 1994).

E. The cost of buying workers' compensation insurance is based on a complicated formula of previous claims, types of workers insured (e.g., clerical personnel have less risk of injury than do truck drivers), and an element calculated by the state based on annual costs (*Survey of Workers' Compensation Laws,* 1999).

F. The only factor that can be effectively modified by the employer is the cost associated with the number and severity of workplace injuries.

G. Workers' compensation insurance carriers also have a stake in decreasing costs of claims submitted to them. A competitive marketplace in the insurance field demands that companies sell their product for workers' compensation programs at the lowest possible price.

H. Many strategies are employed in keeping claims costs low, but none is being more aggressively used than management of medical costs.

■ **FITTING THE PIECES TOGETHER: MEDICAL CASE MANAGEMENT IN THE WORKERS' COMPENSATION SYSTEM**

A. Medical management processes have been involved in the periphery of workers' compensation programs for a number of years, both medically and vocationally.

B. Societal changes and escalating medical costs have placed a larger burden on employers required to provide workers' compensation coverage for their employees. Case management strategies are used as tools to lower medical costs, maintain a stable workforce, and decrease cost.

C. Case managers working in the workers' compensation field encounter a greater number of stakeholders than in other areas. Additionally, a workers' compensation claim can be a complicated, often protracted process in which case managers can become involved at any time.

D. Workers' compensation laws demand the case management process be adapted to work within that structure.

■ **HISTORICAL APPLICATION OF MEDICAL CASE MANAGEMENT IN WORKERS' COMPENSATION**

A. Claims processors have attempted to provide some degree of medical management for a number of years using various legal maneuvering to limit overuse of medical services and bring compensation claims to closure.

B. The services of medical professionals in the claims-handling process were usually limited to catastrophic accidents and other injuries that would severely limit an injured worker's prospects of returning to gainful employment.

C. In the decade between the mid-1980s and the mid-1990s, the costs of worker' compensation exploded in American industry (Stoddard, 1998).

   1. The National Council of Compensation Insurance published data indicating that the nationwide cost of compensation claims was $69 billion, with about 45% of the cost in medical care.

   2. Medical costs have tripled in workers' compensation in a decade. This

is illustrated in the cost of self-insurance costs for 1983 to 1993 (Stoddard, 1998) (Fig. 11–1).

3. Some of the reasons for the escalating medical costs are thought to be:
   a. Health care inflation
   b. Aging of the workforce
   c. Coverage expanding in repetitive use injuries, stress, psychological injuries, and aggravation of usual diseases of life and coverage of occupational diseases
   d. Cost shifting from other areas of health care
   e. Lack of ability to impose medical utilization standards (Douglas, 1994)

■ ADAPTING CASE MANAGEMENT PRACTICES TO WORKERS' COMPENSATION STRUCTURE

A. Enumerating the stakeholders in workers' compensation case management
   1. Adapting usual case management techniques and practices to the workers' compensation field requires the practitioner to recognize the responsibilities of the various people and organizations with a role in mediating a work-related injury claim (Fig. 11–2).
      a. Employer—reports claim and monitors claim; may have a risk manager or other representative to assist with a claim.
      b. Claims adjuster—has the responsibility of investigating the claim, applying laws, and making the first determination about compensibility, paying indemnity, paying medical bills, and directing case management.
      c. Attorneys—plaintiff if retained by injured worker; defense for insurance carrier and employer.

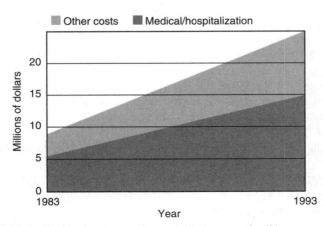

FIGURE 11–1 Workers' compensation costs for a group of self-insurance companies.

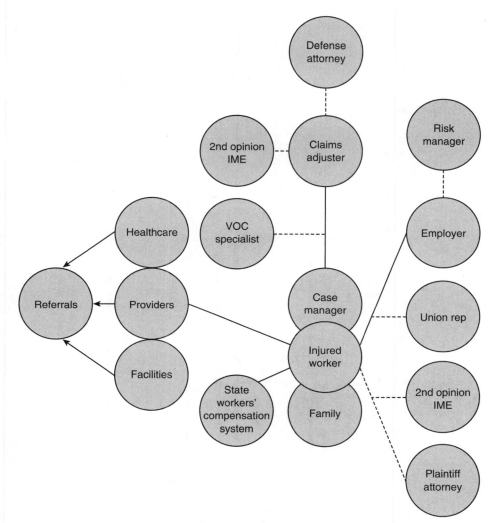

FIGURE 11–2   Coordinating the stakeholders. The presence of multiple players in a single worker's compensation claim requires case managers to coordinate the activity of those involved.

    d. Union representative—can assist in protecting worker's rights and also has input into return-to-work issues.

    e. State administrative agency—body at state level with jurisdiction over workers' compensation claims.

2. A workers' compensation claim can be protracted for the typical flow of a workers' compensation claim from date of injury through date of settlement (Fig. 11–3).

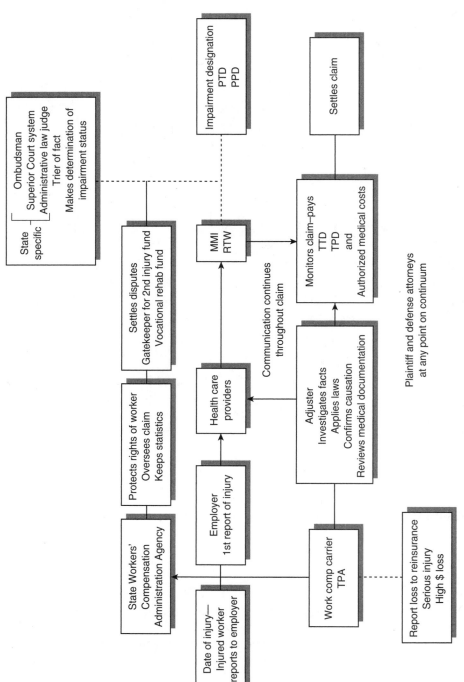

FIGURE 11-3 Life of a worker's compensation claim.

■ WORKERS' COMPENSATION LAWS THAT DIRECTLY AFFECT CASE MANAGEMENT PRACTICE

A. Laws governing workers' compensation administration are enacted by each state and territorial legislature and administered by state agencies.

B. The U.S. Congress legislates development of regulations for federal workers and all other workers in the District of Columbia. Programs that are also overseen on the federal level include:

1. Longshore and Harbor Workers' Compensation
2. Black Lung Act

C. Laws are written and amended frequently. Because case managers must comply with the laws in order to practice legally and ethically, a source for learning about them is essential. Comprehensive compendia of state and federal laws can be found in:

1. Annual editions of *Analysis of Workers Compensation Laws* prepared and published by the U.S. Chamber of Commerce
2. *Survey of Workers' Compensation Laws* (1999) prepared and distributed by the Alliance of American Insurance

D. Workers' compensation laws dealing with claims issues have only a peripheral impact on medical management. However, knowledge of laws creating the medical system has a direct effect on the ability of the case manager to accomplish goals (Mullahy, 1998).

E. Workers' compensation case mangers have a responsibility to be familiar with applicable laws but must exercise caution to avoid the appearance of giving legal advice to injured workers or employers.

■ STATE WORKERS' COMPENSATION LAWS THAT DIRECTLY IMPACT CASE MANAGEMENT PRACTICE

A. Arguably the most challenging laws for workers' compensation medical managers are those that dictate the selection and use of health care providers. Each state mandates the manner in which providers can be chosen (*Survey of Workers' Compensation Laws*, 1999).

1. The initial choice of a health care provider can be made by
   a. The injured worker without restriction
   b. The employer or insurance company by
      (i) Directly selecting a provider for the injured worker
      (ii) Posting a panel of providers from which the injured worker selects
      (iii) Belonging to a medical care organization (MCO) with preferred provider (PPO) lists from which the injured worker may choose

2. State laws also control changes of providers during the course of treatment. These guidelines for changes are quite complex in many states, and the claim handler can guide the case manager.

3. State laws may also regulate the use of independent medical examinations (IMEs). This is an evaluation generally arranged by the payor

to confirm, rebut, or supplement medical findings offered by the injured worker's chosen physician or other provider (Douglas, 1994).

   a. Regulations might limit the number of such examinations.
   b. There may be a specific time interval required between IMEs.
   c. State regulations can limit the type of practitioner who performs IMEs.
   d. Administrative agencies can require the payor and the injured worker to abide by the findings of specific physicians on a "designated doctor" list.

B. State regulations pertaining to use of health care services by injured workers often reflect efforts to contain medical costs. MCOs for workers' compensation health care providers are allowed or required in a few states. Guidelines for case managers working for or with an MCO vary by state and are available either from the state administrative agency or from the MCO.

   1. States that do not allow MCOs often have some mechanism for regulating cost-containment efforts by payers.
      a. Use of health care services can be regulated by:
         (i) Type of provider
         (ii) Number of visits
         (iii) Duration of visits
         (iv) Cost of treatment
         (v) Peer review
         (v) Practice parameters
      b. Precertification or preauthorization of the following are required in some states:
         (i) Inpatient or outpatient surgery (nonemergency)
         (ii) High-dollar durable medical equipment, diagnostic tests, costly or extensive therapies and procedures (such as MRIs, epidural injections, and work-reconditioning programs)
         (iii) Treatment for specific diagnoses (such as a second opinion for spinal surgery)
      c. Medical bill reviews and repricing services are allowed in most states. State regulations indicate whether repricing at so-called usual and customary rates (payments are based on a data base reflecting standard charges for geographic area) or a fee schedule (published schedule of reimbursement allowed for charges for health care related to on-the-job injury) is allowed. The repricing is based on uniform data bases.

C. Almost all states and territories set up second injury funds for injured workers to assist the injured worker and provide a financial offset for the employer. Conditions covered include:

   1. Previously rated permanent impairment resulting from an on-the-job injury
   2. Medical disability

3. Diseases that substantially impact recovery from work-related injury (U.S. Chamber of Commerce, 1997)

D. Vocational rehabilitation as provided by workers' compensation regulations is sometimes coordinated concurrently with medical management. Each state regulates the parameters concerning vocational rehabilitation for injured workers who are unable to return to previous employment. A complete listing of state and territorial programs is available in the annual *United States Chamber of Commerce Analysis.*

■ PRACTICING THE CASE MANAGEMENT PROCESS WITHIN A WORKERS' COMPENSATION STRUCTURE

A. The entire range of case management practices can be applied in a workers' compensation industry setting. The skills and knowledge described are among those identified as critical for case managers by Chan and colleagues (1999).

B. There are customary requirements for employment as a workers' compensation case manager.

C. The settings in which a case manager might practice these processes are varied.

D. The organization or facility paying for these services often determines the scope and duration of case management.

E. The case management process as described by Mullahy and other authors can be applied to the most frequently encountered workers' compensation claims.

■ MEDICAL CASE MANAGEMENT PROCESSES USED IN WORKERS' COMPENSATION

A. Case finding and targeting
   1. "Lost time" claims (cases in which the injured worker has not returned to work within the time frame that triggers wage replacement benefits) are far more likely to be referred for case management than "medical only" cases, implying the injury has not prevented the injured worker from working at his usual job.

B. Evaluating and assessing
   1. Case managers in workers' compensation settings assess the injured worker's needs through claim file and medical record review; direct contact with the injured worker and his family, medical providers, employer, and others; and evaluation of current treatment plan and setting for that treatment.
   2. Part of the assessment process in workers' compensation case management is to evaluate the extent of injuries, probable treatment plan, expectation of complete recovery, and estimated time out of work. This information is reported to the claims handler so that appropriate reserves can be set. Reserves are the sum of money the insurance com-

pany or self-insured funds set aside to pay all costs associated with a claim. This process is an important one for claims handling, and the case manager's assessment can be critical.

C. Planning, identifying, and solving problems
   1. Case managers in workers' compensation have the special task of recognizing the problems that have resulted from an on-the-job injury. The payer cannot address other health concerns and social problems unless these have a direct impact on the patient's recovery from injuries.
   2. Workers' compensation laws actually proscribe offering benefits for nonrelated care and activity. Case managers can direct injured workers and their families to appropriate agencies and services.
   3. Plans for addressing related problems are written and provided to appropriate parties.

D. Coordinating multiple health care providers
   1. In the current workers' compensation atmosphere, there are likely to be a number of health care providers involved.
   2. Recognition of state laws governing selection of care providers, including the use of MCOs, is essential.
   3. Highly developed communication skills are involved in monitoring health care progress, making recommendations based on it, and then assisting the injured worker in receiving the most effective care available.

E. Utilization review activities
   1. Because workers' compensation laws regulate health care service selection and utilization, the case manager must practice these activities within that framework.
   2. The workers' compensation system now contains utilization review (UR) companies and MCOs used by insurance companies, large employers, and self-insureds. Case managers from these settings often have the responsibility of coordinating UR activities with the cost-containment companies.

F. Precertification, preauthorization activities
   1. In the workers' compensation mosaic of state laws, preauthorization and precertification of procedures, services, and equipment can be mandatory, allowed, or forbidden. Therefore, it is necessary that the case manager be knowledgeable about the requirement in the state with jurisdiction for the claim.
   2. MCOs and other cost-containment companies often have the responsibility for the processes in states with an allowance or requirement for them.
   3. Because providers of health services and equipment are accustomed to securing preauthorization, a workers' compensation case manager is often requested to make decisions on authorization.
   4. The basic premise in all of workers' compensation health care allowance is that payment will be made for services that are "reasonable and necessary" to treat work-related injuries. The case manager is of-

ten called on to evaluate the reasonableness and necessity of various health care providers' services and charges.

G. Negotiation and contracting

1. The payment structure in workers' compensation in almost all states is based on a fee schedule or an acceptance of "usual and customary" costs listed in data bases. The case manager must be aware of allowable charges before negotiating prices with health care providers or risk negotiating at higher costs.

2. Some services or equipment that are seen infrequently in dealing with injured workers are considered "off-record" and not on fee schedules or in data bases. These items need to be negotiated on a case-by-case basis or through the use of PPOs.

3. Establishing a network of providers is part of most case managers' responsibilities, whether on a formal or informal basis. When provider selection is allowed by the payer, there is an increasing trend toward using established workers' compensation PPOs for both health care services and equipment. Some of the largest of these PPOs are:

   a. FOCUS
   b. MEDVIEW/CNA
   c. HOMELINK

4. When there is no statutory guidance for regulating charges and the selection of health care providers is strictly the injured worker's choice, there is often little incentive for the providers to negotiate for reduced cost or utilization.

H. Reporting

1. The great majority of case management services in the workers' compensation field are performed at the request of the payer in the system (insurance company, TPA, employer), and reporting needs to be concise and clear.

2. Reporting of all assessment, planning, intervention, and outcome activities documents the worth of the case management services and the usefulness of maintaining these services when appropriate (Box 11–1)

3. All case management reports are part of legal records. In the workers' compensation arena, there is a likelihood that case management reports will appear in litigated cases.

■ **FREQUENTLY ENCOUNTERED REQUIREMENTS FOR WORKERS' COMPENSATION CASE MANAGERS**

A. A degree or registration in a health care–related field with a strong clinical background

B. National case management certification (a number of certification programs are considered acceptable)

C. Background in emergency care, occupational health, rehabilitation, or orthopedics

CASE STUDY ONE

ASSESSMENT

Mr. M is a 45-year-old Hispanic man who has immigrated from his native Mexico. He lives in one Northeastern state and works in another state some distance from his home. His employer (a food preparation plant) provides transportation to and from work, but otherwise Mr. M relies on public transportation. Mr. M's family remains in Mexico, but some extended family members live and work with him. Mr. M was injured at work when he accidentally got his nondominant hand stuck in a machine, causing a crush injury, fracturing fingers and producing a degloving of the hand. A degloving injury is one in which the skin and other tissue is peeled away from the hand and fingers. The injured worker had already had surgeries, spent 3 days in the hospital, and was discharged before the first report of injury was made to the workers' compensation insurance company.

PLAN

Because the injured worker had been sent to his home and already had a treatment team and treatment plan established before referral, the case manager assigned had to backtrack to get the information and then assess the feasibility of that plan. Using an interpreter, the case manager found the injured worker's support system somewhat unstable, and the fact he was treated near his workplace, which was at a distance from his home, complicated arranging treatment options. The case manager found a hand therapist whose credentials met the hand surgeon's criteria, located near the injured worker's home and on a bus line. The case manager established that Mr. M had a friend who could provide transportation to and from the physician's office for periodic visits. The friend was also able to interpret for the injured worker. The case manager visited with the employer, who was anxious about his worker, eager to provide assistance, and motivated to bring him back for modified work.

COORDINATING AND IMPLEMENTING

This case was managed by the collaborative efforts of internal and external case managers. Costs were kept in check by meeting the injured worker at selected physician appointments and using telephonic case management techniques otherwise. Each physician visit was coordinated for the injured worker. When it was noted that the friend interpreting for Mr. M was failing to understand and explain some of the medical concerns, a bilingual health professional was provided for that task. The case manager obtained information about the essential functions of the modified job from the employer and a commitment to allow the injured worker to return as soon as possible. The physician approved of the modified job, and the injured worker returned to work 4 months after his injury.

MONITORING, OUTCOMES, AND EVALUATING

Although the injured worker was allowed to return to work, it was necessary to continue case management activities because Mr. M continued therapy with the

CASE STUDY ONE

hand surgeon for almost a year. He had three additional surgeries for tendon repair and scar revision. After each surgery, the case manager reactivated the hand therapy and coordinated a return to work on modified duty. Mr. M complained (through a union attorney!) that working in the cold environment of the food preparation area caused an exacerbation of symptoms; the case manager went to the plant and observed the hand after his shift. She was able to document that there were no external changes noted, and the injured worker was able to wear a glove whenever necessary.

The goals of case management were well met because the injured worker's successful treatment allowed him to regain function to such an extent that his permanent impairment was about a third of the expected rating.

■ MOST COMMON SETTINGS FOR WORKERS' COMPENSATION CASE MANAGERS

A. Insurance companies and workers' compensation carriers

B. TPAs

C. Risk management consulting companies

D. Independent case manager companies
   1. National companies
   2. Small local companies
   3. Individual case managers

E. Employers
   1. Usually large companies with many employees
   2. May be part of complete disability management system
   3. May be done in conjunction with occupational nursing duties

F. Providers
   1. Occupational medicine practices
   2. Orthopedic or other medical practices treating large numbers of workers' compensation patients
   3. Physical medicine and rehabilitation clinics and facilities

G. Government entities
   1. State and local government employees
   2. Large government institutions such as universities and hospitals
   3. State funds
      a. State-funded workers' compensation program that directly competes with insurance companies writing business within the state (e.g., California)
      b. Monopolistic state fund that writes workers' compensation insur-

ance exclusively in a state and does not allow competitive insurance (e.g., North Dakota, Nevada, Ohio) (Douglas, 1994)

4. Federal government
   a. Case management conducted through the U.S. Department of Labor
   b. Case managers usually contracted independent practitioners
   c. Program started in 1994

H. MCOs

■ SCOPE OF MEDICAL MANAGEMENT IN WORKERS' COMPENSATION SETTINGS

A. Referrals for most case management services come from the payor; therefore, the payer decides whether services are required.
   1. Internal case managers are those working directly for the payer.
   2. External case managers are those, generally in independent case management companies, from whom the payer purchases case management services.
   3. Case managers with providers and MCOs derive their income from the payer.

B. At present, medical management services are being performed in three different ways:
   1. Telephonic case management
      a. In workers' compensation, this method of case management restricts the three-point contact (injured worker, employer, physician) to telephone calls, faxes, E-mail, and letters.
      b. This method allows a case manager to oversee a high volume of open cases from a single location, making it a less costly way to apply medical management services.
      c. Effective telephonic case management requires adequate computer software designed for the purpose of monitoring medical procedures, physician appointments, therapy schedules, compliance, and the various complexities of workers' compensation medical management.
      d. Anecdotally, case management activities that are performed only through electronic communication are perceived to be less effective in achieving the same level of positive outcomes for injured workers as other forms of case management, but to date no studies have been performed to verify it.
      e. Relying on telephonic case management for catastrophic and serious work place injures is of limited value.
      f. Case managers doing solely telephonic medical management must be knowledgeable in the case management process and skilled communicators in order to be effective managers and not merely observers and reporters.
   2. On-site case management
      a. The "traditional" method of workers' compensation case manage-

ment in which the injured worker is visited in his home setting for an initial assessment, a workplace visit is made, a job analysis is performed, and most physician appointments are attended by the case manager.

b. On-site case management performed by an external case manager adds to the cost of file handling.

c. Internal case managers usually have too large a caseload to perform on-site case management effectively.

d. Although on-site case management is thought to be effective in producing positive outcomes for injured workers, few studies directly address cost-benefit ratios (Akasbas, Gates, & Galvin, 1992).

e. Case selection is an important component in measuring the benefit of on-site case management. In general, the more potentially expensive the claim might be, the more cost-effective on-site case management can be.

3. Collaborative case management services is an amalgamation of telephonic and on-site activity. It combines techniques of both types of case management to offer appropriate services in the most cost-effective manner.

a. Insurance carriers and large employers manage cases in this manner.

b. The Office of Workers' Compensation for federal employees has been established with Department of Labor nursing staff coordinating case management activities with field nurses. Although other factors are involved, case costs have decreased dramatically as this program grows (Box 11–2).

■ APPLYING THE CASE MANAGEMENT PROCESS

A. Conventional wisdom accepted in the workers' compensation industry is that 10% of injury cases generate 90% of the cost (Douglas, 1994; Akabas, Gates, & Galvin, 1992). Whether that formula is scientifically accurate, a small percentage of workplace injuries consume large amounts of money and attention. These are the cases most frequently referred to medical case managers. The vast majority of referrals are lost time cases.

B. As illustrated in Figure 11–3, a workers' compensation claim can be prolonged and complex. A case management referral can occur at any time in that continuum, and the case management process needs to be adapted to meet the needs of the injured worker and the payor at that level.

C. Because relatively few categories of injury cases are referred for case management, the case management process can be modeled to describe the most common types.

1. Catastrophic and serious injury cases

a. Catastrophic injuries include severe head injuries, spinal cord injuries, severe burns, limb amputation, multiple fractures, and major organ and tissue damage. These cases are the easiest to identify

CASE STUDY TWO

ASSESSMENT

Mr. P is a 47-year-old man working as a clerk in a retail store located in a residential area in a Southern city. He is married and the father of four school-aged children. Mr. P was working with others in the store during the day when the store was robbed. The robber had a gun and, before leaving the store, deliberately aimed the gun at Mr. P and shot him in the lower abdomen. Mr. P was taken to a medical center and was found to have injuries involving the bowel, bone, and nerves; however, the major structures in the pelvis were intact. The insurance carrier was notified within a day and a case manager was assigned; she went to the hospital immediately. Because of the early intervention, the case manager was able to make a thorough assessment and immediately begin a case management plan to provide the family and employer with much-needed support.

PLANNING

The injured worker remained in the hospital for about 2 weeks recovering from wounds and surgeries to repair them. His post-hospital needs were not extensive, and it was decided that he could convalesce at home because his wife did not work outside of the home. Some minor durable medical equipment was needed for safety and comfort. The case manger arranged all outpatient appointments and services. The owners of the retail business were elderly and very troubled by their worker's injuries. They were kept informed and were agreeable to the injured worker returning to work at any level of activity restriction.

COORDINATING AND IMPLEMENTING

Mr. P had four physicians providing care while in the hospital, and all required outpatient follow-up. Because of these multiple providers, it was decided that a physiatrist would be involved to coordinate medical needs. After the specialists completed their treatment, the physiatrist remained as the treating physician.

Mr. P's recovery was complicated by his teen-aged son's extreme reaction to the workplace violence. His behavior was erratic, and his psychotic-like episodes disrupted the family and Mr. P's recovery. Because workers' compensation insurance must specifically address the needs of the injured worker, the case manager found a counselor for Mr. P, and she (the counselor) suggested family counseling as a method of dealing with Mr. P's own post-traumatic issues and his concern for his son. The son's mental health deteriorated, and the family counseling was not adequate to meet his needs. The case manager helped the family identify appropriate community resources, including a local victims' aid fund to help address the son's mental health needs.

Mr. P continued in therapy for several months because of his orthopedic and neurologic injuries. He continued in counseling, and the plan for returning to work became an increasing stressor for him, his family, and his employer. The case manager and the counselor worked on strategies to ease Mr. P back into his regular job. Because there was little physical demand in the job and Mr. P's

continued

CASE STUDY TWO

coworkers volunteered to assist him, there only remained the psychological barriers to returning to work. The injured worker was ultimately successful, and the strategy of working a few hours and being able to leave whenever he felt it necessary appeared to have been the key.

MONITORING, OUTCOME, AND EVALUATION

Most of the case management activities were finished when the injured worker was able to resume full-time employment. Because his physical injuries had healed before his emotional injuries, there were no outstanding medical issues. Mr. P was able to resume most of his preinjury hobbies and duties. The case management goals were met and exceeded as the injured worker returned to full duties and had little residual physical or psychological impairment. The aftermath of workplace violence, however, was not as smooth. The injured worker's family had a difficult time in regaining its equilibrium, the son was hospitalized for a time, and the family's functioning was troubled. Preinjury issues (such as possible abusive episodes) were identified. Mr. P's employer also began to have serious health problems, and he and his wife sold their business within a year of the episode.

---

and are usually referred to case management services soon after notice of the injury is received.

b. Each referral source might have a different definition of what kinds of injuries are deemed serious, such as potential high-dollar loss or potential for severe impairment.

c. Goals for case management are to ensure high-quality, effective medical care for the injured worker while containing costs and attempting to limit impairment.

2. Case management process model—catastrophic and serious cases

  a. Assessment

    (i) Begin the assessment immediately after the referral is received. Discuss expectations for case management with the referral source.

    (ii) Identify and contact the facility case manager or discharge planner and establish credentials and responsibility.

    (iii) Determine the nature and extent of the injuries, current treatment plan, and prognosis.

      (a) Review the chart and all medical records available.

      (b) Speak to physicians and other caregivers to understand the patient's current status.

      (c) Interview the injured worker and family members.

        (i) Determine the understanding of injuries, prognosis and treatment.

        (ii) Identify the strength of the patient's support system.

(iii) Identify any critical needs (such as lodging, child care).

(iv) The home environment is assessed by establishing where the injured worker lives, with whom, the structure (in case home modification is contemplated), and any safety concerns.

(v) Question the availability of transportation for outpatient visits when appropriate.

(iv) Contact the employer to identify any source of support by employer and coworkers, including options for the patient's return to work. During this contact, a rapport is developed with the employer that will be maintained throughout the case management process.

b. Analyzing and planning

(i) Determine whether the current setting is appropriate for the injured worker's medical needs and its accessibility for family members. (It is not uncommon for an injured worker to be injured at a remote job site or to be transported to a facility that is a distance from family members.)

(ii) After assessment of the diagnosis and treatment plan and monitoring of medical progress, formulate the expected time frame before discharge.

(iii) Establish whether the injured worker can be dismissed directly to home or will need to be admitted to another facility for a different level of care.

(a) Knowledge of home environment and support system is critical in making determination on level of care.

(b) Cost of home care versus institutional care is a strong factor. If the injured worker needs multiple health care services or is unable to safely perform activities of daily living, these needs can often be met more economically at a subacute or skilled nursing facility.

(iv) The case management plan reflects knowledge of the concurrent plans of medical providers, family members, and facility case manager. The case management plan deals with health care needs and optimum recovery of function expected, including a return to work.

c. Implementing and coordinating

(i) The facility discharge planner is made aware of PPOs, special contracts, and other cost-containment issues at the outset in states where this is allowed.

(ii) If there are not PPOs or other contracts in place, the case maager seeks out appropriate providers for needed services and negotiates the best service at the best price with each of them.

(iii) The case management plan is shared with the injured worker, family, claims handler, employer, medical providers, and hospital discharge planner. The plan is then adjusted until agreement on the plan is reached.

(iv) Coordination with the facility discharge planner is necessary to set up transportation needs, home care providers, durable medical equipment providers, and outpatient appointments for follow-up care.

(v) When the injured worker is not ready for discharge to home, coordination with the discharging and the admitting facilities is the workers' compensation case manager's responsibility.

(vi) When needs are identified that seem to be outside the scope of workers' compensation coverage, the claims handler is consulted. If it is determined that concurrent medical or social service needs do not arise from the injury and do not significantly impact recovery from injuries, the injured worker or the family and the facility discharge planner are informed. The workers' compensation case manager can provide limited assistance in referring the injured worker and his family to appropriate providers and agencies.

d. Monitoring, evaluating, and reporting of outcomes

(i) The case manager receives and reviews reports from all health care providers.

(ii) If the injured worker is treated in a rehabilitation or other extended stay facility, the case manager attends team conferences.

(iii) The case manager maintains contact with the injured worker and family through telephone calls and visits.

(iv) Physician visits are monitored either by attending appointments when treatment decisions are anticipated or through telephonic management procedures.

(v) Medical services are evaluated, coordinated, and changed to meet the goals of recovery of health and function.

(vi) The injured worker's recovery is usually monitored until he or she is stated to be at MMI.

(vii) Assistance is made to return to regular or modified work whenever possible. When a work-related injury results in permanent disability, with ongoing needs for medical care and equipment, the case management plan often includes a life care plan and recommendation for case manager involvement.

3. Prolonged treatment, multiple providers, overuse of service cases

a. These cases are referred for case management often out of the frustration of the injured worker, the claims handler, or the employer over a lack of case resolution. The case manager is likely to receive this referral later in the claims process.

b. This category of cases might include:

(i) Prolonged treatment for an injury with unrelated complications

(ii) Development of complex injury sequela such as regional causalgia (formerly identified as reflex sympathetic dystrophy [RSD]), chronic pain, fibromyalgia, or chronic myofascial syndrome

(iii) Longer-than-expected recovery from injuries without known complications

(iv) Prolonged disability from a minor injury with insufficient medical causation

(v) Inability to communicate successfully with medical providers or a noted lack of clear diagnosis, treatment plan, or work status

(vi) Multiple treatments with physical therapy, chiropractor, and other practitioners without documented progress

c. Claims-handling issues or litigation may be involved or imminent.

d. The goals for case management are to determine appropriate and effective medical care, coordinate timely delivery of that care, communicate goals to all stakeholders, and assist in the patient's return to work when possible.

4. Injury claims with known barriers to recovery and rehabilitation, "red flag" cases

a. Claims adjusters recognize that some injured workers have innate or acquired barriers to achieving optimum recovery from injuries and rehabilitation, and refer them to case management.

(i) Injured workers with concurrent disability or disease that may or may not be associated with a work-related incident.

(ii) Injured workers who do not speak or understand English will have difficulty understanding and complying with medical regimens.

(iii) Injured workers with a perceived lack of incentive to comply with medical treatment and return to work.

(iv) Goals for case management are to address specified problems, identify achievable solutions for problems, coordinate medical care that will help the injured worker recover from injuries, and assist in the patient's return to work.

5. Case management process model—prolonged treatment with complications and complicating factors

a. Assessment

(i) Discuss case management expectations with the referral source.

(ii) Review the claim file thoroughly.

(a) Understand the mechanism and causation of injury.

(b) Review all medical bills and find matching medical reports.

(c) Determine the treating physician or other practitioner (such as chiropractor) who is directing care.

(d) List all health care providers since the injury.

(e) Identify what medical records are needed to complete a medical record review.

(iii) Interview the employer to gather his or her understanding of injury, treatment, and barriers that are preventing the injured worker from returning to work. Determine the availability of modified work to address activity restrictions.

(iv) Interview the injured worker and the family. If the worker is represented by an attorney, permission is sought from the attorney before directly contacting the injured worker or the family. If the worker is represented and contact allowed, the interview might be scheduled in the attorney's office or in other controlled surroundings.

    (a) Determine the injured worker's understanding of the injury; any diagnoses, treatment including medication, barriers to a return to work; and additional treatment that he or she feels might be helpful.

    (b) Determine whether language or culture is a barrier to understanding medical treatment and the return-to-work process.

    (c) Ask about concurrent medical problems, family dynamics, the home environment, and the potential for job placement if necessary.

    (d) Interview the worker and the family to understand whether the prolonged treatment and time off work is meeting some other needs such as caring for children, other family members, or any other financial disincentives to returning to work.

    (e) The injured worker or his or her attorney might not allow all questions to be answered.

b. Planning and analyzing

    (i) The case management plan focuses on the patient's achieving the goals of return to optimum health and recovery of function, including a return to work.

    (ii) Through the detailed review of medical records, the case manager determines the most appropriate provider to achieve these goals.

    (iii) The plan will include suggestions for diagnostic procedures to confirm diagnoses, if appropriate (e.g., if a diagnosis of regional causalgia is suspected, electrodiagnostics, three-phase bone scan, and ganglion blocks are standard procedures in this condition).

c. Implementing and coordinating

    (i) The case management plan is shared with all stakeholders and revised as needed. Examples of workable communication tools for telephone calls and letters can be found in Chapter 7 of *The Case Manager's Handbook* (Mullahy, 1998).

    (ii) Communicate with all medical providers to get the patient's updated records, along with current diagnosis, treatment plan and activity restriction, including restrictions for work.

    (iii) Ideally, the injured worker (and attorney) will cooperate in trying to achieve the goals of optimum recovery of health and function, but should an adverse reaction occur, the claims adjuster will be consulted.

(iv) Selecting the appropriate provider to help in achieving goals can be accomplished with the cooperation of the injured worker by scheduling a second opinion or a change of physician. If an adverse situation exists, an IME will be scheduled with approval from the adjuster.

(v) Communication with the employer continues, and efforts are made to assist the injured worker in his or her return to work.

(vi) Coordination of the delivery of appropriate medical care continues until there is a physician-issued MMI date.

d. Monitoring, evaluating, and reporting of outcomes

(i) Follow up with the injured worker and employer to evaluate success of medical treatment and return to work.

(ii) If a full duty release is anticipated soon after the injured worker has returned to work on modified duty or shortened hours, monitoring of status will continue until that release.

(iii) A report of case management activity and outcomes will be given to the adjuster.

6. Workplace violence, a growing concern, results in physical and psychological injuries that are referred for medical case management.

a. The issue of workplace violence is prominent in the United States, and the number of workers affected is increasing. As reported in *Business Insurance* (1996), violence in the workplace contributes a cost to business of up to $75 billion annually.

(i) There are 15 deaths a week, with homicide being the leading cause for women of occupational deaths and the third leading cause for men.

(ii) There are 3000 assaults each day.

(iii) Fifteen percent of American workers report being a victim of workplace violence.

b. The sources of workplace violence are varied.

(i) Internal conflicts and disruptions such as assaults, fistfights, labor unrest, disgruntled employees, family members, "horseplay," and arson or bomb

(ii) External criminal activity such as aggravated robberies, effect of a fellow worker's homicide, physical assaults outside the workplace (fire personnel, service and delivery employees)

c. The workers' compensation aftermath of workplace violence can be very challenging for the medical manager.

(i) Physical injuries that result from gunshots, stabbings, and beatings are often complex and require multiple providers for treatment.

(ii) Many workplace violence injuries result in some post-traumatic stress symptoms for the injured worker and other personnel.

(iii) The aftereffects of violence complicate the return-to-work process for the injured patient and his or her family, coworkers, and employer.

d. Goals for the case manager are to identify the effects of violence on the injured worker and others; coordinate timely delivery of health care, including psychological support when it is determined to be necessary; and assist in the patient's return to work.

7. Case management process model—violence in the workplace—aftermath

   a. Assessment

      (i) Medical records are reviewed and providers consulted to determine nature and extent of the patient's injuries, treatment plan, and prognosis.

      (ii) Review police and newspaper reports, if available.

      (iii) The injured worker and family are interviewed.

         (a) Determine their understanding of injuries, treatment plan, and prognosis.

         (b) Understand family structure and support system.

         (c) Assess the injured worker's ability to remember and discuss the details of the injury.

         (d) List any preexisting mental and physical health concerns that might affect the patient's recovery from injuries.

         (e) Identify barriers to recovery of health and function, including signs of post-traumatic stress in injured worker or family members, or both.

      (iv) Interview the employer to discuss the events of the injury and determine plans for the patient's return to work.

         (a) Discuss the impact of the patient's injuries on the employer and coworkers.

         (b) Identify the employer's ability to modify the patient's job for return to work, including changes of hours and addressing safety concerns.

   b. Planning and analyzing

      (i) The case management plan focuses on achieving goals of return to optimum health and recovery of function, including a return to work.

      (ii) Determine appropriate health care providers for physical and psychological care.

      (iii) If post-traumatic stress signs are noted to be present, the case management plan includes an opportunity for the injured worker to be evaluated by an appropriate mental health care professional.

      (iv) The case management plan is shared with all stakeholders and modified as needed.

   c. Implementing and coordinating

      (i) Gather medical records.

    (ii) Coordinate all health care provider visits for timely delivery of services.

    (iii) Whenever possible, attend physician appointments that will include decision-making activity with the injured worker.

    (iv) Communicate with the employer.

        (a) Discuss progress of injured worker in return to health and function.

        (b) The employer may identify other workers who are having difficulty coping with the episode of workplace violence. An external case manager can offer services only to an employee who has filed a claim. Therefore, the employer needs to be directed toward other resources such as EAPs (employee assistance programs) for these workers.

        (c) Address concerns in regard to the injured worker's return to work.

    (i) Check on availability for modifications to meet physical restrictions resulting from injuries.

    (ii) Implement plan for modification of job duties, task assignments, hours of work, and other workplace concerns in coordination with mental health recommendations if available.

    (v) Facilitate a return to work by communicating with appropriate health care providers.

  d. Monitoring, evaluating, and reporting of outcomes

    (i) Monitor and review all medical records.

    (ii) Communicate with injured worker, providers, and employer until MMI statement is received and the injured worker has returned to optimum functioning.

    (iii) A report of case management activity and outcomes is given to the adjuster.

8. Workers' compensation referrals to assist in return-to-work activities

  a. Regaining all functional activities by an injured worker is important, but the activity most central to the process is a return to work.

  b. Studies show that only 50% of injured workers return to their jobs after being off for 6 months, 25% after 12 months, and the percentage drops to single digits after 24 months (Douglas, 1994).

  c. The case manager integrates a return to work in all assigned cases for workers' compensation medical management unless instructed to do so otherwise. (Because case managers in employer settings usually have precise guidelines and procedures to follow in assisting a return to work for injured workers, only the role of external case managers is considered here.)

  d. Goals of case management are to assess barriers to return to work; communicate with the employer and educate him or her, if necessary, on the positive effects of returning injured worker to work; address medical concerns that may prevent a return to work; and coordinate the return to work process.

9. Case management process model—return to work referral

a. Assessment
  (i) Discuss case management expectations with referral source.
  (ii) Ascertain whether the assignment includes a need for comprehensive interview with injured worker.
  (iii) Identify any claims-handling issues involved in the failure of the injured worker to return to work.
     (a) Extraneous employment issues
     (b) Plaintiff attorney involvement
  (iii) Review the claim file thoroughly.
     (a) Understand the mechanism and causation of injury.
     (b) Review all medical records to determine what restrictions on activity have been identified.
     (c) Determine treating physician or other practitioner (such as chiropractor) directing care.
     (d) Identify the barriers preventing the injured worker from returning to work.
  (iv) Interview the employer to gather his or her understanding of injury, treatment, and barriers preventing the injured worker from returning to work.
  (v) Communication with the employer includes
     (a) A review of the employer's return-to-work policy
     (b) If no formal policy exists, the case manager will ask about usual practices in allowing an injured worker to return to work before being released for full, unrestricted, duties.
     (c) A discussion about modified or "light" duty
     (d) Any union rules affecting return to work
     (e) An understanding of the injured worker's preinjury position and essential tasks
  (vi) If it is part of the case management assignment, interview the injured worker and the family, if approved by plaintiff attorney of a represented worker.
     (a) Determine understanding of injuries and treatment.
     (b) Identify barriers to returning to work.
b. Planning and analyzing
  (i) The case management plan focuses on barriers to returning to work and possible solutions to these identified problems.
  (ii) The case management plan is shared with all stakeholders and is modified as required.
c. Implementing and coordinating
  (i) The case manager determines whether the treating physician has identified appropriate activity restrictions, and if not, communicates with the physician to determine specific restrictions.
  (ii) The case manager coordinates the medical care identified by the physician as necessary to release the injured worker for work.

(iii) Communication with the employer about the return to work includes:

(a) Education on the positive effect on both the injured worker and the workers' compensation claim process when the worker returns to work as soon as possible (Pimentel, 1995).

(b) An understanding of modifying usual job duties to meet activity restrictions as stated by the treating physician.

(c) Discussion of short-term employment in another job for the employer to meet the stated activity restrictions.

(d) Referral to a claims adjuster to discuss partial temporary payments (PTDs) if wages or hours are less than usual wage.

(iv) The case manager derives from communication with the employer an understanding of the physical activity involved to do the injured worker's usual job.

(a) A job description is requested from the employer.

(b) If no job description is available or if the physical requirements of the job are not detailed, the case manager may opt to conduct a job analysis that will provide the treating physician with a clear idea of the physical abilities necessary to return the injured worker to his or her usual job.

(c) Information included on a job analysis includes (Douglas, 1994):

(i) Job title

(ii) Tools, machines and equipment used regularly

(iii) The usual work cycle and number of hours worked weekly

(iv) Specific essential physical demands regarding lifting (including amount lifted in pounds), bending, reaching, crawling, climbing, and kneeling

(v) Hours typically spent sitting, standing, and walking

(vi) The frequency each essential function occurs in a work day

(vii) Repetitive activity, including physical action and duration of activity in a work shift

(viii) Environment (temperature, air quality, uneven surfaces for walking)

(ix) Return-to-work options and modifications available

(v) The case manager will recommend using the services of an ergonomic specialist for job analysis and activity recommendations if the physical demands are particularly complex or the return-to-work issues are critical in the claim-handling process.

(vi) The case manager will communicate with the treating physician and present the completed job analysis for review.

(vii) If a clear diagnosis is present, appropriate treatment has been rendered, and all barriers for recovery of health and function have been addressed, but the injured worker has not been released for work, the case management plan will include a request for a Functional Capacity Evaluation (FCE). This evaluation objectively identifies the injured worker's current level of functioning and provides the physician objective testing to assist in determining activity restrictions and possible impairment.

(viii) When all activity fails to return the injured worker to work, a referral to vocational rehabilitation may be made in accordance with individual state laws. The case manager's involvement with vocational rehabilitation will be directed by paying source.

d. Monitoring, evaluating, and reporting of outcomes

    (i) Follow up with the injured worker and employer to evaluate the success of medical treatment and return to work.

    (ii) If a full duty release is anticipated soon after the injured worker has returned to work on modified duty or shortened hours, monitoring of status will continue until that release.

    (iii) Vocational rehabilitation is monitored if requested.

    (iv) A report of case management activity and outcomes will be given to the adjuster.

10. Cases assigned to a case manager for scheduling IMEs and second opinions

a. An IME is a frequently used tool to resolve medical issues and questions in a workers' compensation claim (Douglas, 1994).

b. As previously discussed, the frequency and number of IMEs and the practitioner used may be regulated by state workers' compensation laws.

c. Whether the case manager is arranging an IME as a specific task or whether it is part of an ongoing management file, general guidelines are as follows:

    (i) IMEs are often a claims-handling maneuver and are coordinated with the claims adjuster or manager to ensure that appropriate goals are set and met.

    (ii) Because an IME can be viewed as an adversarial action, a careful explanation of the reasons for scheduling the evaluation is made to the injured worker if direct communication is allowed.

    (iii) The selection of the practitioner to do the evaluation is key to the outcome.

    (iv) The physician selected (or other practitioner required) will be well qualified and credentialed, usually with board certification in the specialty.

    (v) Many physicians do not perform IMEs, and the ones who do perform them as part of their practices generally have specific guidelines and requirements that must be followed.

(vi) The claims adjuster may have input into selection as part of the overall claim-handling process.

(vii) The communication between stakeholders is vital both for the success of resolving medical questions and as a legal responsibility of the case manager.

(viii) It is essential both as a process component and a legal responsibility that the case manager get all accumulated medical records, including x-ray studies, to the independent examiner for review.

    d. The final case manager task following an IME is to secure a report and provide it to the claim adjuster for distribution.

■ ETHICAL AND LEGAL CONSIDERATIONS FOR WORKERS' COMPENSATION CASE MANAGERS

A. Case managers have the responsibility of developing a personal code of ethics, promoting ethical standards in the workplace, and establishing ethical standards in their profession.

B. Case managers apply ethical standards to their practice.

C. Legal issues in workers' compensation claims challenge both the practice and the professionalism of case managers.

■ CASE MANAGERS ARE GUIDED BY ETHICAL PRINCIPLES (CASE MANAGEMENT SOCIETY OF AMERICA [CMSA], 1995)

A. General ethical principles as defined by a number of ethicists are
    1. Patient advocacy
    2. Beneficence versus maleficence (strive to do good, but do not do harm)
    3. Justice
    4. Truthfulness

B. Individual case managers develop their own personal ethical guidelines by study and research and have a responsibility to assist others in the profession in establishing ethical standards in the workplace and for the profession as a whole (CMSA, 1995).

■ APPLYING ETHICAL PRINCIPLES TO CASE MANAGEMENT

A. Case managers in any practice find themselves in daily struggles to address patients' rights while fulfilling responsibilities for which they are paid (Mullahy, 1998).

B. Case managers involved in workers' compensation claims practice in an inherently difficult area because there are many stakeholders, often with sharply competing interests.

C. The case manager in workers' compensation establishes and communicates ethical standards that guide the practice.

D. Patient advocacy:

1. Goals for advocating for an injured worker include recommending and coordinating the most effective medical care to treat injuries that will lead to an optimum recovery of function.

2. The principle of promoting patient autonomy is tempered by state laws and claims considerations. However, the case manager communicates to the injured worker rights and responsibilities of all concerned in the coordination and delivery of medical care.

3. It is imperative that the case manager inform the injured worker when the payer is providing the services and clearly define the expectations of the payer for activity and reporting.

E. Striving for promoting good and preventing harm in workers' compensation case management:

1. Medical management in workers' compensation system is based on promoting good medical care for the injured worker, working within the laws of the state.

2. A positive outcome for the injured worker in achieving maximum medical improvement and a return to the highest possible level of function, including work, is an application of the principle (Purtillo, 1998).

F. Justice:

1. This area is one with the most potential ethical dilemmas for a worker's compensation case manager.

2. The entire workers' compensation system came about as a result of unfair treatment of an injured worker, and one of the established goals of the present-day system is to provide a safer workplace.

3. The injured worker has the right to expect confidentiality in the handling of medical records and other personal information; however, workers' compensation laws give access to the records to a number of stakeholders. The use of electronic mail and other Internet communication is opening new areas of concern (Putillo, 1998).

4. As noted earlier, the cost of workers' compensation is borne by the employer and by society as a whole in the price of goods and services. Taxes are used to provide workers' compensation coverage to local, state, and federal government employees. Overuse or abuse of the system by any participant does an injustice to all members of society.

5. Some examples of conflict in the application of the principle of justice are:

   a. The injured worker has an agenda that does not include recovering from his or her injuries and returning to work.

   b. The employer's dealings with the injured worker are not consistent with either the letter or the spirit of employment laws.

   c. The claims handler fails to inform the injured worker of pertinent facts and rights that might affect the outcome of his or her injury claim.

   d. The case manager consistently overbills or prolongs medical management of a claim unnecessarily.

G. Truth:
   1. Telling the truth is the underlying principle for the case manager to gain trust and, therefore, cooperation from the injured worker, the employer, the adjuster, and all medical providers (Mullahy, 1998).
   2. Telling the truth is the basis for the case manager to be a patient advocate for the injured worker in a system that has many competing interests.
   3. Truthfulness is necessary when medical records are presented to a medical provider for review so that all interests are represented fairly.

■ LEGAL ISSUES FOR THE WORKERS' COMPENSATION CASE MANAGER

A. The case manager's role, while primarily medically focused, is linked to the legal issues in a claim.
   1. The case manager has the responsibility of knowing and following state laws dictating medical care providers in a workers' compensation claim.
   2. The case manager cannot contact an injured worker directly when he or she is represented by an attorney without permission and needs to abide by the instructions of the plaintiff attorney in matters concerning communication with the injured worker.
   3. Laws in some states restrict the flow of information between medical providers and the case manager.
   4. Failure to adhere to laws can result in penalties against the payer with substantial fines.

B. The case manager is legally accountable to practice case management within the scope of her or his professional license.
   1. The case manager has the responsibility of knowing about applicable laws dealing with workers' compensation practice, and to fail to do so falls below professional standards (CMSA, 1995).
   2. Case law is developing that increases the case manager's accountability for referrals to health care providers when an unanticipated negative event occurs (Guido, 1997).
   3. The case manager has a responsibility to report accurately on case management activity and provide the report to appropriate parties.

■ TRENDS IN WORKERS' COMPENSATION CASE MANAGEMENT

A. The effort to contain costs in workers' compensation claims continues to promote innovative programs.

B. Federal legislation in the 1990s has impacted case management practice.

C. Outcome-driven quality assessment is a tool for case management practices.

■ COST-CONTAINMENT PROGRAMS

A. Managed care companies
  1. A number of state legislatures are considering application of additional managed care principles to their workers' compensation systems.
  2. Managed care companies are forming to meet current and anticipated needs in the various states.
  3. Case management is a vital part of all managed care legislation.

B. Early intervention by case managers
  1. Historically, claims by injured workers (except for catastrophic or serious cases) have been referred to case management after the worker fails to respond to medical treatment or is unable to return to work.
  2. Today, the trend is to allow both internal and external case managers to become involved soon after the injury is reported (Chan, 1999).

C. Twenty-four-hour coverage
  1. The concept of 24-hour coverage by combined health and workers' compensation insurance or for self-insured employers has long been considered. The basic premise is that health insurance would cover all injuries and illnesses to American workers without regard to causation. Therefore, the resources spent in investigating causation and related health care needs would be saved.
  2. Although pilot programs have been tested in several states and by major employers, there is no clear consensus on its applicability for larger populations or how the issue of indemnity is addressed.

■ RELATING WORKERS' COMPENSATION CASE MANAGEMENT TO 1990S FEDERAL LEGISLATION (PIMENTEL, 1995)

A. The American with Disabilities Act (ADA)
  1. The act went into effect on July 26, 1992.
  2. The intent was to prohibit employers from discrimination against qualified individuals with a disability in many areas of employment.
  3. Nearly 3 years after the law was enforced, the Equal Employment Opportunities Commission reported that 85% of charges received involved existing employees, many of whom reported work-related impairment.
  4. Case managers involved in any part of return-to-work activities of an injured worker are responsible for knowing the basic tenets of ADA.
  5. The case manager does not give legal advice concerning protection of injured workers' rights in respect to the ADA, but refers the employer to his or her employment attorney for that advice.

B. The Family Medical Leave Act (FMLA)
  1. This act was signed into law in 1993.
  2. The intent of the act is to provide employees with an option to take up to 12 weeks of unpaid leave for a serious illness of the worker or a family member with job restoration (or equivalent) guaranteed.

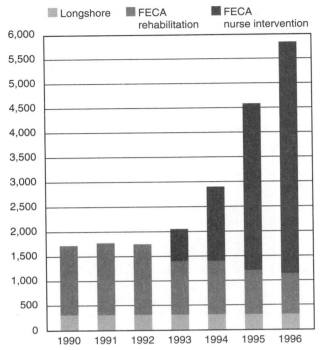

FIGURE 11–4   OWCP vocational rehabilitation programs return people to work. (Source: U. S. Dept. of Labor Office of Workers' Compensation Programs Annual Report 1996.)

3. Most workers' compensation claimants are eligible for FMLA as a result of their work-related injury.
4. Employees are not obligated to return to work on modified or "light duty" when claiming benefits under the FMLA.
5. Although an injured worker might not be eligible for indemnity payments if he or she does not return to work while claiming FMLA ben-

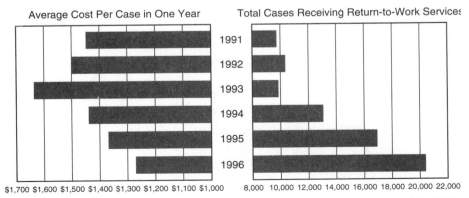

FIGURE 11–5   Federal Employees' Compensation Act return-to-work costs. (FY 1991–FY1996).

efits, he or she cannot be dismissed from employment during the 12 weeks.

■ DOCUMENTING QUALITY OF SERVICES BY OUTCOME MEASUREMENTS

A. For legal and ethical protection, the case manager will make referrals to health care providers who offer outcome measurements as proof of their competency.

B. Case managers document the success of their interventions by the outcomes they achieve.

1. Although there is a great deal of anecdotal evidence of the benefit of case management in the workers' compensation system, there are few objective data to confirm it (Akabas, Gates, & Galvin, 1992).

2. There is not yet general agreement on what data are measured and what measurements are needed to make comprehensive statements about positive outcomes.

3. It is estimated that case management activities toward the return-to-work process can reduce the cost of a claim by 50% (Pimentel, 1995).

4. A model for reporting outcomes is presented by the Office of Workers' Compensation Programs in its annual report to Congress (U.S. Department of Labor, 1996); this illustrates the value of workers' compensation case management. As previously noted, the case management program was inserted into a system already established to meet the goals of returning injured workers to their jobs. The dramatic changes in both returning injured workers to preinjury productivity and case cost savings can be attributed to the efforts of case managers (Figs. 11–4 and 11–5).

REFERENCES

Akabas, S., Gates, L., & Galvin, D. (1992). *Disability management.* New York: American Management Association.

Case Management Society of America (CMSA) (1995). *Standards of practice.* Little Rock, AR: CMSA.

Chan, F., et al. (1999). Foundation knowledge and major practice domains of case management. *The Journal of Care Management, 5*(1),10–28.

Douglas, J. (1994). *Managing workers' compensation.* New York: John Wiley and Sons.

Guido, G.W. (1997). *Legal issues in nursing.* Stamford, CT: Appleton & Lange.

Mullahy, C. (1998). *The case manager's handbook.* Gaithersburg, MD: Aspen Publications.

Pimentel, R. (1995). *The return to work process.* Chatsworth, CA: Milt Wright & Associates.

Purtilo, R. (1998). Rethinking the ethics of confidentiality and health care teams. *Bioethics Forum 14,* 3(4), 29–37.

Staff. (1996). Steps to stem workplace violence. *Business Insurance, 30,* 51.

Stoddard, S., et al. (1998). *Chartbook on work and disability in the United States.* Washington, DC: Institute on Disability Rehabilitation Research.

Survey of workers' compensation laws (1999). Downers Grove, IL: Alliance of American Insurance.

United States Chamber of Commerce (1997). *Analysis of workers' compensation laws.* Washington, D.C.: U.S. Chamber of Commerce.

United States Department of Labor, Office of Workers' Compensation Programs (1992, 1996). *Annual report to Congress.* Washington, D.C.: United States Department of Labor.

CHAPTER 12

• • • • • • • • • • • • • • •

Disability Case Management

LESLEY WRIGHT

MARTHA HEATH EGGLESTON

DEBORAH V. DiBENEDETTO

LEARNING OBJECTIVES

Upon completion of this chapter, the reader will be able to:

1. Describe the history of the disability management movement.
2. Define important terms and concepts relating to disability management.
3. List the driving forces that led to disability management programs.
4. Discuss important components to building a successful disability management program.
5. Describe factors that are important in the development and design of a disability management program.
6. Identify the stages of the case management and disability process.

IMPORTANT TERMS AND CONCEPTS

Alternate Dispute Resolution Program
Americans with Disabilities Act (ADA)
Bargaining Unit
Claims Administrator
Continuity of Care
Disability Management
Ergonomics
Early Intervention

Elimination Period
Employee Assistance Program (EAP)
Family Medical Leave Act (FMLA)
In-House Case Management
Integrated Disability Management
Integrated Benefits
Labor Code
Line Management

Long-Term Disability	Temporary Total Disability
Managed Care	Third-Party Administrators (TPA)
Modified Duty Team	Time Loss Management
Occupational Injury Versus	Transitional Work Duty
Nonoccupational Injury	Treating Physician, Primary Care
Permanent Partial Disability	Provider, and Attending Physician
Productivity Experts	24-Hour Program
Risk Management	Vocational Rehabilitation
Return-to-Work Program	Wellness Program
Short-Term Disability	Workers' Compensation

■ INTRODUCTION AND HISTORY OF THE DISABILITY MANAGEMENT MOVEMENT

A. History of the disability movement

  1. Early America

    a. In early America, the settler's primary goal was one of survival. "Laws in the Thirteen Colonies excluded settlers who could not demonstrate an ability to support themselves independently. Immigration policy forbade people with physical, mental, or emotional disabilities to enter the country" (United States Commission on Civil Rights, p. 18)

  2. Nineteenth-century America

    a. The advancement of financial assistance from state governments occurred in the 19th century with virtually no support from the federal government.

    b. The 19th century was a time of humanitarian religious influence that stressed the need for the successful to assist the unfortunate.

  3. Post–Civil War era

    a. The United States was moving from an agricultural society to a country focusing on industry and manufacturing.

    b. Eugenics, "the science which deals with all influences that improve inborn qualities of a race," as described by the theorist Sir Francis Galton, began during this period. The growing interest in this theory provides insight into the climate of "genetically perfect" members of society.

  4. World War II

    a. After the devastating factors resulting from the Great Depression, World War II had an incredible effect on the economy, industry, and growth. This explosive movement created a demand for workers. Because these workers comprised women and disabled and retired individuals, the rehabilitation movement significantly changed.

    b. The Vocational Rehabilitation Act Amendments of 1954: Public Law 565 was enacted after President Eisenhower recognized the contributions made during wartime by persons with disabilities.

This law provided for vocational rehabilitation for persons with a disability. The legislation increased the federal share of the funding of the federal–state vocational rehabilitation programs from 50% to 3 federal dollars for every 2 state dollars.

5. Vietnam era to present
   a. By the 1970s society's scholars were beginning to question the rationale in the continuation of the heavily funded vocational rehabilitation programs in an era of marked unemployment.
   b. The Vietnam War resulted in a staggering number of disabled soldiers being released to the civilian work force. This created more of a need for vocational rehabilitation.
   c. Employers have been providing health care benefits and compensation for work-related injuries with no real coordination of benefits. Employees may receive varying degrees of medical treatment based on the reimbursement schedule.

B. Influence of the rehabilitation process and concepts
   1. Caseload management is a systematic process merging counseling and managerial concepts and skills through the application of techniques from intuitive and researched methods, thereby advancing efficient and effective decision-making for functional control of self, client, setting, and other relevant related factors for anchoring a proactive practice.
   2. Essentials of managing case flow are the ability to maintain a relationship with an individual and assist with the medical issues, as well as vocational and personal aspects of a case. The case manager has the ability to analyze and understand occupational and industrial trends, as well as legislation relative to disability program.
   3. The vocational rehabilitation process from the case manager's perspective includes planning, organizing, directing, coordinating, implementing, and controlling.

■ KEY DEFINITIONS

A. Disability management is the process of managing occupational and nonoccupational illnesses and disease.

B. Integrated benefits is the integration of short-term disability (STD) and long-term disability (LTD), workers' compensation, group health, and other related benefits under a single medical management plan whose focus is providing quality, timely, and cost-effective medical care, and successful return to work and productivity.

   This model provides the basis for managing a person's occupational (work-related) and nonoccupational (off-the-job) health and productivity.

   Owing to disparate benefit programs and information management systems, the marketplace provides for several variations of integrated benefits. This includes integrated disability management.

C. Integrated disability management is the coordinated management of STD and LTD. In some limited situations, it may also include the coordinated management of workers' compensation along with STD and LTD claims.

D. The return to health and productivity model is the driving force of integrated disability management. Without effective and efficient methods to return the patient to work, the integrated process cannot succeed.

E. Integrated disability management combines the management of STD, LTD, WC, and when feasible, group health benefit programs by streamlining handling of claim reporting, administration, medical management, and return-to-work activities.

F. Disability management focuses on returning the injured or ill employee to productive work. This process uses transitional work or modified work programs and assignments that are developed by interdisciplinary teams, which generally include risk management, human resources, operations and line management, occupational health, safety and health promotion, labor, and case management professionals.

This team develops, coordinates, and supervises modified and transitional work assignments for individuals with temporary disabilities regardless of cause (occupational or nonoccupational).

Some companies may use transitional work in compliance with the Americans with Disabilities Act (ADA) for persons with permanent disabilities or permanent limitations, regardless of their causation.

G. Transitional work assignments can be identified by trained vocational counselors; medical, occupational, or physical therapists; and human resource professionals. Transitional work may accommodate an individual's temporary or permanent disability, thus allowing that individual to re-enter and successfully manage productive employment.

H. Disability management relies on transitional work assignment programs that are modified work assignments identified by qualified professionals to facilitate effective return to work for the temporarily disabled worker.

The return-to-work model is the cornerstone of the disability management program. Case managers should seek to develop a job bank of all typical, modified, and transitional work assignments that an employer manages. This job bank is then a resource for available work assignments and can be used to facilitate an injured worker's successful re-entry into the employer's work setting.

Proactive education of the employee in the organization's total benefits program can promote employee morale; reduce lost time, malingering, litigated costs, and training and production costs; and foster a supportive work environment.

Benefit programs, commonly referred to as 24-hour care, combine traditional group health, workers' compensation programs, and STD and LTD disability programs, while being mindful of each state's statutes and laws, federal regulations, and indemnity benefits.

I. The Disability Management Employers Coalition Inc. (DMEC), a national organization that focuses on education and training employers, promotes an integrated approach to disability and health management by a controlled approach to providing benefits regardless of the origin. DMEC recognized that many large employers already provided health, disability, and life insurance benefits to their employees and realized that an integrated approach meant combining the existing coverage to create the same benefits. Therefore, the process of providing medical care, lost time income, and permanent disability compensation to anyone who was injured simplified the benefits program package.

In association with the Insurance Educational Association (IEA), DMEC developed the Certified Professional in Disability Management (CPDM) Program, training industry-specific personnel in the integrated process. The DMEC advocates two types of case managers—the administrative case manager and the clinical case manager.

■ IMPORTANT TERMS AND CONCEPTS

A. Disability management—What is it?

1. Disability management is the process of limiting a disabling event, providing immediate intervention once an injury or illness occurs, and returning the patient to work in a timely manner.

B. Disability management program

1. A program with a primary mission to reduce the financial costs associated with all disabilities, while fostering an open, honest, nonadversarial environment of claims administration through the development of a coordinated disability management program with the focus on ability rather than disability.

   a. Services included in a disability management program are coordinated access to all employer-provided benefit plans and services that impact on the disability, including workers' compensation, health care, sick leave, state disability, STD and LTD, salary continuation, pension and retirement plans, union plans, medical leaves of absence, and Social Security Disability.

   b. Internal departments that typically have responsibility for the design and administration of one or more programs, or play a key role in the process, are human resources, risk management, occupational health, safety finance, legal, bargaining units, and operations.

   c. External sources or departments that may be involved are the workers' compensation carrier, health care provider, third party administrators, life insurance carriers, reinsurers, disability carriers, and managed care providers.

C. Cost-of-disability survey

Employers may spend up to 17% of payroll on the total cost of disability to their corporation (DiBenedetto, 1998) (see Chapter 13, Occupational Health Case Management).

A cost-of-disability survey must be made, because without this information it is impossible to determine the extent of potential savings to the organization.

1. When preparing a cost-of-disability survey, an organization should identify all direct and indirect costs associated with the employer's disability programs. Direct costs include:

   a. Workers' compensation indemnity payments

    b. Extended sick leave and salary continuation

    c. STD and LTD payments

    d. Medical costs for a condition that would require wage replacement

    e. Pension and retirement benefits paid under a disability clause

    f. Life insurance benefits under a premium waiver

    g. Life insurance benefits under an accelerated death benefit

    h. Benefits paid pursuant to a disability clause in a union contract

    i. Other costs to be considered include those indirectly associated with the cost of disability and lost time, including overtime payments, lost employee productivity, broken equipment, related training, and the cost of replacement or temporary workers.

■ DRIVING FORCES THAT LED TO DISABILITY MANAGEMENT PROGRAMS

Several factors, including financial, administrative, and clinical, led to the development of the integrated disability management program and integrated delivery systems.

A. The rising costs of medical care, lost time, and litigation are just a few of the financial concerns that gave rise to solutions such as managed care, integrated delivery systems, and capitated costs. Employers, particularly self-insured employers, sought the benefit of integration from the delivery aspect, and in turn sought to blend the administration and management of these costs.

B. The costs of workers' compensation and LTD were escalating and adding to loss of production and loss of time. Although the initial treatment for work-related injuries was traditionally aggressive, dollars were lost because temporarily or permanently injured workers were not brought back to work in a timely fashion. There was a severe lack of modified or transitional duty jobs available for displaced workers. Ultimately, workers were less likely to return, further increasing both hard and soft dollar costs.

    The development of a good return-to-work program and a supportive work environment ultimately led to increased success rates in return-to-work activity and work production.

    This process then was sought for nonoccupational injuries. If the benefits derived from in-house rehabilitation, transitional work, and modified job duties were seen in patients with occupational injuries, why were they not used for those individuals who had suffered the same injury outside of the workplace?

    The recognition that both nonoccupational and occupational disability could be managed effectively and efficiently in this manner with supportive employers, supervisors, and caregivers gave rise to managed integrated disability.

    Laws protecting those individuals with disabilities—that is, through the ADA—have mandated that employers make employment available to "qualified individuals with disabilities" and make "reasonable accommodations" to ensure that those persons have the opportunity to be gainfully employed.

C. A variety of certifications have been developed that focus on disability management of injured workers. Many of these certifications have been discussed throughout this book. The development of specialized certifications and credentials has encouraged the idea of specialization. Certifications include the certified disability management specialist (CDMS), certified case manager (CCM), certified occupational health nurse specialist and case manager (COHN/CM and COHN-S/CM), and others.

D. DMEC began in 1992, when a small group of employers came together to discuss the issues associated with developing disability management programs. The group incorporated in 1995, has chapters in many states, and is looking to expand internationally.

   DMEC recognizes that the effort to bring legislative change is slow and seeks to educate and train its members in the disability management processes and principles. Therefore, in association with the IEA, DMEC helped develop the position entitled certified professional in disability management (CPDM) (DMEC, 1996).

E. Streamlined vendor relationships or managed care may not necessarily have driven the disability movement, but it surely has encouraged the speed and efficiency of the process. An integrated delivery system, or managed care system, has immense benefits for both group health and workers' compensation claims. Having immediate access to a medical history is of enormous benefit to the claims administrator and treatment team in a work-related injury. Ensuring that the primary care physician is knowledgeable in job-related functions is of equal benefit to the group health provider and administrator.

   This level of access enhances the vendor–employer relationship and promotes efficient communications that allows for one source to administer claims for workers' compensation, group health, and STD and LTD programs.

F. Clinical pathways, clinical protocols, and utilization review practices have educated administrators and employers about the benefits of quality, time-effective access to medical care. Use of these resources may also be accountable for the integrated disability system and acceptance of the return-to-work program. Ultimately, cost containment is the underlying driving force of this and most other health- and occupation-related movements.

G. Employers' attitudes toward individuals with disabilities and return-to-work programs cannot be discounted as one of the leading factors that have driven the disability management movement in the quest for "managed results."

H. The mission of the Integrated Benefits Institute (located in San Francisco, California) is to "provide research, discussion and analysis, data services and legislative receive to measure and improve integrated benefits programs, enhance efficiency in delivery of all employment-based benefits and promote effective return-to-work" (Parry & Molmen, 1996).

I. Washington's Business Group on Health, which coordinates an annual national conference on disability management, has taken a pivotal role in educating the industry on this topic.

J. The American Association of Occupational Health Nurses (AAOHN) and the American College of Occupational and Environmental Medicine (ACOEM) provide disability management and return-to-work services in addition to occupational health programs for employers' populations.

■ BUILDING A SUCCESSFUL DISABILITY MANAGEMENT PROGRAM

A. Identify internal departments involved with disability
1. Bargaining units
2. Operations
3. Human resources
4. Risk management
5. Occupational health
6. Safety
7. Finance
8. Legal and labor relations

B. Identify external departments
1. Workers' compensation carrier
2. Third-party administrators
3. Health care providers
4. Life insurance carrier
5. Disability carriers
6. Managed care providers

C. Once the programs and departments are identified, comparisons made, and costs of programs charted, determinations of modifications should be made to meet disability goals.
1. Changes usually made are
   a. Implementation of or increased safety and wellness programs
   b. Coordination of benefits
   c. Uniform definition of disability
   d. Transitional or modified return-to-work program
   e. Integrated medical treatment
   f. Single or coordinated case management programs
   g. Single-source application process
   h. Employee advocate or gatekeeper
   i. Use of disability duration guidelines
   j. Networked systems
   k. Coordinated vocational rehabilitation

■ FACTORS IMPORTANT IN THE DEVELOPMENT AND DESIGN OF A DISABILITY MANAGEMENT PROGRAM

A. Know your organization's benefits program

It is important to know the programs within your company that provide benefits to employees. In addition to workers' compensation, STD and LTD, and sick pay programs, monetary benefits often can be obtained through life insurance programs, pension programs, retirement, and union and state disability benefits. This information usually can be accessed through the human resources or benefits departments, which is why members from these disciplines make good return-to-work program team members.

B. Know your organization's primary illness or disability

It is beneficial for the safety or occupational health nurse to identify the most common types of injuries or illnesses so that clinical pathways or established modified jobs can focus on these frequent disabilities. If the in-house case manager does not have a medical background, this information should be sought from a medical case manager, occupational health nurse, or established primary treating physician.

C. Selecting vendors

1. Select a network of providers that not only covers tertiary care but that specializes in the core area that your company predominantly needs. Maintain a provider data base that lists both their addresses and specialties.

2. Select vendors that are invested in your employees and will assist in the implementation of the return-to-work program.

3. If possible, implement a software program that will enhance communications between the organization and its vendors.

D. Education

1. The case manager, in collaboration with the employer's representative or team, will need to educate all parties involved in the return-to-work program. Education should begin before implementation so that all divisions associated with the program have become thoroughly acquainted with it and understand their role in its success and purpose.

2. Education is ongoing for the case manager who is managing individuals' care both proactively and after disability.

3. Providing employees information on company policies can prepare them in the event of a disability or disease. Proactively, providing the access channels, corporate policy, and structure can minimize many of the traditional obstacles that prevent people with a disability from returning to gainful activity.

E. Accessibility

1. The case manager must remain accessible. Delegation is an important skill that the case manager can learn. He or she should be prepared to guide employees to the appropriate division to obtain the information they are seeking.

2. State and federal laws and statutes often have minute changes that can affect individuals' benefits significantly. Although informed case managers are aware of much of this information, it is usually best if it is provided by an individual in that discipline, that is, benefits, human resources, or union.

F. Modified or transitional duty team

1. Productivity management is the goal driving the return-to-work program. To maximize productivity management, an organization needs to minimize costs associated with it. From a disability perspective, these costs can encompass "hard dollar" savings by minimizing loss time, training time, and medical costs, or "soft dollar" savings by improving employee morale.

2. The team should meet routinely and should be led by case management, because the case manager may often be the primary coordinator of the return-to-work program. In other cases, the team may be chaired by representatives of the company (e.g., human resources and occupational health).

G. Clinical aspects

1. The program may benefit from an assigned precertification program.

2. Thorough clinical communication and documentation should be made so that administrative personnel can make informed decisions.

3. A case manager with related credentials and experience in occupational illness or injuries, and return-to-work clinical, vocational, and psychological aspects of injury and disease would likely be best suited for this position. The reader is directed to Chapters 11 and 13 for additional information.

4. A return-to-work support group would provide avenues for shared experiences and peer assistance.

H. Administration

1. A bill review process can be considered to monitor providers' bills. Many managed care providers are self-contained with this delivery system and can review bills from several providers.

2. Bill review, clinical documentation, and interface systems can minimize fraudulent activity on behalf of participants and providers.

3. Legal departments have direct access to claims to advise when to file for subrogation or other third-party payors.

4. Use network providers. If the providers are not part of a managed care module or do not offer partnerships with companies that provide durable medical equipment, therapy, pharmaceuticals, or other supplies, then obtain a network provider for those items.

5. The program should be equipped with an established method of reporting claims. There should be a time frame for claims reporting and one call-in line or claims reporting number. Early intervention allows for immediate care and, if necessary, the dissemination of patients' records between clinical and medical providers in a timely fashion to maximize your results-oriented approach to care.

6. Forward accident reports and other related reports to safety and the occupational health nurse so that informed adjustments to the work site or worker can be implemented.

7. Have an avenue and policy for grievance complaints. Third-party mediators or arbitrators are available to provide alternative dispute resolution. Case managers can be equipped with this training and certification.

■ STAGES OF THE CASE MANAGEMENT AND DISABILITY PROCESS

A. Development of the program

1. Development of a transitional work or modified duty team. This team will assist in the development, coordination, and implementation of the return-to-work process. The team should meet routinely to keep abreast of disabled workers and their progress in their medical–return-to-work continuum.

2. Develop a job bank. If the in-house case manager does not have a vocational or occupational health background, assistance from a vocational professional is desirable. The job bank should include descriptions and analyses of all regular, transitional, and modified duty jobs. This function may well be ongoing in that job changes and job development occur for various reasons and needs, for example, downsizing, uncommon illness, disease, or disability.

3. Develop a relationship with your selected vendors. Be sure that the selected vendors are vested in the interest of your employees and will be willing and accessible to discuss and learn the return-to-work program.

4. Implement an appropriately designed software program that will aid in the facilitation of necessary documentation both within and outside of the company. It is necessary to have direct access to the claims administrator or adjuster so that benefits can be coordinated in a timely fashion, and in the case of catastrophic injuries, excess carriers can have immediate knowledge of the progression of the claim.

5. Implement an early intervention program. Many employers have adopted a call-in or reporting line. Timely access through one source can minimize lost and delayed reported claims. It may be of benefit to standardize the intake format so the emergency or treating physicians become familiar with the specific information you need or how to ask for information they need to document the claim appropriately.

6. Develop a communications protocol. Often, losing or displacing employees arises from a lack of communication between the employer and the injured employee. Traditional workers' compensation field case managers have reported that one of their primary obstacles in returning an injured worker back to his or her place of employment is the worker's perception that the employer lacks interest in the worker and does not wish for his or her return—that he or she may somehow now be "labeled." In-house case management facilitates effective communication skills and can accomplish this goal. Also, with the case manager's trained ear, the patient can be referred to an Employee As-

sistance Program (EAP) should concerns arise about his or her emotional well-being.

7. EAP programs are excellent resources for case managers and can provide confidential counseling services for a variety of needs. Case managers need to be aware of other problems that can arise from an individual's disability—financial difficulties (e.g., reduced income), dependency difficulties (e.g., single parent), or addiction (e.g., prescription drugs),

8. If your company has the capability, establish a wellness program. This program can be in house or can be in partnership with a local facility. These programs have the capacity to facilitate on-site extended physical and occupational therapy, or allow a specially devised program to combine both therapy and job functions in the return-to-work process. Implement proactive wellness incentives and programs. Coordinate with the wellness division for routine health screens and education on routine aging illnesses and concerns (e.g., high-cholesterol diets, high blood pressure). Encourage corporate physical activities (e.g., walks, aerobics, softball team) that are designed to provide your employees the recommended weekly exercise regimens.

B. Coordination of program
   1. The case manager is ultimately the return-to-work (RTW) coordinator in the absence of an RTW coordinator at the employer's site. As the RTW coordinator, the case manager maintains regular contact with all key stakeholders:
      a. Injured or sick worker and family
      b. Treating physician
      c. Other treatment providers
      d. Worker's supervisor and management
      e. Medical, occupational health, and wellness departments
      f. Human resources and employee benefits
      g. External case management (as appropriate)
      h. Claims adjuster or TPA
      i. Modified or transitional duty team
      j. EAP (as appropriate)
   2. Establishing protocols. The case manager is advised immediately of the claim filed. If the claim warrants specialty care, the case manager can advise of the referral and submit to the treating physician a description of the worker's job functions. The case manager should expect from the physician time frames for medical or rehabilitation intervention and estimates on the duration of the patient's treatment and rehabiliation, and what, if any, physical limitations may be permanent. This information is then provided to the team.
   3. The case manager is responsible for providing the treating physician with a description of a modified duty job for authorization to release the patient back to work on either a limited or full-time basis.
   4. The case manager is responsible for disseminating the physician's projections to the benefits division so that benefits providers can be informed.

5. The case manager coordinates with the team on the return-to-work process. Implementation is achieved through supervision, documentation, and communication. The case manager executes the process and follows it through documenting progress, addressing pitfalls, and consulting with administration, precertification, managed care, health care, or any other outside provider who is not part of the internal modified duty team.

6. The case manager's knowledge is instrumental in reporting satisfaction with the providers of service. The case manager has an ethical and professional obligation to ensure that his or her client—the "injured person"—receives appropriate, quality medical intervention and is not placed at risk for further injury. Cost-contained quality medical care can be afforded to all employees who require it by systematically streamlining access to quality care and monitoring standards and progress of care or service provided.

   Case managers can assist in the availability of quality care for all people by eliminating providers or participants recognized for abusing, relying, or defrauding the system. Having access to all medical files improves the chances that fraudulent or "laissez-faire" practices are identified.

7. Continuity of medical care and its proper sequencing is key to promoting the patient's early return to work. The case manger must promote effective, intensive medical care to bring about healthy outcomes.

C. Corporate policy

   Corporate policy and pressures are frequently focused on productivity and finance. The case manager must sensitively meet the needs of both the employer and the employee when coordinating the return-to-work program. Juggling personalities and problems is what effective case managers are often recognized for, despite their intensive training within their own discipline. For example, accessing ergonomic specialists who can make work-site accommodations for modified duty or injury prevention programs is an excellent tool for combining productivity management with employee needs.

   The case manger has the responsibility to keep both the employee and the business healthy (Flynn, 1998).

D. Integrating systems

1. The integration process can be taken in small steps. Often, the first group of benefits to integrate are STD and workers' compensation.

   a. Establishing clinical guidelines and expectations can assist significantly with the medical management of these disabilities.

   b. Employing a managed care network can minimize time lost to shuffling medical records and accessing specialty physicians and treatment providers.

   c. Using one source to provide medical equipment, pharmaceuticals, and other supplies can promote efficiency of delivery and containment of costs.

   d. Having on-site wellness programs benefits all areas of health and disability management, but if qualified professionals are readily accessible, then creative, therapeutic return-to-work protocols can be established.

   e. Information technology is key and necessary when one is truly integrating all systems.

   f. The transitional work and modified-duty programs are essential to successful return to work and productivity of the workforce.

   g. Disability management should encompass both occupational and nonoccupational disabilities and be fully integrated with the STD, LTD, and WC programs.

     Integrated disability case management strategies ensure that injured workers have timely intervention, medical, disability, and return-to-work management. Other chapters in this book that discuss other aspects of disability management include Chapters 12 and 13.

     "If we are to achieve managed results we need to effectively manage our surroundings." Integrated disability management is a step in this direction.

REFERENCES

Caston, S. & Wright, L. (1997). The returning worker. *Rehab Management,* October/November, 52–56.

DiBenedetto, D. V. (1998). Total health and productivity management: Foundation for integrating benefit programs. *OEM Report, 12,*6.

DiBenedetto, D. V. (1999). Benchmarking the effective of integrated disability management strategies. *Total Health Management, 1*(1). Park Publishing, MO.

DiBenedetto, D. V. (1997–2000). *Principles of workers' compensation and disability case management* (2nd ed.). Yonkers, NY:DV Di Benedetto & Associates.

Disability Management Employer Coalition (1996). *Building a modified duty return to work program.* San Diego, CA: DMEC.

Eggleston, M. & Wright, L. (1997). Disability management: Catastrophic case management. *Case Review, 3*(3), 59–61.

Flynn, B. (1998). Benefits integration: 24 hour coverage. *Case Review,* May/June, 47–60.

Fong, C., Leahy, M., McMahon, B., Mirch, M., & DeVinney, D. (1999). Foundational knowledge and major practice domains of case management. *The Journal of Care Management, 5*(1), 10–30.

Laszewski, R. (1998). The myth of managed disability. *The Rehabilitation Professional,* July/August, 19–34.

Parry, T., Molmen, J.D., & William, P. (1996). *Return to productivity.* San Francisco: Integrated Benefits Institute.

Strickland, T. (1999). Integrated disability management. *The Case Manager, 10*(1), 51–53.

United States Commission on Civil Rights. (1983). *Accommodating the spectrum of abilities.* Washington, D.C.: U. S. Government Printing Office.

CHAPTER **13**

• • • • • • • • • • • • •

Occupational Health Case Management

DEBORAH V. DiBENEDETTO

LEARNING OBJECTIVES

Upon completion of this chapter, the reader will be able to:

1. Determine the scope of occupational health (OH) case management practice and its relationship to employer benefit programs and workforce initiatives.
2. Define important terms related to OH case management.
3. Define key concepts of OH case management.
4. State the economic cost of disability to employers and the potential savings associated with OH case management services.
5. Identify the similarities and differences between occupational and nonoccupational benefits.
6. List the characteristics of specific integrated benefit models being implemented by employers.
7. Identify the goals of integrated benefits programs.
8. State at least three regulations that impact OH case management services and return to work.
9. Identify the base of knowledge required for OH case managers.
10. Describe key tools used in delivering OH case management services.
11. State key characteristics of return-to-work programs and at least two examples of reasonable accommodations.

IMPORTANT TERMS AND CONCEPTS

24-Hour Programs and Managed Care
Cost Effectiveness
Disability Duration Guidelines
Functional Capacity Assessment
Functional Job Analysis
Independent Medical Examinations
Integrated Benefits
Integrated Disability Management
Occupational Health Case
   Management
Occupational Health Case
   Management Process
Occupational Medicine Practice
   Guidelines

Paid Time Off Arrangements
Reasonable Accommodation
Rehabilitation
Return-to-Work Programs
Second Opinion Examinations
Service Effectiveness
Service Efficiency
Service Integration
Work Hardening
Workers' Compensation Managed
   Care
Workforce Management

■ INTRODUCTION

A. Occupational health (OH) case management is a basic component of OH health nursing practice.

B. OH nursing practice is the specialty practice that provides for and delivers health care to workers and worker populations. Optimizing health, preventing illness and injury, and reducing health hazards are the foundational core for the practice base (Salazar, 1997).

C. OH health nurses and physicians play an integral role in determining, facilitating, and expediting the appropriate return to work of employees who are absent from work due to occupational or nonoccupational injuries or illnesses, or both.

D. Whenever case management services are provided to workers, worker populations, or persons whose care is financed by an employer's benefit program, the implications of their health status and functional recovery must be coordinated with OH and return-to-work goals and objectives.

E. OH case management is the process of coordinating the individual employee's health care services to achieve optimal quality care delivered in a cost-effective manner.

F. OH case management involves the management of occupational (workers' compensation [WC]) disability, nonoccupational disability, and incidental absence.

G. In addition to assessing, planning, directing, coordinating, implementing, managing, and evaluating care, the OH case manager establishes or qualifies a provider network, recommends treatment plans, monitors outcomes, and maintains a strong communication link among all the parties (American Association of Occupational Health Nursing [AAOHN], 1996).

H. The OH case manager coordinates the proactive efforts of the health care team to facilitate an individual's health care services from the onset of injury or illness to a safe return to work or an optimal alternative.

I. OH case management includes the development of preventive systems and the mobilization of appropriate resources for care over the course of the health event.

J. OH case management and medical care is delivered with the ultimate goal of returning the worker to pre-illness or pre-injury function or to the highest level of functioning achievable in the most cost-effective and time-efficient manner.

K. Comprehensive OH case management is ideally provided by OH nurses; because of the emphasis on return to pre-injury function, OH nurses are well positioned to support an appropriate return-to-work plan as part of the overall OH case management plan (AAOHN, 1996; American Board for Occupational Health Nursing [ABOHN], 1999).

L. OH case managers are most often registered professional nurses. Professional certifications for OH nurse case managers include:
1. Certified case manager (CCM)
2. Certified OH nurse (COHN)
3. Certified OH nurse specialist (COHN-S)
4. Certified OH nurse case manager (COHN/CM)
5. Certified OH nurses specialist/case manager (COHN-S/CM)
6. Certified disability management specialist

M. OH case managers generally belong to AAOHN, the Case Management Society of America (CMSA), or a similarly oriented professional organization.

■ KEY CONCEPTS OF OCCUPATIONAL HEALTH CASE MANAGEMENT

A. Goals of OH case management programs include (DiBenedetto, 1998–2000; Shrey & Lacerte, 1997):
1. Facilitate the employee's return to work in a timely manner.
2. Assist employees in navigating the benefit and medical care arenas.
3. Minimize lost time in the workplace.
4. Decrease the cost of lost time benefit programs such as short- and long-term disability, salary continuation, and WC.
5. Facilitate employer control of disability issues.
6. Improve corporate competitiveness.
7. Maximize use of employer resources.
8. Reduce human cost of disability.
9. Enhance morale by valuing employee physical and cultural diversity.
10. Protect the employability of the worker.
11. Ensure compliance with relevant laws and organizations, such as the Americans with Disabilities Act (ADA), Family Medical Leave Act

(FMLA), Occupational Safety and Health Administration (OSHA), and Department of Transportation (DOT).

12. Reduce the adversarial nature of disability and litigation.

13. Improve labor relations.

14. Promote joint labor–management collaboration.

15. Facilitate direct workers' involvement in planning.

B. The economic cost of disability and lost time

1. The economics of occupational and nonoccupational injuries and illnesses deplete the financial assets of employers, insurance companies, persons with disabilities, and the nation.

2. Decreased workplace productivity costs millions of dollars, which results in higher consumer prices for goods and services and insurance premiums. The cost of disability impacts the entire nation.

3. Employers may spend as much as 18% to 20% of payroll on the cost of lost time due to worker disability, injury, and illness (Table 13–1).

4. The costs of disability (as depicted in Table 13–1) can be categorized as direct, indirect, or disability management costs. These costs entail:

   a. Direct costs: Those "out-of pocket," first dollar payments for sick days, indemnity and lost wages paid, short-term disability (STD), long-term disability (LTD), WC, salary continuation programs, and medical care (paid under group health plans and the medical care portion of WC)

   b. Indirect costs: Overtime payments, the cost of temporary or replacement workers, broken equipment, supervisory oversight of the replacement workers, and lost productivity

TABLE 13–1
Cost of Disability

Direct Costs	Indirect Costs	Administrative Costs	Total Cost of Disability
• Sick leave	• Replacement workers	• Claim management	⇩
• Salary continuation	• Training	• Communication	
• Workers' compensation	• Supervisory oversight	• Loss prevention	
• Short-Term disability	• Repair of broken equipment	• Occupational health and safety	⇩
• Long-Term disability	• Overtime payments	• Case management	
• Related medical costs	• Lost productivity	• Return-to-work programs	⇩
		• Employee assistance programs	
		• Wellness	
8–12 % of payroll	1–4% of payroll	1% of payroll	8–17% of payroll

(D.V. DiBenedetto & Associates Ltd., New York, 1998)

    c. Disability management costs: Claims management, communication, loss prevention, return-to-work programs, employee assistance, and health promotion and wellness programs

C. As more emphasis is placed on controlling costs across the organization, management is now taking a closer look at the cost of lost time in the workplace. Companies are beginning to have a much broader definition of "disability" in the workplace. This broader definition includes both occupational (WC) and nonoccupational (STD and LTD) disability.

D. Lost workdays doubled due to disabling conditions between 1972 and 1992. The federal General Accounting Office reports that three out of 10 persons eligible to return to work do not, owing to a lack of disability management, and on any given day, 25 to 33% of the typical workforce is not at work and receiving wages (Abbott, 1997).

E. Companies can spend up to 17% of payroll for total disability, that is, the sum of all costs—direct, indirect, and administrative—for occupational and nonoccupational benefit programs (see Table 13–1). This expense reduces a company's ability to spend money on research, investment, and return on shareholder value (DiBenedetto, 1998).

F. There are many similarities between nonoccupational and occupational (WC) programs (Table 13–2). Employers are moving toward integrated models to manage lost time due to disability because of the similarities between occupational (WC) and nonoccupational/group benefit programs.

    As we look at the various benefits an employer provides to its employee populations, WC, short- and long-term disability, medical (including WC medical care) and other paid time off (PTO) benefit components, including salary continuation, are generally rich in composition yet managed by different organizations within a company. Much like the pieces of a puzzle, each benefit is a separate and distinct program. Each program is managed by either the benefit or human resource function (generally nonoccupa-

TABLE 13–2
Comparison of Occupational and Nonoccupational Benefits

Nonoccupational Benefits	Occupational Benefits (WC)
• Medical care	• Medical care
• Short-term disability	• Temporary disability
• Long-term disability	• Permanent disability
• Vocational rehabilitation (under LTD)	• Vocation rehabilitation
• Life insurance	• Death benefit
• Accident, death, and disability insurance	
• FMLA coverage	• FMLA coverage
• ADA accommodation	• ADA accommodation
• Return to work	• Return to work

(DV DiBenedetto & Associates Ltd., New York, 1998)

tional benefits—STD, LTD, group health) or risk management for occupational program components (WC). The totality of benefits provided to employees gives a worker "24-hour coverage" in terms of lost wage replacement and coverage for medical care. That is, if an employee were injured on the job, he or she would receive medical and indemnity payments under the WC system. If the employee is ill or injured off the job, he or she can collect benefits under STD or LTD and medical benefits from group health arrangements. This leads to fragmentation, duplication, and extra cost to the company. In some cases, employees are also eligible for salary continuance, based on company policy and seniority (DiBenedetto, 1998).

When we compare occupational and nonoccupational benefit program components, we see that there are many similarities (see Table 13–2) between the two. Both provide for medical care, wage replacement for the short or long term, vocational rehabilitation, and death benefits. ADA and FML compliance issues surround both benefits: injured workers may be eligible for job-protected leave under the FMLA, and those with a permanent disability may be eligible for reasonable accommodation under the ADA. Return-to-work issues abound for both occupational and nonoccupational lost time (DiBenedetto, 1998).

G. The models for disability management include:
  1. Integrated benefits and integration of all indemnity and medical benefit programs. This approach integrates all benefit programs into one integrated program, merging STD, LTD, WC, and medical care into one comprehensive program.
  2. Integration of STD and LTD benefits. This is one of the more common integrated products available in the marketplace today. Nonoccupational disability is managed in a coordinated fashion with an eye on LTD. Should the person remain disabled past the period of STD, actions are taken early in the process to facilitate claim administration and movement of the patient into LTD.
  3. Integrated disability management. This approach coordinates STD, LTD, and WC claim administration, usually with a single intake and claim reporting process, coordinated case management, and emphasis on managing total disability to return a person to work.
  4. Managed care for WC. Implementing managed medical care arrangement for WC is a growing trend.
     a. More than 40 states allow some form of managed medical care for occupational injuries or illnesses.
     b. WC managed care is characterized by the use of preferred providers; negotiated fee schedules or payments for medical care; capitated rates; aggressive, facilitated return-to-work efforts; the use of treatment protocols and disability duration guidelines; and case management.
  5. 24-hour programs and managed care. Although health care reform died out a few years ago, market-driven reform continues. This approach focuses primarily on a single source for both occupational and nonoccupational medical benefits, with characteristics similar to those of managed WC arrangements.

  a. It may or may not be directly managed with the claim for indemnity payments for STD, LTD, or WC.

  b. Employers provide 24-hour medical coverage but do not coordinate WC care and group health care.

6. PTO arrangements. More employers are moving toward PTO arrangements, in which employees are given a bank or savings account of time that they can use for a variety of reasons, such as sick days, vacation, personal time, and so forth. Generally, PTO benefits are implemented using the same policies that direct an employer's incidental absence, sick time, and FMLA programs.

■ MAXIMIZING WORKFORCE HEALTH AND PRODUCTIVITY

A. The goals of the integrated benefit model are focused on increasing the health and productivity of the workforce.

B. Goals of the integrated model include improved benefit delivery; increased quality; greater employee satisfaction; higher workforce productivity; timely, accurate, and appropriate benefit payments; and decreased plan administration costs and efforts secondary to improved efficiencies.

C. To date, 25% to 50% of employers have implemented or are considering an integrated approach to employee benefit programs. Of those who have integrated programs or approaches, savings of up to 30% to 50% of direct costs for total disability (occupational and nonoccupational) have been demonstrated (DiBenedetto, 1999).

D. Companies should set the following integrated benefit program goals for their programs (DiBenedetto, 1999):

  1. Improved quality and access to medical care
  2. Timely and appropriate return to work of the injured or ill employee
  3. Increased productivity at the work site
  4. Reduced cost of benefits and lost work time
  5. Mitigation of employee confusion about benefit program components
  6. Timely benefit administration and benefit payment
  7. Decreased litigation
  8. Increased ease of administration
  9. Consolidated information management and record keeping
  10. Improved employee morale
  11. Better use of a critical resource—the employee

E. The ultimate goal of an integrated benefit program is to manage all forms of absence from work consistently by improving employee access to appropriate medical care and promoting workforce productivity through facilitation of return to work.

F. Workforce management centers on the concept of managing all aspects of occupational disability and proactive health and safety information and training, aggressive management (including case management) of occupational and nonoccupational lost-time cases and effective return to work within the regulatory arena specific to the employer (DiBenedetto, 1997–2000) (Fig. 13–1).

G. Workforce management is concerned with (DiBenedetto, XXXX):
1. Demographics of the employer's worker populations
2. OH and non-OH management
3. Health and productivity programs, metrics, and outcomes
4. Benefit plan design that augments the needs of the worker population
5. Consideration of work, life, and family impacts on the worker population and the impact on their ability to be at work
6. Integrating benefit programs such as integrated disability management, case management, and coordinated return to work programs

H. Goals of the integrated health and productivity model include improved benefit design and delivery of services; increased quality; greater employee satisfaction; higher workforce productivity (i.e., being at work); timely, accurate, and appropriate benefit payments; and decreased plan administration efforts and costs (DiBenedetto, 1997–2000).

■ REGULATIONS THAT IMPACT OH CASE MANAGEMENT AND RETURN TO WORK

A. WC

B. Statutory STD

C. FMLA

D. ADA

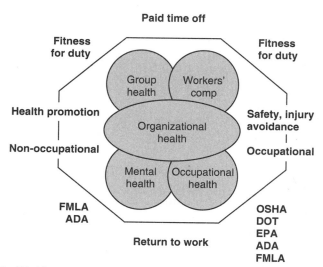

FIGURE 13–1 Workforce management: total health and productivity model concept. (Source: DV DiBenedetto & Associates Ltd, reprinted with permission from OEM Health Information, June 1998.)

E. DOT
   1. Commercial driver licensing (CDL) requirements
   2. Mandatory drug and alcohol testing

F. OSHA

G. Health Insurance Portability Act (HIPPA)

H. Consolidated Omnibus Reconciliation Act (COBRA)

I. Employee Retirement Income Security Act (ERISA)

J. Social Security Disability Income (SSDI) and the new Ticket to Work Act

■ PURPOSES OF THE OCCUPATIONAL HEALTH CASE MANAGEMENT PROGRAM

A. To provide high-level, quality professional case management services to promote access to and use of quality medical care, in the appropriate setting, at an appropriate cost, with the ultimate goal of effective and efficient return to function and work.

B. The scope and role of the OH nurse providing case management services varies depending on the nature of the business setting, expectations of the employer, role assignments, and philosophy of the OH program. Case management has generally been an integral component of the OH program but is becoming more formalized as a specialty within the field of practice.

C. OH case management services may focus on clients with occupational or nonoccupational injuries or illnesses, or both. It may also include the delivery of case management services to the worker's dependents.

D. OH case management may focus on large loss cases, that is, high-cost, prolonged recovery or those with multiple providers and fragmented care.

E. OH case management is designed to prevent fragmented care and delayed recovery while facilitating the employee's recovery and appropriate return to work in a full-duty or modified work capacity.

■ MODELS OF OH CASE MANAGEMENT

A. OH case management is generally provided by OH nurses and physicians who are familiar with the employee's job tasks, conditions of work, work processes, benefit programs, supervisors, and community providers.

B. OH case managers are primarily registered professional nurses with knowledge of OH nursing, OH and safety practice, relevant work conditions, health promotion, regulatory issues, benefit programs, and return to work requirements.

C. OH case management service delivery models include:
   1. On-site case management services: Services are provided by the employer's own staff or designee (i.e., vendor) at the actual workplace. These services may involve actual client contact in the workplace, by phone, or through field visits.

2. Telephonic case management: Services are coordinated through electronic communication. Services may be provided on an interstate or intrastate basis.

3. Off-site or field case management services are provided outside of the employer's workplace, generally by a third-party administrator (TPA), insurance company, or case management vendor. In some cases, the employer's OH case managers may make field visits to the employee, provider, or carrier to facilitate appropriate case management services and return to work.

D. OH case management settings include acute care hospitals and systems; corporations; social insurance programs; public and private insurance sectors; fee-for-service, managed care, and case management organizations; government, the military, and government-sponsored programs; and provider agencies and facilities.

■ FUNCTIONS OF OH CASE MANAGEMENT

A. The functions of the OH case manager mirror the steps of the OH nursing case management process, for example (AAOHN, 1994):
   1. Client identification, outreach by the case manager, and verification of eligibility for services
   2. Individual assessment and diagnosis to determine level of function and service needs of client
   3. Service planning and resource identification
   4. Linking the client to the needed service within the community or service network
   5. Service implementation and coordination of care
   6. Monitoring the service delivery process and utilization by the client
   7. Advocacy for the client within the service network
   8. Evaluation of the service delivery, client status, satisfaction, and desired case management outcomes

■ STRUCTURAL ELEMENTS OF THE OH CASE MANAGEMENT PROCESS

A. The following structural elements are client focused, dynamic, and facilitated desired OH case management outcomes (AAOHN, 1994):
   1. Service effectiveness—choosing the appropriate provider and the most effective diagnostic and therapeutic interventions for the client to speed recovery
   2. Service efficiency—timely OH case management and medical management during the acute phase of the client's injury or illness
   3. Service integration aims to avoid multiple providers and reduce fragmented medical care. The OH case manager uses his or her communication and negotiation skills during this structural part of the case management process.
   4. Cost effectiveness considers the cost of services when choosing the provider, setting, or intervention for the level of injury or illness.

5. Standards of Practice for Occupational Health Nurses have been established by AAOHN. They may be obtained by the reader by contacting AAOHN at *www.aaaohn.org* or by calling 800-241-8014.

■ CHARACTERISTICS OF INTEGRATED DISABILITY PROGRAMS

A. OH case management programs focus on providing case management services to workers regardless of the nature or case of injury and absence from work due to medical reasons.

B. OH case managers provide integrated disability case management services to increase workforce health and productivity.

C. Characteristics of integrated disability management programs involve:
1. Coordinated WC and STD and LTD claim administration
2. Single-intake and claim reporting process
3. Coordinated case management of both occupational and nonoccupational disability
4. OH case management is integrated or coordinated with managed care arrangements.
5. Information management systems and reporting are integrated.
6. Administrative processes are streamlined and automated.
7. Disability definitions and regulatory compliance issues are consistently defined and managed across all programs that meet the organization's needs and objectives.

■ THE OH CASE MANAGEMENT PROCESS (ABOHN, 1999)

A. Assessment
1. Establishes criteria and uses case finding and screening to identify workers who are appropriate candidates for case management.
2. Conducts comprehensive assessment of employees.
3. Assesses informal and formal support systems.
4. Assesses community, workplace, and vendor resources.
5. Assesses essential functions of job (physical and mental demands) to facilitate hiring, proper placement, and return-to-work activities.
6. Identifies gaps that exist in the service continuum.
7. Periodically reassesses the health status of the worker.
8. Assesses the need for safety, accident prevention, and health promotion programs.
9. Conducts comprehensive assessment of all disability-related expenses and benefit utilization.
10. Assesses workplace policies on return-to-work and job accommodations.
11. Identifies legal, labor, and regulatory implications.
12. Assesses disability plans, policies, procedures, and communication links.
13. Identifies roles and responsibilities of the worker, supervisor or man-

ager, case manager, benefits–risk manager, health care providers, TPAs and insurers, and others, as needed.

14. Recognizes challenges to successful outcomes.

B. Planning

1. Reviews worker's goals and expectations.
2. Reviews employer and corporate goals.
3. Prepares analysis and synthesis of all data to formulate an appropriate plan of care.
4. Uses appropriate components of employee benefits plan or plans.
5. Analyzes and synthesizes data to formulate appropriate diagnoses and interdisciplinary problem statements.
6. Plans the worker's timely and appropriate return to work.
7. Coordinates service providers responsible for furnishing services.
8. Participates in special provider arrangements, for example, preferred provider organizations (PPOs), health maintenance organizations (HMOs), point of service organizations (POSs), and managed care contractors.
9. Collaborates with community, workplace, and vendor personnel.
10. Develops a plan of care, including health care and medical treatment goals, through an interdisciplinary and collaborative group process, which includes the employee and his or her caregivers.
11. Participates in development of programs for safety, accident prevention, and health promotion to prevent future occurrence of injury and illness cases.
12. Coordinates administration of case management among benefit plans, including WC.
13. Applies principles consistent with the ADA in preplacement and ongoing job placement activities.
14. Participates in disability plan design and policy and procedure development.

C. Implementation

1. Links the worker with the most appropriate community resources.
2. Acts as a liaison with health care providers.
3. Coordinates access to quality, cost-effective care and services.
4. Coordinates clinical and medical management of cases.
5. Implements early return to work/modified duty programs.
6. Facilitates rehabilitation and job accommodation for WC and nonoccupational disabilities.
7. Provides appropriate education for the worker, family, providers, and community resources.
8. Assists the worker to negotiate the health care system.
9. Develops and maintains standards, policies, and protocols to support the case management process.
10. Participates in interagency groups and community agencies to support or represent the case management program.

D. Evaluation

1. Manages data and information systems for the purposes of research, trend analysis, program modification, and continuous quality improvement.
2. Evaluates quality of management efforts, teamwork, and workflow design.
3. Monitors and modifies the return-to-work plan.
4. Monitors the worker and others to ensure a smooth transition to work and continued progress.
5. Evaluates and monitors the plan of care to ensure its quality, efficiency, timeliness, and effectiveness.
6. Ensures that services are appropriate, cost effective, and supportive of worker independence.
7. Monitors the worker's decision-making abilities regarding choices, utilization, and consequences.
8. Evaluates worker outcomes to determine case disposition.
9. Evaluates effectiveness of safety, accident prevention, and wellness programs.
10. Evaluates disability-related expenses and programs for program or benefit enhancement and refinement, as well as for areas of duplication.
11. Tracks and evaluates program outcomes periodically for success of case management activities (e.g., reduced cost, reduced accidents, reduced severity of injury or illness, efficiency of process, and customer satisfaction).
12. Evaluates due diligence of providers and provider networks.

E. Overall, the OH case manager (ABOHN, 1999):

1. Functions as an employee advocate.
2. Balances the needs of the workplace with the needs of the worker.
3. Communicates effectively throughout the case management process.
4. Ensures confidentiality and complies with established codes of ethics and legal or regulatory requirements.
5. Documents case management activities.
6. Monitors and encourages appropriate use of health care resources.
7. Participates in public speaking, marketing, and research related to case management services and the programs provided.

■ BASE OF KNOWLEDGE REQUIRED FOR OH CASE MANAGERS

A. The following knowledge, skills, and abilities are needed to function effectively as an OH nurse case manager (ABOHN, 1999):

1. Case management process, including assessment, planning, intervention, and evaluation
2. Rehabilitation principles (e.g., work hardening and conditioning, functional capacity evaluation

3. Vocational rehabilitation (e.g., labor market survey, transferable skills analysis)
4. Prevention and wellness promotion
5. Federal regulatory programs (e.g., FMLA, ERISA, ADA, Social Security Insurance [SSI], COBRA, DOT, OSHA)
6. State regulatory programs (e.g., WC, statutory disability)
7. Liability issues in case management
8. Legal and ethical issues (e.g., confidentiality)
9. Knowledge of and access to appropriate community resources
10. Life-care planning concepts
11. Statistical and data analysis (e.g., cost–benefit analysis, return on investment, trends analysis, economic analysis)
12. Tracking and measuring costs
13. Conflict management skills
14. Negotiating skills
15. Oral and written communication skills
16. Decision-making ability
17. Problem-solving ability
18. Adult learning principles
19. Principles of quality improvement (e.g., continuous quality improvement [CQI], total quality management [TQM], International Standards Organization [ISO] 9000, ISO 14,001)
20. Protocol development and utilization
21. Understanding of the role and function of case management participants (i.e., human resource personnel, benefits managers, insurance carriers, TPAs, risk managers, safety director, line managers, external providers, and legal counsel)
22. Use of information technology
23. Sociocultural influences
24. Principles of utilization review and precertification
25. Alternative treatment modalities
26. Job analysis
27. Principles of management
28. System abuse (e.g., fraudulent practices by worker, employer, or vendor)
29. Health care delivery systems (e.g., health insurance, managed care models [HMO, PPO, POS])
30. Trends in case management (e.g., disability, WC, rehabilitation, integrated models)
31. Labor relations
32. Disability plan designs (e.g., STD, LTD, WC)
33. Disability terminology and concepts (e.g., independent medical examination [IME], second opinion, impairment ratings, deductibles, copays, indemnity, reserves)

34. Contractual agreements (e.g., with workers, employers, vendors, TPAs, unions)
35. Disease management
36. Principles of litigation

■ KEY TOOLS AND PROCESSES IN OH CASE MANAGEMENT

A. Clinical practice guidelines: These guidelines are voluntary in nature and may be specific to an institution; some are mandated by state WC laws (e.g., Massachusetts), or they may be voluntary (e.g., New York). There are no nationally promulgated clinical guidelines dictating medical care.

1. The American College of Occupational and Environmental Medicine (ACOEM) has developed clinical practice guidelines for potentially work-related health problems in worker populations. Entitled *Occupational Medicine Practice Guidelines: Evaluation and Management of Common Health Problems and Functional Recovery in Workers,* the guidelines
   a. Are based on the injured workers' presenting complaints
   b. Emphasize prevention
   c. Emphasize proper clinical evaluation
   d. Provide guidance for medical and disability management
2. The ACOEM guidelines are relatively unique in that they address the entire spectrum of management of a presenting problem rather than focusing on a specific diagnosis or procedure, assuming that the diagnosis is correct or that the procedure is warranted.
3. The goals of the ACOEM guidelines include:
   a. Provision of uniform information to a diverse group of practitioners who care for or manage potentially work-related health concerns
   b. Provision of guidance for case management
   c. Speeding functional recovery
   d. Improving the quality of care for potentially work-related health problems, including improvements in appropriateness, efficiency, effectiveness, and reduction of variation in practice
4. It is important for the OH case manager to know the scope of treatment, which will ultimately help the worker return to functionality as soon as possible.
5. Several states have established treatment guidelines for WC injuries, which may be mandated by the municipality (e.g., Massachusetts has 26 mandatory treatment guidelines).
6. Although no one specific national treatment plan exists for the myriad health issues and complaints, the ACOEM guidelines provide a means to evaluate and manage medical care of workers.

B. Disability duration guidelines: Help the provider and case manager to determine a person's potential for return to work within a given time frame.

C. Specified recovery guidelines assist by establishing a benchmark or expected time frame during which a worker recovers from his or her disability.

D. Persons with the same diagnosis or medical condition will recover at different rates and be able to return to work within a general time frame; however, recovery is as variable as a person's individuality.

E. Disability and ability to return to work are also dependent on the worker's healing or adaptation to illness or injury and the scope of his or her job functions.

F. Disability duration guidelines are just that—guidelines that are invaluable as a frame of reference when used in conjunction with other factors of disability, work requirements, values and belief systems, and so forth.

G. A variety of disability duration guidelines are available for determining the potential length of workers' absence due to injury or illness; examples include:
   1. The Medical Disability Advisor
   2. Occupational Disability Guidelines
   3. Milliman and Robertson

H. Functional capacity assessments (FCAs) are used to directly measure a person's functional ability to perform specific work-related tasks. An FCA may be requested by the OH professional, human resources, provider, adjustor, or other key stakeholder.
   1. An FCA involves examining an individual as he or she performs activities in a structured setting. It does not necessarily reflect what the person should be able to do but what he or she can do or is willing to do at the time of the evaluation. Functional capacity depends on motivation, cognitive awareness, behavioral factors, and sincerity of effort, all of which have a major impact on the FCA (AMA, 1995).

I. Functional job analysis is one of the most important tools used to help return the injured worker to his or her pre-injury occupation or job. The job analysis
   1. Defines job requirements
   2. Lists and describes the job's essential and non-essential functions
   3. Should be current and representative of the employee's job responsibilities
   4. Should always be shared with the treating physician or provider and the OH case manager to aid in return-to-work planning

J. Independent medical examinations (IMEs) are used to confirm a person's diagnosis, current medical treatment and care, the scope and nature of disability, the potential for permanent disability and impairment, ability to return to work, and medical information and testing outcomes. The IME provider never becomes the treating physician.

K. Second opinion examinations (SOEs) are used to confirm a person's diagnosis, provide more information, and make recommendations for potential treatment options. Often the employee may choose to be treated by the SOE provider.

L. Rehabilitation: The goal of medical and vocational rehabilitation is to restore the employee's function and return him or her to the pre-injury state. Types include physical, occupational, and vocational rehabilitation.

M. Work hardening is physical therapy that mimics actual work demands. Exercises and work-simulated activities are monitored by professionals to allow the injured worker to build up his or her work task tolerance gradually. Work hardening activities may be provided at the work site under the supervision of physical therapists and the OH case manager (DiBenedetto, 1997–2000).

■ RETURN-TO-WORK PROGRAMS

A. In OH case management, case managers are not only concerned about ensuring appropriate medical care but must also address, from the initial assessment on the date of injury or illness, the goal of returning an individual to productive work at the earliest possible time in either a transitional, modified, or full-duty capacity.

B. The ultimate goal of OH case management is to assist the ill or injured person to achieve the highest level of medical improvement and to facilitate his or her successful return to work in the most cost-effective and efficient manner (DiBenedetto, 1997).

C. Companies should have in place formal return-to-work policies and procedures to expedite the injured worker's effective return to work in a timely manner.

D. Employer return-to-work programs should allow for the following types of work assignments:
1. Full duty
2. Temporary, alternative, or transitional work
3. Modified duty assignments

E. Return-to-work assignments that are to other than full duty must be reviewed on a regular basis by both the OH case manager and company to ensure the employee is progressing as planned.

F. If an employee requires permanent accommodation owing to a permanent disability or medical condition that precludes him or her from performing essential functions of his or her job, then reasonable accommodation under the ADA must be considered.

G. According to the Job Accommodation Network, the facts about job accommodation include:
1. Job accommodations are usually not expensive.
2. Job accommodations may be as simple as the rearrangement of equipment.
3. Job accommodations can reduce WC and other issuance costs.
4. Job accommodations can increase the pool of qualified candidates for an employer.

5. Job accommodations can create opportunities for persons with functional limitations.

H. Examples of reasonable accommodation include (DiBenedetto, 1997–2000):
1. Facility renovations
2. Job restructuring
3. Part-time or modified work
4. Reassignment to a vacant position
5. Acquisition or modification of equipment
6. Adjustments or modifications of training, examinations, training materials, or policies
7. Other similar accommodations, including leaves of absence

■ IMPORTANCE OF OH CASE MANAGEMENT TO BUSINESS AND THE NATION

A. OH case management involves the prevention of lost time in the workplace, management of WC and disability lost-time cases, and an employee's effective and timely return to work.

B. Lost time in the workplace costs employers millions of dollars in lost productivity and, ultimately, customer sales.

C. OH case management activities, along with integrated approaches to both benefit programs and disability management, have yielded significant savings to employers and the overall cost of disability to the nation.

D. Keeping employees healthy, safe, and productive (i.e., being fit for work) ensures the economic status and workforce productivity of the nation.

REFERENCES

Abbott, R. (1997). The business case for integrating benefits. *Journal of Compensation and Benefits, 58,* 63.

American Association of Occupational Health Nurses (1994). *Case management advisory.* Atlanta, GA: AAOHN.

American Association of Occupational Health Nurses (1996). *Position statement: The occupational health nurse as case manager.* Atlanta, GA: AAOHN.

American Board for Occupational Health Nursing (1999). *Case management certification blueprint.* Hinsdale, IL: ABOHN.

American Medical Association (1995). *Guide to the evaluation of permanent impairment* (4th ed.). Chicago: AMA.

DiBenedetto, D. V. (1997–2000). *Principles of workers' compensation and disability case management course.* Yonkers, NY: DV DiBenedetto & Associates.

DiBenedetto, D. V. (1999). Benchmarking the effectiveness of integrated disability management strategies. *Total Health Management, 1,* 1. Park Publishing, MO.

DiBenedetto, D. V., et al. (1990–1998). *The OEM occupational health and safety manual.* Beverly Farms, MA: OEM Press.

DiBenedetto, D. V. (1998). Total health and productivity management: Foundation for integrated benefit programs. *OEM Report, 12,* 6. Beverly Farms, MA: OEM Press.

DiBenedetto, D. V., & Hall, J. C. (1995). Workers' compensation and disability case management. *OEM Report, 9,* 12. Beverly Farms, MA: OEM Health Information, pp. 93–100.

Salazar, M. K. (1997). *AAOHN core curriculum for occupational health nursing.* Philadelphia: W.B. Saunders.

Shrey, D. E., & Lacerte, M. (1997). *Principles and practices of disability management in industry.* Boca Raton, FL: CRC Press.

CHAPTER 14

· · · · · · · · · · · · ·

Behavioral Health Case Management

SUSAN GREGORY

Upon completion of this chapter, the reader will be able to:

1. Identify commonly occurring behavioral health care conditions.
2. Describe the most commonly used methods of treatment.
3. Assess for high-risk behavioral health care disorders.
4. Evaluate treatment effectiveness in behavioral health care.
5. Understand the role of alternative and complementary medicine in treatment of behavioral health disorders.
6. Identify community agencies.

Behavioral Health Care
DSM-IV
Substance Abuse
Substance Dependence

Personality Disorder
Psychopharmacology

■ INTRODUCTION

A. The incidence of behavioral health disorders (*Diagnostic and Statistical Manual of Mental Disorders*, 4th ed. [DSM-IV], 1994)—Incidence rates of various disorders are estimates only. Estimates depend on accurate reporting, the definitions used by clinicians and other reporting entities, associated disorders, and the population being studied. Often, a disorder is observed infrequently in a specific setting but quite frequently in another, and these observations affect estimation and reporting.

1. Disorders of childhood
   a. Mental retardation—1%, no apparently familial pattern, 50% heredity
   b. Attention deficit disorder (ADD; with and without associated hyperactivity)—3% to 5% in school-age children, male-to-female ratio 4:1 in the general population; positive familial patterns
2. Dementia
   a. Alzheimer's type—2% to 4% of the population older than 65 years of age
   b. Alzheimer's type and vascular—20% older than 85 years of age
3. Schizophrenia—0.5% to 1.0% of general population, male-to-female ratio not clear
4. Major depressive disorder—male-to-female ratio 1:2, 10% to 25% females, 5% to 12% males; 1.5 to 3 times more common in individuals who have a first-degree biological relative with the disorder
5. Bipolar disorder—equal male-to-female ratio; 0.4% to 1.6% of population; positive familial pattern
6. Anxiety disorders and post-traumatic stress disorder
   a. Panic disorder—male-to-female ratio 1:2–3; 1.5% to 3.5% of population; 50% of patients diagnosed have associated agoraphobia; 4 to 7 times more common in individuals who have a first-degree biological relative with the disorder
   b. Post-traumatic stress disorder—1% to 14% of population; 3% to 58% of at-risk individuals
   c. Obsessive-compulsive disorders—male-to-female ratio is equal; 2.5% incidence in the general population; more common in individuals who have a first-degree biological relative with the disorder
   d. Generalized anxiety disorder—male-to-female ratio 1:2 to 3; 5% incidence; familial patterns are unclear
7. Pain disorder—10% to 15% of adults; women appear to experience some chronic pain conditions, such as headache and musculoskeletal pain, more often than men
8. Eating disorders
   a. Anorexia nervosa—greater than 90% female; 0.5% to 1%, positive familial pattern
   b. Bulimia nervosa—at least 90% female; 1% to 3% in females, 0.1% to 0.3% in men
9. Adjustment disorders—male-to-female ratio is equal; 5% to 20% of patients are seen in outpatient clinics
10. Personality disorders—11 types have been identified
    a. Paranoid—more common in men; 0.5% to 2.5% of general population; 2% to 30% in clinic or hospital settings
    b. Schizoid—uncommon
    c. Schizotypal—more common in men; 3% of general population
    d. Antisocial—men, 3% of the general population; women, 1% of the general population

    e. Borderline—male-to-female ratio 1:3; 2% of general population; 10% to 20% of clinic or hospital settings

    f. Histrionic—2% to 3% general population; 10% to 15% in treatment settings

    g. Narcissistic—50% to 75% diagnosed are men; less than 1% in general population; 2% to 16% of patients in treatment settings

    h. Avoidant—male-to-female ratio is equal; 0.5% to 1% in general population; 10% in treatment settings

    i. Dependent—more frequently diagnosed in women; the most frequently reported personality disorder in the treatment setting

    j. Obsessive-compulsive—twice as common in men; 1% of general population; 8% to 10% in treatment setting

B. Incidence of substance-related disorders

  1. Alcohol dependence—male-to-female ratio 5:1; 8% to 14%, positive familial pattern

  2. Alcohol abuse—male-to-female ratio 5:1; 5%, positive familial pattern

  3. Other substance-related disorders

    a. Cannabis abuse—more frequent in men; 4% of general population

    b. Amphetamine-related disorder—male-to-female ratio 1:3 to 4; 2% of general population

    c. Cocaine-related disorder—male-to-female ratio equal; 0.2% of general population

    d. Hallucinogen-related disorder—male-to-female ratio 3:1; 0.3% of general population

    e. Opioid-related disorder—male-to-female ratio 3 to 4:1; 0.7% of general population

    f. Phencyclidine-related disorder—75% more prevalent in males; accounts for 3% of deaths and 3% of emergency room visits

    g. Inhalant-related disorders—70% to 80% more common in adolescent boys; dependence and abuse occur in only a small portion of individuals who use inhalants

C. Co-morbidities

  1. Any general medical or surgical condition may coexist with a psychiatric or substance-related disorder.

  2. The presence of a psychiatric or substance-related disorder may complicate the diagnosis or treatment of general medical conditions.

    a. Patient's inability to identify or report physical symptoms

    b. Patient's exaggeration of physical symptoms

    c. Patient's ability to comply with treatment regimens

  3. Some general medical conditions may cause psychiatric symptoms (Kaplan & Sadock, 1990).

    a. Connective tissue diseases

    b. Endocrine and metabolic

    c. Gastrointestinal

    d. Hematologic

    e. Infections

   f. Neoplasias
   g. Neurologic
   h. Nutritional
D. The role of prescription and over-the-counter medications in causing psychiatric symptoms
   1. Anxiety
   2. Depression
   3. Delirium, hallucinations, paranoia
   4. Sexual dysfunction
E. Screening for behavioral health disorders (Small, 1991)
   1. General medical evaluations to rule out physiologic causes of symptoms. Tests recommended are specific to the behavioral health symptoms.
      a. Computed tomography (CT) and positron-emission tomography (PET) scans
      b. Electroencephalography (EEG)
      c. Evoked potential studies, computerized topographic brain mapping
      d. Endocrinologic studies
   2. Psychological and neuropsychological tests
      a. Beck Depression Inventory
      b. Hamilton Depression Inventory
      c. Thematic Apperception Test
      d. Rorschach Test
      e. Minnesota Multiphasic Personality Inventory
      f. Sentence Completion Tests
      g. Self-Administered Alcoholism Screening Test
      h. Conners Parent-Teacher Rating Scale
      i. Child Behavior Checklist
   3. Community screening
      a. PrimeMD—a tool developed by Pfizer Pharmaceuticals to assist primary care providers in screening for depression, anxiety, and other behavioral health disorders.
      b. SF-36—a tool to determine the severity of behavioral health symptoms and their effects on functionality and the sense of well-being.
F. Sources of case management referral
   1. Forensic and legal—e.g., domestic violence
   2. Payors and managed care
      a. Primary care ("carve in")—a system wherby health care services are managed within the network of practitioners and providers who supply all other health care services.
      b. Specialty care ("carve out")—a system whereby behavioral health care services are managed separately from other health care services under a separate and distinct insurance benefit allowance.
      c. Disease management programs

3. Employers and employee assistance programs (EAPs)

4. Community agencies

G. The need for case management in behavioral health care—Stigma concerning severe psychiatric and substance-related disorders still exists. Behavioral health case managers coordinate care among various caregivers, treatment providers, and practitioners and identify community resources available.

■ KEY DEFINITIONS

A. Behavioral health care—Evaluation and treatment of psychological and substance abuse disorders (National Committee for Quality Assurance, 1997)

B. Dependence—A cluster of physiologic, cognitive, and behavioral symptoms caused by repeated self-administration of substances, resulting in tolerance, withdrawal, and compulsive drug-taking behaviors (*DSM-IV*, 1994)

C. Substance abuse—A maladaptive pattern of substance use manifested by recurrent and significant adverse consequences within a 12-month period. Adverse consequences may include failure to fulfill major role obligations, using substances despite obvious physical hazards (e.g., driving under the influence), legal problems resulting from substance use, or recurrent social or interpersonal problems (*DSM-IV*, 1994).

D. Personality disorder—An enduring pattern of experience and behavior that deviates significantly from the expectations of the individual's culture; is pervasive, inflexible, and stable; and leads to distress or impairment. There are 11 personality disorders identified in *DSM-IV*.

E. *DSM-IV* (*Diagnostic and Statistical Manual of Mental Disorders,* 4th ed.)—Manual that describes the various psychiatric, psychological, and substance-related disorders categorically. The *DMS-IV* identifies diagnostic and associated features, differential diagnoses, and incidence and prevalence of disorders, and describes the course of illnesses. The *DMS-IV* codes and terms are compatible with ICD-9-CM and ICD-10. This manual promotes the multiaxial system of diagnosis that includes the clinical disorder that is the focus of treatment, associated personality disorders, general medical conditions, psychosocial and environmental problems, and a Global Assessment of Functioning for each patient (*DSM-IV*, 1994).

F. Psychopharmacology—The use of drugs and medications specifically prescribed to reduce, control, or eliminate the symptoms of a psychiatric or substance-related disorder (Calandra, 1995).

■ COMMONLY OCCURRING BEHAVIORAL HEALTH CARE CONDITIONS AND THEIR IMPLICATIONS FOR CASE MANAGEMENT

A. Disorders of childhood—attention deficit/hyperactivity disorder (ADD/ADHD)

1. Subtypes may be inattentive type or hyperactive-impulsive type. These patients display inattentiveness or hyperactivity, or both, that frequently causes disruption in family, school, or occupational settings.

Fidgeting and other inappropriate activity in a school setting can cause academic problems. Behavioral dysfunction and other symptoms tend to worsen in situations that demand sustained attention or mental effort or that lack novelty or stimulate interest for the patient. Behavioral dysfunction can be disruptive to others and result in frustration on the part of parents, teachers, and other caregivers. The low self-esteem created by this illness can cause patients to act out in the home, school, work, and social settings. This disorder often coexists with conduct disorders, oppositional defiant disorder, and certain developmental disorders.

2. ADD/ADHD is usually diagnosed in the early elementary school years. Symptoms typically lessen in the adolescent and early adult years but may continue into mid-adulthood.

3. This condition is primarily seen in the primary care setting and can often be adequately managed by the pediatrician. Medications such as psychostimulants reduce symptoms in about 75% of patients, causing improvement in self-esteem and enhanced rapport with parents and teachers. Antidepressants, antipsychotics, or lithium are used if other medications fail and if symptoms are very severe or in cases of acutely aggressive behavior. Psychiatric care is generally sought in more severe cases and almost always involves behavioral therapy for both the patient and the family for support, education, and structure. The school must be alert to the needs of the child with respect to medication administration, consistency, and limit setting.

B. Mood disorders

1. Major depressive disorder

   a. Patients with this condition display a depressed mood or loss of interest or pleasure in almost all activities for at least 2 weeks. Additional symptoms such as weight changes, changes in sleeping patterns, changes in psychomotor activity, persistent feelings of guilt or worthlessness, difficulty concentrating or thinking, impairment of social or occupational role expectations, or suicidal ideation may also be present. The depressed patient may present for evaluation or treatment following a suicide attempt, and all depressed patients should be considered "at risk" for suicide. Depression in children is often seen as irritability rather than a sad mood.

   b. Major depressive disorder is diagnosed by a careful interview, including personal and family history. At present, there are no laboratory findings diagnostic of major depressive disorder. Alcohol or other substance abuse can mask symptoms of this disorder. Patients may abuse substances in an attempt to "self-medicate" symptoms.

   c. Major depressive disorder can last 6 months or longer if left untreated. Once the diagnosis has been established, treatment generally consists of a combination of antidepressant medications and supportive psychotherapy. Some patients find the support and structure of group psychotherapy beneficial, especially if social dysfunction has occurred as a result of depression. The patient's family members should be educated about the disease and alerted to signs of recurrence. Clinicians and case managers should be vigilant about the suicide risk in these patients and be watchful of signs that a patient is considering suicide. Clinicians should not hesitate to ask patients if they are considering suicide or self-harm. Patients may demonstrate increased suicide potential by giving away belongings, making a will, saying goodbye to loved ones, or hoarding medications. In many patients, suicidal ideation is not predictable, and there is no mechanism available to determine which patients will attempt or complete suicide. Some patients act on suicidal ideation after initiating treatment for depression, when energy levels begin to improve.

2. Bipolar disorders

  a. Recurrent and episodic experiences of hypomanic or manic episodes, during which patients may be hyperactive, hyperverbal, irritable, insomniac, distractible, agitated, and grandiose, and experience flight of thoughts and ideas, characterize this class of disorders. Sixty to seventy percent of manic episodes occur following an episode of major depression in a cyclical fashion. Psychotic symptoms may develop in some patients.

  b. This disorder is diagnosed by careful interview and history, as are most psychiatric disorders. These patients are at risk for suicide or self-harm during either the depressed phase or the manic or hypomanic phase.

  c. Treatment consists primarily of symptom control with mood-stabilizing medications such as lithium carbonate. Patients whose symptoms are not controlled by lithium carbonate may respond to antipsychotic or anticonvulsant medications. Compliance with medical therapy should be monitored and addressed by case managers. These patients may not like the loss of euphoria produced when mood is stabilized and may fail to comply with treatment. Many of the drugs prescribed for bipolar disorder must be carefully monitored by blood level determinations, which can be disruptive to patients.

C. Substance abuse disorders

1. Alcohol-related disorders

  a. Alcohol dependence is physiologic dependence characterized by evidence of tolerance (needing more of the substance to produce a desired effect) and withdrawal when administration of the substance is discontinued (a syndrome that may include sweating, tachycardia, hand tremor, insomnia, nausea or vomiting, agitation, anxiety, hallucinations, or grand mal seizures). Delirium tremens may be considered a more severe form of withdrawal and is considered to be a medical emergency.

  b. These disorders are diagnosed by history, physical examination, and interview. The condition can go undiagnosed if the patient continues to use alcohol and no withdrawal symptoms are observed. Over time, the patient may be increasingly unable to fulfill occupational or social expectations, which may cause distress.

  c. Treatment consists of abstinence from alcohol, supportive psychotherapy and education, and community support services such as Alcoholics Anonymous. Patients whose withdrawal symptoms are severe may need to be hospitalized or observed by trained clinicians during initial alcohol detoxification to achieve abstinence safely. Some patients respond well to the administration of disulfiram (Antabuse), which promotes enforced sobriety by producing a very unpleasant reaction when used in conjunction with alcohol and is a deterrent to alcohol abuse for some patients. Antidepressants, mood stabilizers, and antipsychotics are not indicated unless the patient presents with symptoms of other mental disorders when abstinent and sober.

2. Cocaine-related disorders
   a. Cocaine and its derivatives are available in a variety of forms. Crack cocaine, or rock cocaine, is smoked. Cocaine powder can also be inhaled or "snorted" or mixed with water and injected. Cocaine may be used with other drugs such as heroin. Cocaine is a powerful euphoric and can produce dependence very quickly. Because of the rapid onset of dependence and associated tolerance, individuals who use cocaine may become involved in criminal activities in order to acquire the drug. Chronic use may lead to paranoid ideation, anxiety, weight loss, sleep disturbances, depression, and a variety of psychosocial disturbances. Withdrawal symptoms are associated with high-dose use and are generally transitory. Dysphoria is the most common withdrawal symptom observed.
   b. Diagnosis is made by interview and history. Physical examination may reveal damage to nasal passages in patients who snort cocaine.
   c. Treatment involves abstinence, education, and support. Patients typically do not require detoxification, but occasionally patients may experience acute depression during withdrawal. These patients should be observed for suicidal ideation. Occasionally, a patient will require antidepressant medications.

D. Anxiety disorders/panic disorders/post-traumatic stress disorder
   1. Generalized anxiety disorders
      a. Anxiety is a pathologic state characterized by a pervasive feeling of dread accompanied by somatic signs. This disorder is characterized by chronic, generalized anxiety. Anxiety is differentiated from fear, which is a response to a known cause or threat.
      b. Anxiety disorders are diagnosed by interview and history. Psychological testing is occasionally helpful. There are no laboratory tests for anxiety. Clinical evaluation should include examination to rule of general medical conditions such as angina pectoris, hyperthyroidism, hypoglycemia, and hyperventilation syndrome, which can mimic anxiety.
      c. Treatment involves psychopharmacology. Anxiolytics and some antidepressant medications are effective. Psychotherapy is useful in patients to improve insight into anxiety-producing conflicts. Cognitive-behavioral therapy and group therapy provide support, symptom relief, and behavior change. Patients with anxiety often experience depression as well. These patients should be observed for suicidal ideation.

2. Post-traumatic stress disorder (PTSD)

   a. This disorder is a type of anxiety disorder produced by an extraordinary life stress. This event is relived in dreams and intrusive thoughts. These patients may experience sleep disturbances, hypervigilance, exaggerated startle response, or psychogenic amnesia for the event.

   b. Diagnosis is made by interview and history.

   c. Treatment is similar to that used for patients with generalized anxiety disorder.

3. Obsessive-compulsive disorder

   a. Recurrent intrusive ideas, impulses, obsessional thinking, and repetitive, compulsive behavior patterns are the hallmark of this disorder. If the patient attempts to ignore the intrusive thought or to curb compulsive behavior, his or her anxiety becomes intolerable.

   b. The disorder is diagnosed by interview and history. Patients often recognize that their behaviors or obsessions are unreasonable but feel powerless to stop them. Distress occurs when these activities and behaviors become excessively time consuming or interfere with the person's ability to function in role-appropriate situations.

   c. Treatment is the same as that used for patients with generalized anxiety disorder.

4. Panic disorders

   a. This disorder is characterized by spontaneous attacks of overwhelming anxiety and dread. Panic attacks may be associated with agoraphobia. During a panic attack, the patient may experience such severe autonomic hyperactivity that he or she fears that death will occur. These attacks are so frightening to patients that anticipatory anxiety may occur because the patient fears the attack.

   b. Diagnosis is made by interview and history.

   c. Treatment is the same as that used for patients with generalized anxiety disorder.

E. Eating disorders

   1. Anorexia nervosa

      a. This disorder is characterized by an intense fear of gaining weight or of becoming fat, which results in a body weight 15% or more below expected normals. The patient's perception of his or her actual body weight is disturbed to a significant degree. Women may experience amenorrhea. Anorexics are rigid, self-deprecating, obsessional, and anxious. Anorexia seems to be a reaction to demands for independence or social and sexual functioning in adolescence. This disorder is potentially fatal (5% to 12%) secondary to starvation.

      b. The diagnosis is made by history, interview, and physical examination to rule out general medical causes.

      c. Treatment modalities may depend on the degree of weight loss and associated physical conditions. Inpatient treatment may be necessary for reversal of potentially life-threatening effects of starvation. These patients resist medications, and, in fact, no drugs have proved effective with anorexics. Antidepressants or anxiolytics may relieve depression or anxiety. Cognitive-behavioral therapy seems to be the most promising when it is aimed at changing attitudes and habits concerning food, eating, and body image. Family therapy is helpful, especially when the identified patient is an adolescent.

2. Bulimia nervosa

   a. This disorder is characterized by recurrent episodes of binge eating; a feeling of lack of control over eating behaviors; overconcern with body shape and body weight; and episodic purging with laxatives, self-induced vomiting, laxatives or diuretics, dieting, or excessive exercise.

   b. This disorder is diagnosed by history, interview, and physical examination. Many patients have signs of self-induced vomiting, including lacerations of fingers, dental abnormalities, and often severe abnormalities of electrolytes. The patient may actually have normal, or near-normal, body weight on examination. Depression, anxiety, shoplifting (food), and alcohol abuse are often associated with bulimia.

   c. Treatment for bulimia nervosa may include hospitalization for patients with extreme metabolic disturbances. Psychopharmacology is generally more effective for bulimics than for anorexics. Antidepressants are the agent of choice for most patients. Psychological treatment is aimed at normalizing eating habits, attitudes about food, and perceptions of the "ideal" body image. Patients respond best to a combination of individual cognitive-behavioral therapy and group psychotherapy.

F. Schizophrenia

   1. This disorder is characterized by psychotic symptoms that impair functioning and involve disturbances in feeling, thinking, and behavior. The patient may experience delusions, hallucinations, loosening of associations, social withdrawal, absence of motivation, inappropriate affect, agitation or catatonia, and disorientation.

   2. This condition is diagnosed by observation, history, and interview. Five different types of schizophrenia have been identified. They are differentiated by the predominant symptom clusters.

   3. Treatment for schizophrenia may involve hospitalization for acute management, antipsychotic medications, psychosocial treatments to improve social skills, and rehabilitation. Antipsychotics are often required life-long for maintenance. Some antipsychotics are available in "depot" form requiring an intramuscular injection every few weeks. This form is most widely recommended for patients who may not be compliant with daily dosing regimens. Most antipsychotics have side effects, and some schizophrenic patients discontinue medication if the side effects are intolerable, causing relapse. Some side effects abate over time and must be tolerated by the patient in the short term. Other side effects can be life threatening, and patients and caregivers must be educated about them and about how to access emergency treatment, if necessary. The goal of antipsychotic treatment is to give the

smallest dose of the medication that relieves symptoms with the fewest possible side effects. Compliance with treatment and reintegration of schizophrenic patients into the community is a challenge for case managers.

G. Adjustment disorders

1. This disorder is characterized by an abnormal behavioral response to a psychosocial stressor. The stressor, occurring within 3 months before the onset of symptoms, is an otherwise normal life experience such as the birth of a child, marriage, illness, divorce, or job loss. The patient may experience depression, anxiety, occupational or academic problems, disturbance of conduct, physical complaints, or social withdrawal. Symptoms do not persist longer than 6 months.

2. Adjustment disorder is diagnosed by history and patient interview.

3. Treatment involves psychotherapy to provide support, to teach new or alternative coping skills, and to help the patient understand the meaning of the stressor to him or her. Infrequently, the patient who experiences debilitating depression or anxiety may benefit from short-term pharmacotherapy.

H. Personality disorders (Raderstorf, 1995)

1. These disorders are characterized by enduring maladaptive patterns of behavioral, emotional, cognitive, perceptual, or psychodynamic functioning. Eleven personality disorders have been identified, and each disorder has different psychodynamics and presenting symptoms. The implications for case managers vary by type of disorder. The group of odd or eccentric personality disorders (paranoid, schizoid, schizotypal) includes patients who avoid others, are mistrustful, and describe odd or "magical" belief systems. The group of dramatic, emotional, and erratic personality disorders (histrionic, narcissistic, antisocial, borderline) includes patients who do not recognize the rights of others, demonstrate impulsivity and disturbances of conduct, have poor or absent interpersonal relationships, may self-mutilate or engage in suicidal threats or gestures, and present as highly dramatic or grandiose. The anxious, fearful personality disorders (obsessive-compulsive, avoidant, dependent, passive-aggressive) include patients who are perfectionistic and inflexible, shy and submissive, and who demonstrate procrastination, obstructionism, and stubbornness.

2. These disorders are diagnosed by history, interview, and, occasionally, projective or neuropsychological testing.

3. It is extremely difficult to treat these patients owing to the ingrained behavior and thought patterns and their general resistance to treatment. Noncompliance or marginal compliance may result. Treatment may include pharmacology such as low-dose antipsychotics (especially in the odd, eccentric groups and patients with borderline personality disorder). Individual psychotherapy may be supportive or insight-oriented, depending on the type of disorder observed and the patient's ego strength. Some patients respond well to group therapy; however, individuals with paranoid personality disorder do not do well in a group setting. Hospitalization is sometimes necessary as a cri-

sis intervention methodology, especially with borderline patients who self-mutilate or make suicidal gestures. Patients with antisocial personality disorders may experience legal and other societal sanctions.

■ TREATMENT METHODOLOGY

A. Hospitalization—Used for treatment of acute conditions in which the patient is in danger of harming himself or herself or others, or is unable to care for himself or herself owing to psychiatric symptoms. Hospitalization is the most restrictive type of treatment for behavioral health conditions. Hospitalization is occasionally used to initiate new medications when the patient must be observed closely for potentially life-threatening side effects. This treatment modality is used for acute detoxification from substances with which the potential for severe withdrawal symptoms exists. Laws governing involuntary short- or long-term confinement differ from state to state, and case managers must be aware of individual state laws and restrictions. The case manager's role during and following hospitalization is identifying the patient's needs for post-hospital follow-up and maximizing the potential for patient compliance.

B. Partial hospitalization—This treatment modality involves the patient for 4 hours or more per day in a structured setting. Patients receive milieu therapy, psychoeducation, and individual and group therapies. Partial hospitalization may be used as an alternative to inpatient hospitalization for the patient who has a strong community support system, is not deemed to be an acute suicidal risk, and who requires close supervision of medication effects. Case management's role in patients enrolled in a partial hospital program includes knowledge of how to access emergency treatment for the patient and development and implementation of an aftercare plan.

C. Ambulatory care—Outpatient and intensive outpatient treatment are effective for patients whose conditions can be managed outside of a structured setting. Individual, group, family, and couples therapy are delivered in this setting. Patients' medications can be monitored effectively on an ambulatory basis once dosages are stabilized. Case management's role in ambulatory care may be minimal. The case manager and patient should be aware of how to access emergency services if the patient's symptoms should worsen, if he or she experiences suicidal thoughts or impulses, or if intolerable or potentially dangerous medication side effects occur.

D. Pharmacotherapy—Medications are prescribed by a physician to treat or relieve symptoms of behavioral health disorders. The role of case managers in pharmacotherapy is to ensure that the patient has sufficient access to medications (benefits, pharmacy availability, finances), to be alert for possible noncompliance with medication administration, and to be cognizant of potential side effects that may not be observed by the patient or caregiver. The case manager must be aware of which side effects require emergency treatment, which should be reported to the physician, and which might be dose or duration related (Puzantian & Stimmel, 1994).

E. Support groups—Community support services are available in many communities. Alcoholics Anonymous, Narcotics Anonymous, CHADD (support services for families of patients with attention deficit disorder), and others are available. Access to support services is often available at no, or minimal, cost to the group member. Support groups provide education, emotional support, socialization skills, and empathy for patients and families experiencing behavioral health problems. The advent of the Internet and World Wide Web has made some support systems available on-line. This is useful when no such support exists in the community; however, patients who tend to isolate themselves from others should not be encouraged to use on-line support services when community services are accessible.

■ ASSESS FOR HIGH-RISK BEHAVIORAL HEALTH DISORDERS

A. Suicidality—Potentially, all patients with psychiatric and substance-related disorders are at risk for suicide. Suicide tends to occur in clusters in the spring and summer and with media attention. At present, the population at highest risk for suicide is the elderly white man who is a widower. Although women attempt suicide more often than men, men are more often successful suicides. Men tend to use more violent methods than women. The most predictive suicide risk is a past history of a suicide attempt; approximately 50% of patients will repeat an initial attempt and 10% of patients will eventually succeed. Other predictive risk factors include nationality (Eastern Europeans, Scandinavians, Japanese), psychiatric diagnosis (major depression, bipolar disorder, psychosis and schizophrenia, substance-related disorders, antisocial and borderline personality, organic disorders, panic disorder), and age, with elderly patients being most common. Recent stressors, illnesses, unemployment or job stress, and positive family history of suicide increase the risk. The most conservative approach is to admit the patient who is at risk for suicide when there is any doubt about his or her safety. The implications for case management with these patients are the need to develop an effective support system within the family and community to manage emergency situations, and to provide support and safety for the patient.

B. Violence—Closely related to suicidality is the patient who is at risk for violence. Signs of impending violence include a recent violent act, alcohol or substance intoxication, verbal or physical threats, presence of a weapon, patients responding to command hallucinations, paranoid patients, patients with organic mental disorders affecting the frontal lobe, certain patients with mania or agitated depression, and patients with personality disorders prone to rage or impulse dyscontrol. These patients require crisis intervention in order to protect themselves and others. The involuntary placement of these patients on locked psychiatric units, when necessary, can increase the patient's anger and aggressivity. Physical restraints, medications, and avoidance of provocative situations are helpful. Behavioral disorders can sometimes lead to domestic violence. Victims of domestic violence may not report behaviors for a variety of reasons (Cole, 1999). Some clinicians feel reluctant to question possible victims of domestic violence because of the ongoing threat of violence to the victim, powerlessness to provide services, lack of knowledge about community services, or overburdened community support services.

C. Recidivism—Relapse and return to acute care occurs when the patient is noncompliant with treatment, when the patient's support system is unable to manage his or her needs, or when a stressor exacerbates a chronic condition. Some illnesses, such as substance-related disorders, mood disorders, and the psychoses, are characterized by relapse and recurrence. These episodes can be devastating to the patient and the family, who experience a sense of failure and loss of self-esteem. The noncompliant patient who repeatedly relapses generates anger and frustration, not only in the family, support system, and other caregivers but also in his treatment staff. The implications for case management are to manage the acute phase of illness and treatment, monitor compliance with aftercare plans, be aware of the needs of the patient for independence, and be aware of the needs of the patient who seeks the comfort and security of an acute care setting. Mobilizing frustrated and exhausted support services for a patient with a history of recidivism may be a challenge for the case manager (Curtis, Millman, Struening, & D'Ercole, 1994–1995).

D. Dual diagnosis—Assessment and diagnosis of patients with dual diagnosis (psychiatric and substance-related disorders) can be difficult. A patient who presents for treatment under the influence of mind-altering substances may not be accurately diagnosed until the effects of the substance have been eliminated. Until this is possible, the patient must be treated symptomatically and conservatively, with the health care staff providing a safe environment while observing for symptoms of psychiatric disorders. Common dual-diagnosis situations include the patient with generalized anxiety disorder or panic who abuses alcohol to reduce feelings of anxiety, or the depressed patient who uses cocaine to relieve symptoms of depression. The patient, once accurately diagnosed, must receive treatment for both disorders concurrently. Many dual-diagnosis treatment programs have been established in clinics to meet the needs of these patients. The psychiatrist who prescribes anxiolytic medications for a dually diagnosed patient must be aware of the potential for abuse of the medication. The addictionologist must be cognizant of the "normal" sad affect experienced by some patients who are recovering from alcohol or drug dependence, or both, and be able to distinguish this condition from an acute mood disorder that may require pharmacologic intervention. All treatment practitioners must be alert to the potential for suicide in this population.

■ **EVALUATE TREATMENT EFFECTIVENESS IN BEHAVIORAL HEALTH**

A. Prevention
   1. Grief counseling following death or divorce may lessen the patient's pathologic reaction to this "normal" stressor and provide preventive

treatment. Supportive treatment helps to provide patients experiencing prolonged grief with an emotional outlet. The goal of case management in these circumstances is early identification of cases and to mobilize and provide access to resources.

2. Emergency evaluation and counseling following "disaster"—Evidence suggests that emergency assessment and treatment of victims of disasters and extraordinary stressors, such as hurricane, rape, or fire that destroys a home, can alleviate or minimize resultant inappropriate behavioral, emotional, or cognitive reactions. Short-term use of antidepressants may be indicated in certain situations. Ongoing supportive therapy is indicated after initial crisis resolution. The goal of case management in these situations is early identification of circumstances that may require this type of intervention and to mobilize and provide access to necessary resources.

3. The role of psychopharmacology—Most clinicians agree that the majority of patients suffering from a psychiatric or substance-related disorder cannot fully benefit from pharmacology alone. The long-term effects on occupational, familial, and social roles of a behavioral disorder need to be managed. The patient may need social skills retraining and supportive therapy to prevent relapse or develop a support network, develop adequate coping skills, and improve confidence and trust. Pharmacologic interventions alone may be used when the patient has not experienced any disruption in his or her role behaviors, but this is uncommon. Pharmacology in conjunction with supportive individual or group follow-up or cognitive behavioral therapies has shown to produce the best outcome. The case manager's role in pharmacotherapy is to evaluate for noncompliance and to intervene if noncompliance does occur. The patient who dislikes the side effects of a medication may be tempted to discontinue it without permission of the prescribing physician. The patient may need education about short-term side effects that are likely to dissipate or may need referral back to the physician for a medication adjustment or change.

4. Awareness programs (DARE, MADD)—These types of programs create awareness of behavioral health disorders in the general community. Some groups raise and provide funds for educational programs and government lobbying efforts. The purpose of these programs is to reduce the incidence of new cases.

B. Acute care, including psychopharmacology, hospitalization, partial hospitalization, brief psychotherapy, and intensive group psychotherapy, is considered effective if a patient is prevented from committing suicide, is adequately and effectively matched with appropriate resources for follow-up care, and has symptoms under sufficient control to move to the next least restrictive treatment setting.

C. Long-term care, including psychopharmacology, state hospitalization, support groups, and community agencies, is effective if the patient's potential for recidivism is minimized. This process requires the coordinated efforts of case managers, support services, practitioners, and caregivers, as well as the patient himself or herself.

- **UNDERSTAND THE ROLE OF ALTERNATIVE AND COMPLEMENTARY MEDICINE (ACM) IN THE TREATMENT OF BEHAVIORAL HEALTH DISORDERS**

    A. Causative factor—The use of ACM in some patients can actually cause certain psychiatric symptoms such as euphoria, anorexia, agitation, or depression. Herbs, minerals, and other compounds can easily be purchased at the local nutrition center. Patients who present with psychiatric symptoms should be asked about the use of ACM and other over-the-counter products that are known to cause psychiatric symptoms.

    B. Self-care and self-help—Because of the increasing availability of medical advice via the Internet, popular media, and direct-to-consumer advertising by pharmaceutical companies, patients are increasingly more knowledgeable about treatment alternatives. Often, the patient presents to the physician and requests a particular drug or therapy regimen before being examined. The patient who is already "sold" on the notion of one type of treatment may be reluctant to accept an alternative type, even when presented with medical evidence to support the advantages of one treatment over another. Similarly, patients who are averse to the use of pharmacotherapy because of their known potential for side effects may not accept a recommendation to try pharmacotherapy.

- **INSURANCE COVERAGE AND FINANCIAL ASSISTANCE**

    Employer-funded insurance plans, managed care plans, and other types of health insurance plans may offer different benefits for behavioral health care than for other general medical conditions. The number of visits allowed may be limited, or there may be a dollar limitation on coverage imposed. The pharmacy benefit or the formulary used by the individual carrier may not include the patient's drug regimen. The implications for the case manager in this type of payment arrangement are to maximize the use of scarce resources. Most managed care plans require that proposed treatment be "medically necessary and appropriate" for the diagnosis. Long-term treatment that is not aimed at relieving symptoms, promoting return to premorbid functioning, or effecting the development of a coordinated support and aftercare system may not be approved. Palliative treatment or treatment that is for the convenience of the practitioner or family members may not be considered medically necessary. Occasionally, however, caregivers need respite from the care of a chronically ill patient. The case manager should explore resources to provide such a respite, as well as supportive services and community resources for the caregivers.

- **THE BEHAVIORAL HEALTH PATIENT AND THE EMPLOYER**

    A. Ninety percent of substance abusers are employed.

    B. Americans with Disabilities Act

    C. Employee assistance programs

REFERENCES

Calandra, J. (1995). New frontiers in psychopharmacology. *American Journal of Continuing Education in Nursing, 7,* 46–56.

Cole, T. B. (1999). Case management for domestic violence. *Journal of the American Medical Association, 282*(6), 513–514.

Curtis, J. L., Millman, E. J., Struening, E., & D'Ercole, A. (1994–1995). Effect of case management on rehospitalization and utilization of ambulatory case services. *Hospital and Community Psychiatry, 43*(9), 895–899.

Diagnostic and statistical manual of mental disorders (4th ed.}. (1994). Washington, D.C.: American Psychiatric Association.

Kaplan, H.I. & Sadock, B.J. (1990). *Pocket handbook of clinical psychiatry.* Baltimore: Williams & Wilkins.

National Committee for Quality Assurance. (1997). *Accreditation guidelines for managed behavioral healthcare organizations.* Washington, D.C.: NCQA.

Puzantian, T. & Stimmel, G. L. (1994). Review of psychotropic drugs. *Pharmacy Practice News.*

Raderstorf, M. (1995). *Personality disorders and their impact on case management.* Minneapolis, MN: Mark Raderstorf and Associates

Small, S. M. (1991). *Outline for psychiatric examination.* Buffalo, NY: State University of New York at Buffalo.

CHAPTER 15

• • • • • • • • • •

Maternal-Infant Case Management

LORI A. DAVIS
PAT ORCHARD

LEARNING OBJECTIVES

Upon completion of this chapter, the reader will be able to:

1. Identify components of maternal-infant case management.
2. Define important terms in maternal-infant case management.
3. Identify specific skills for case managers in maternal-infant case management.
4. Outline essential knowledge areas for case managers in maternal-infant case management.

IMPORTANT TERMS AND CONCEPTS

Betamethasone
Fetal Heart Rate Monitoring
Gestational Diabetes
Health Maintenance Organizations (HMO)
Home Uterine Activity Monitoring (HUAM)
Hyperemesis Gravidarum
Multifetal Pregnancies
Placenta Previa
Predisposing Factors to Preterm Labor
Preeclampsia
Pregnancy

Premature Rupture of Membranes
(PROM)
Preterm Birth
Prostaglandin
Tocolytic Therapy
Total Parenteral Nutrition (TPN)
Trimester
Vaginal Birth After Cesarean Section
(VBAC)
Viable

■ INTRODUCTION TO MATERNAL-INFANT CASE MANAGEMENT

A. Maternal and newborn care are two of the leading health plan expense categories in the United States, accounting for an estimated 27% of hospital admissions, 25% to 33% of hospital costs, and 10% to 49% of health plan costs.

B. Maternal-infant case management is not care management of an individual but of a family unit, more specifically a mother-child unit.

C. In maternal-infant care management, our task begins at conception and continues throughout pregnancy, birth, and the post-delivery phase.

D. The quality of a child's future depends on many factors, not the least of which include the physical and psychological conditions of pregnancy.

E. Identifying women at risk for the development of problems can begin with care from a primary care physician, but often care is not sought until pregnancy is determined. This is where the role of the maternal-infant case manager begins.

■ KEY DEFINITIONS

A. Betamethasone—A steroid given to a pregnant woman to aid in fetal lung development in anticipation of preterm birth.

B. Gestational diabetes—A carbohydrate intolerance that is diagnosed during pregnancy in which the blood sugar levels are elevated. The condition is usually controlled by diet; however, insulin may also be required. The condition usually resolves after delivery.

C. Home uterine activity monitor (HUAM)—A portable and compact monitor that records uterine activity and transmits data via telephone to the perinatal home care provider. Normally, this is not a continuous activity but is done intermittently at frequencies prescribed by the physician or when the mother feels the presence of contractions.

D. Hyperemesis gravidarum—Excessive vomiting during pregnancy; may lead to dehydration and possible starvation.

E. Multifetal pregnancies—A pregnancy of more than one fetus.

F. Placenta previa—A condition in which the placenta is implanted near or covering the cervix, which can result in bleeding and hemorrhage.

G. Preeclampsia—A complication of pregnancy, characterized by increasing hypertension, proteinuria, and generalized edema (toxemia).

H. Premature rupture of membranes (PROM)—Spontaneous rupture of the membranes that occurs more than 1 hour before the onset of labor. The term "premature" here only refers to the relationship with labor and not with gestational age.

I. Preterm birth—A birth occurring before the 37th week of gestation or 21 days before the estimated date of conception (EDC).

J. Preterm labor—Uterine activity accompanying cervical change, occurring between the 20th and 37th week of pregnancy.

K. Prostaglandin—A naturally occurring substance that causes strong contractions of the smooth muscle and dilation of certain vascular beds. It can be used in a gel form to soften the cervix before the induction or in suppository form (as a means of labor induction) for second-trimester pregnancy terminations.

L. Tocolytic therapy—Drug regimen given to decrease uterine activity and arrest the progression of preterm labor. May be given continuously through subcutaneous infusion or orally, although the oral route is usually given a trial before the subcutaneous method.

M. Trimester—Pregnancy is commonly broken down into trimesters: the first, second, and third months equal the first trimester; fourth, fifth, and sixth months are equal to the second trimester; and seventh, eighth, and ninth months are equal to the third trimester.

N. Vaginal birth after cesarean section (VBAC)—Vaginal delivery in a patient who has previously had a cesarean section.

O. Viable—Capable of sustaining life, usually a fetus that is 24 to 28 weeks of gestation; able to sustain life outside of the uterus.

■ ROLE OF THE MATERNAL-INFANT CASE MANAGER

A. The role of a case manager in the scope of maternal-infant health care can be a contributing factor to the well-being of a community.

B. A case management program that functions within the definition of case management as "a collaborative process which assesses, plans, implements, coordinates, monitors, and evaluates options and services to meet an individual's health needs through communications and available resources to promote quality, cost-effective outcomes," maternal-infant health care can have a significant impact on the health status, resource utilization, and future health care needs of a community.

C. The outcome of a healthy infant born to a healthy mother integrated successfully to a community with sufficient resources can validate a successful case management program.

D. With the proper tools, defined core competencies, and clinically experienced case managers, a maternal-infant case management program can be developed and implemented.

■ ASSESSMENT

A. When the case manager demonstrates the basic skills of understanding the physiologic and psychosocial events that occur during the antepartum, perinatal, and postpartum phases, performing the next skill of assessment will be logical and well defined to the case manager.

  1. The assessment phase allows the case manager to collect data through a series of interviews of the client that can be tied to the knowledge of the basic physiology and psychosocial events of the antepartum, perinatal, and postpartum phases of maternal-infant health care. There are many components of a maternal-infant assessment.

  2. Some behavioral components of the assessment process for a maternal-infant case management program should not be disregarded.

  3. These behaviors include the competencies of:

   a. Interviewing skills for collecting subjective data for the data base

    b. Listening and observation (if face to face) skills

    c. Communication and recording skills for a historical data base

    d. Sensitivity to preconceived ideas, languages, and cultural barriers

    e. Awareness of the case manager's personal attitudes and beliefs

4. When the case manager demonstrates successful competencies of the so-called soft skills of assessment, the development of the data base will allow him or her to assess the needs of the client through the gathering of physical, social, psychological, and historical information.

B. The framework of assessment for a maternal-infant case management program is built around the collection of multiple data elements, both historical and current.

C. Gathering of objective and subjective data should be included in the data base collection instrument.

D. Objective data items collected include physician office visit findings, diagnostic and laboratory test results, the client's current health status, family history, psychosocial history, activities of daily living, and review of systems.

E. Subjective data items collected include a client's personal perspective of past history.

F. The subjective and objective data collected allow the case manager to define the perceived issues with the objective findings. This will lead the case manager to the identification phase of any problems, concerns, or interventions, allowing the case manager to begin the planning phase.

■ KNOWLEDGE DOMAINS

A. Five major domains of essential case management knowledge have been identified and recognized as core knowledge areas used by practitioners across the essential activities and functions that constitute case management. These domains are

1. Coordination and service delivery
2. Physical and psychosocial aspects
3. Benefit systems and cost-benefit analysis
4. Community resources
5. Case management concepts

B. A core of any curriculum begins with the understanding and application of the basic components and skills required to apply the knowledge to practice. The defined basic components of a maternal-infant case management program include:

1. Knowledge of the anatomic changes to women that occur during the conception, antepartum, perinatal, and postpartum phases of pregnancy
2. Knowledge of the physiologic changes in women that occur during the conception, antepartum, and postpartum phases of pregnancy
3. Knowledge of fetal development phases during the conception and antepartum period of pregnancy

4. Knowledge of maternal and fetal nutrition
5. Knowledge of the phases of labor and delivery of the birthing process
6. Knowledge of the biologic and behavioral characteristics of the newborn infant
7. Knowledge of newborn nutritional needs
8. Knowledge of the psychosocial components of the childbearing family, including family dynamics, cultural context, and coping skills
9. Knowledge of the various risk factors of the antepartum, perinatal, and postpartum phases of maternal-infant health care
10. Knowledge of the pathophysiology of a high-risk pregnancy, including:
    a. Preeclampsia (toxemia)—occurs in 3% to 6% of all pregnancies
    b. Preterm labor and preterm birth—preterm birth occurs in 7% to 10% of all pregnancies
    c. Multifetal pregnancy—increasing occurrence with prevalence of infertility treatment
    d. Gestational diabetes—occurs in 3% to 12% of pregnancies
    e. Hyperemesis gravidarum—occurs in 0.7% to 2.1% of pregnancies
    f. Placenta previa
    g. Other preexisting physical conditions or diseases
11. Previous pregnancies with pathophysiology
12. Medical chronic disease and the effect of those diseases on pregnancy
13. Current pathologic "states" of pregnancy—hypertensive states, hemorrhage, preterm and post-term labor, and age-related conditions
14. Knowledge of social risks to the pregnancy state, including:
    a. Smoking, drug, and alcohol usage
    b. Community support and available resources
    c. Previous psychiatric disease
C. Many of these knowledge domains are developed through clinical experiences in a variety of health care and provider settings. These clinical experiences allow the development of knowledge of various treatment modes and outcomes.

■ CASE MANAGEMENT CONCEPTS

A. The basic concepts of case management, such as planning, monitoring, coordinating, directing, and evaluating the plan for results-oriented, cost-effective services, form a domain of the case management model.

B. In a maternal-infant case management program, the assessment and the formulation of issues, problems, or concerns lead to an individualized plan for the patient.

C. The case manager's ability to create a plan is included as a competency.

D. Planning requires input and agreement from multiple providers, community service agencies, and the client to set mutual goals.

E. To identify the appropriate interventions to reach the mutual goals, the case manager must translate the problem statements into a positive health statement and establish criteria to meet the mutual goals.

F. The health statements tied to possible interventions for the client will lead to the case management plan.

G. The communication, coordination, organizing, and directing of this plan through intervention remain a major function and required competency of a case manager in a maternal-infant case management program.

H. In a maternal-infant case management program, the case manager must plan for the physical, emotional, and psychosocial needs of the pregnant patient.
   1. Pregnancy affects the entire body of a woman and can produce a very different response from one client to another.

I. The assessment and plan of any pregnant patient must be made in the content of the maternal-fetal unit. The areas for planning include:
   1. Preparation and education of the patient on her physical changes and possible requirements
   2. Discussion of financial issues or concerns related to pregnancy and maternal-infant needs
   3. Review of the present and future effect on the patient in the performance of activities of daily living, including nutrition, exercise, travel, personal hygiene, sexual activity, smoking, alcohol, drugs (prescription, over-the counter, and recreational), and pets
   4. Outline of emotional changes related to changes of pregnancy from physical factors (e.g., hormone changes and body image) to the additional requirements of a new dependent, financial constraints, and family dynamics
   5. Consideration of psychosocial requirements of the pregnancy, such as changes in housing needs, occupational risks and consequences, religious and cultural practices, marital status, and age

J. The maternal-infant case management plan directs the appropriate interventions to direct the actions needed.
   1. A case manager should include in the maternal-infant plan:
      a. Therapeutic interventions
      b. Teaching and counseling interventions
      c. Monitoring and continued assessment interventions
      d. Referral interventions

K. The maternal-infant case manager directs and organizes the interventions for action.

L. There is coordination of activities, collaboration of resources, and monitoring of results from the interventions.

M. On completion of the activities, the maternal-infant case manager must evaluate the results.

1. Have the goals been met throughout the pregnancy?
   a. An example of this evaluation may be seen in the attending of physician appointments during the antepartum phase of the pregnancy.
   b. If the client cannot attend the required monthly antepartum visits, the case manager must be aware of this issue and plan accordingly.
   c. The plan may include several contingency items such as child care, transportation options, and financial resources.
   d. Through the case manager process, the case manager will assess and identify this issue, plan for the problem, and direct, monitor, and evaluate the outcomes of attendance at physician's appointments by the client.
   e. This continuous case management process by the case manager for simple to complex problems, concerns, or identified issues will allow for necessary changes in the plan, utilization of appropriate resources, and results-oriented, cost-effective services.

■ PHYSICAL AND PSYCHOSOCIAL ASPECTS

A. Understanding the interrelationships of the physical and psychosocial aspects of the maternal-infant client is a key competency for the case manager.

B. Previous clinical experience in a variety of settings where maternal-infant health care is delivered is a mandatory competency for the maternal-infant case manager.
   1. Competencies include:
      a. Knowledge of the genetic basis of inheritance, including the conception phase and gene transmission within families
      b. Knowledge of embryonic development and fetal maturation, including the various changes in the maternal anatomic systems
      c. Knowledge of a normal pregnancy and the outcomes that result when normal events do not occur
      d. Knowledge of the family-centered approach to maternal-infant care for the support of the mother and infant
      e. Knowledge of the cultural significance of childbearing for a variety of cultures
      f. Knowledge of the developmental tasks and mental process required for the mother to adapt to the maternal role, from accepting the pregnant state to the mother-child bonding period

C. The maternal-infant case manager's ability to blend the medical, psychological, social, and behavioral knowledge of the pregnant state into an effective plan will benefit the patients, both mother and child.

■ BENEFIT SYSTEMS AND COST–BENEFIT ANALYSIS

A. The outcome of a healthy infant and mother who are integrated into the community, using available and necessary resources that lead to a healthy family, is the goal of a maternal-infant case management program.

1. Unfortunately, the ideal outcome is not always possible.
2. However, with oversight, compliance, and education, positive pregnancy outcomes remain a viable goal of a maternal-infant case management program.
3. Additionally, the maternal-infant case management program can be used to differentiate the high-risk patient from the patient with a normal pregnancy.

B. Knowledge of various benefit plans allows the case manager to tie benefits to identified needs.
1. If there are no benefits available, the case manager will be competent to seek possible alternatives, explore various community resources, or work closely with funding sources for payment of the services needed.
2. The onset of preterm labor and the delivery of low-birth-weight infants has a significant financial impact on health care resources and an emotional impact on the family and community structure.
   a. The family may suffer additional stress if the infant is born prematurely and has congenital defects or develops chronic conditions as a result of prematurity.

C. Benefit analysis is essential for the maternal-infant case manager to provide the highest quality of care within the confines of the mother's resources.
1. Including a variety of educational and behavioral programs complements the case manager's interactions and enhances the potential for a healthy pregnancy and good outcome.
   a. Examples of this can be demonstrated in
      (i) A smoking cessation program
      (ii) A work-adjustment program
      (iii) A nutrition program for the pregnant woman
      (iv) A cost analysis of so-called add-on services, such as home intervention and education to decrease preterm births

D. The easiest way to maximize benefit potential while decreasing expenditures related to pregnancy and birth is through aggressive and consistent use of resources to identify and treat high-risk pregnancies.

■ COMMUNITY RESOURCES

A. A maternal-infant case management program is tied closely to the community.

B. The pregnant patient is encouraged to be involved in the community.

C. A maternal-infant case manager will be competent to:
1. Identify community resources within the neighborhood of the mother
2. Obtain community resource requirements for use by the client
3. Assess every woman for domestic violence, with the ability to provide appropriate counseling and referrals for abuse
4. Determine access to and availability of services for the educational needs of the pregnant patient within the community

5. Evaluate community transportation for access to health care facilities and physician's appointments

6. Determine the employer's involvement in work adaptations for the pregnant worker and the availability of such adaptations

7. Incorporate strategies into the community through educational programs, community volunteer outreach, and community coalitions of persons who seek positive outcomes for future children and families of that community

D. Education of the patient and significant others is another way of increasing the mother's support system and her awareness of ways to ensure a healthy baby.

1. Prenatal education classes are widely produced and available in most areas.

2. Many hospital facilities offer prenatal education as well as childbirth classes for a nominal fee, and often these classes are free.

3. Public health departments offer prenatal education.

4. Many nonprofit organizations within the community offer prenatal education as well.

5. Prepared childbirth classes or Lamaze classes are also offered by many of these groups.

6. For the post-delivery period, there are also centers that offer parenting classes, access to free or low-cost immunizations, car seats, and other services to help ensure a healthy baby.

E. Many health maintenance organizations offer prenatal screening and education programs.

1. Although it is not intended to replace a physician's office visit, prenatal education program, or other health care services, these programs often offer many good booklets, brochures, tapes, and other educational pieces to supplement programs already in place.

2. Many of these programs offer incentives to their plan participants for seeking prenatal care early, keeping monthly or bimonthly visits, or participating in their perinatal wellness program.

3. Incentives are also included for completing either a telephonic or written assessment tool that would help identify mothers at risk.

4. These assessment tools can be useful in obtaining an even more in-depth maternal history and often reveal potential complications or risk factors.

5. Drawbacks to these programs are that health plan participants are already inundated with free educational materials or feel that answering in-depth questions is an invasion of their privacy, even though it would ultimately benefit the pregnancy, mother, and child.

6. Many plan participants enroll in these programs because the incentives can be quite attractive.

   a. Incentives might include any combination of the following:

      (i) Waiver of deductibles or co-payments

      (ii) Gift certificates to local discount stores or specialty stores

      (iii) Coupons for formula or diapers

      (iv) Free homemaker visit following delivery to assist with housework

      (v) Baby blankets, bibs, diaper bags, and bottles

      (vi) Refrigerator magnets for emergency phone numbers

      (vii) Long-distance calling cards

      (viii) Phone hotline access to an experienced obstetrics nurse

■ COORDINATION AND SERVICE DELIVERY

A. Knowledge of perinatal services available is essential for the provision of services and treatment options.

B. Most often, the birth takes place at a hospital or birthing facility.

  1. According to several new laws, both state and federal, length of hospital or facility stay can no longer be mandated or incentivized by third-party payers or facilities for the reduction of health care spending.

    a. These laws mandate that the minimum stay be 72 hours for a routine, uncomplicated vaginal delivery.

    b. The minimum stay following a cesarean section is 96 hours, if it is uncomplicated.

    c. Earlier discharge is possible only if the physician and the mother agree on the discharge decision.

    d. Offering enticements for the mother to leave the hospital early, such as waiving co-payments or deductibles or offering free goods or services, also is not allowed.

    e. These laws were enacted as a direct result of the physician and consumer outcry regarding the movement to discharge mothers and infants within 24 hours after vaginal delivery.

C. When complications arise or a situation becomes high risk, the knowledge of available treatment options becomes key to providing cost-effective, quality care.

  1. Complications arising during pregnancy include:

    a. Hyperemesis gravidarum

    b. Preterm labor

    c. Gestational diabetes

    d. Multifetal pregnancies

    e. Placenta previa

    f. Preeclampsia

E. Treatment for complications does not always require an extended hospital stay.

  1. Some alternatives available that can be used include:

    a. HUAM for those mothers with preterm labor, multifetal pregnancy, or histories of preterm birth

      (i) HUAM—A portable and compact monitor that records uterine activity and transmits data by telephone to the perinatal home care provider.

(ii) Home uterine activity monitoring can be done with or without medication (i.e., tocolytics).

b. Subcutaneous medication therapy can be administered at home for several complications of pregnancy, such as:

(i) Metoclopramide (Reglan) therapy for hyperemesis

(ii) Terbutaline pump therapy for preterm labor (usually used after failure of oral tocolytic therapy)

(iii) Insulin pump therapy for diabetes

(iv) Anticoagulant therapy for coagulation disorders

c. Home nursing visits for administration of injections, nursing assessments, and monitoring, even if provided once daily or several times daily, can be a very cost-effective way of preventing preterm birth and its complications.

d. There are numerous other specialized perinatal services that can be provided at home safely and cost effectively.

e. Such services might not be warranted for most patients, but for a mother who is at high risk or on bed rest, they can be the deciding factor in a preterm or full-term delivery.

f. Examples of other perinatal home services include:

(i) Nonstress testing

(ii) Fetal heart rate monitoring

(iii) Betamethasone therapy

(iv) Dietary analysis

(v) Blood pressure monitoring

(vi) IV hydration therapy for hyperemesis gravidarum

(vii) Total parenteral nutrition (TPN) for severe hyperemesis gravidarum

(viii) Blood testing

g. Many of the services listed can be provided with electronic equipment that has a modem through which data can be transmitted to a center with trained professionals who can update the physician and alert him or her to potential problems.

h. Providers of the services listed should be highly experienced and qualified to provide such services.

(i) All home health providers are not equipped or qualified to take on the responsibility of perinatal care.

(ii) The nurses providing care should have several years of perinatal experience, preferably in labor and delivery, and neonatal and high-risk care, and be well trained to work with the technology at home.

(iii) It is a good idea to know your providers for perinatal care before you need them and be acquainted with the capabilities they have.

2. Coverage for these types of services is not always available; collaborating with the physician, payor source, and patient is essential.

a. It is easy to recognize the cost savings that these programs can establish, but home safety and the mother's ability to self-administer or receive therapies at home must be included in consideration.

   b. The cost savings might not be worth the risk involved; the advantages and disadvantages must be carefully weighed.

   c. A quality perinatal home health provider will also help you make these determinations.

■ PRETERM LABOR AND DELIVERY

A. Because of the prevalence of preterm labor, preterm delivery, and infant mortality and morbidity as a result of prematurity, early diagnosis and treatment is a top priority for the maternal-infant case manager regardless of whether you are a case manager for a health plan or a large birthing facility.

B. Preterm delivery occurs in 7% to 10% of all pregnancies and is a major cause of infant mortality and morbidity.

C. Premature births account for about 70% of infant deaths—about 28,000 each year.

D. Premature births account for about 50% of neurologic handicaps.

E. A study conducted by The Center for Risk Management and Insurance Research at Georgia State University and published by CIGNA in 1992 concluded that improving pregnancy outcomes from "extremely" preterm to "normal" preterm can reduce maternal-newborn charges from $89,426 to $36,134.

   1. Prolonging pregnancy to full term can further reduce charges to $11,209.

   2. The study consisted of 59,000 mother-infant pairs.

F. Predisposing factors to preterm labor include:

   1. Maternal age under 17 years and over 40 years

   2. Smoking

   3. Infections

      a. Chorioamniotis—an inflammatory response in the amniotic membranes, stimulated by organisms in the amniotic fluid, which then becomes infiltrated with polymorphonuclear leukocytes

      b. Pyelonephritis or kidney infection

   4. Previous preterm birth

   5. Placental problems such as abruptio placentae or placenta previa

   6. Lower socioeconomic status

   7. Uterine or cervical anomalies

   8. PROM

   9. Multifetal pregnancy

   10. Previous abdominal surgeries

   11. Chronic maternal conditions or diseases

G. Early detection is the key to preventing preterm birth and prolonging pregnancy.

   1. Many preterm births occur not because the treatment of preterm uterine activity is ineffective but because the early warning signs and symptoms are not recognized.

      a. The early warning signs of preterm labor are:

         (i) Uterine contractions—contractions that occur every 10 minutes or more than five contractions in 1 hour.

         (ii) Menstrual-type cramps—such cramps occur in the abdomen just above the pubic bone.

         (iii) Pelvic pressure—this sensation may feel as if the baby is pushing down and may come and go.

         (iv) Low dull backache—back pain is often a throbbing feeling.

         (v) Increase or change in vaginal discharge

         (vi) Pressure or pain in the lower abdomen, lower back, or thighs

         (vii) Abdominal cramps similar to severe gas pain, which may occur with or without diarrhea

H. Preventing preterm birth requires an effort by health care professionals at all levels, from the telephone triage nurse to the physician, to educate patients regarding preterm labor.

I. Frequent provider contact through office visits and the telephone is key to keeping lines of communication open with the patient throughout the pregnancy.

J. Risk assessments performed in the first trimester and repeated throughout pregnancy can lead to an early diagnosis of preterm labor.

K. If preterm labor is suspected, immediate treatment, lifestyle alteration, and ongoing education can prolong the pregnancy, particularly if these measures are combined with tocolytic therapies.

L. The goal of treatment for preterm labor is to prolong the pregnancy safely, with the end result being a healthy mother and child.

   1. Treatment options include the following in various combinations:

      a. Bed rest—most common and first step in reduction of contractions, although studies are inconclusive as far as efficacy

      b. Fluid overload

      c. Tocolysis with magnesium sulfate, terbutaline, ritodrine, indomethacin, or calcium channel blockers

      d. Restriction of sexual activity

M. General maturity milestone guidelines according to Creasy (1984):

   1. 24 to 27 weeks at birth—long-term intensive care is required and earliest chance of survival.

   2. 29 to 32 weeks at birth—survival rate increases dramatically, but intensive care is still required.

   3. 33 to 37 weeks at birth—suck-swallow reflex matures, body tempera-

ture stabilizes, and lung maturity increases; intensive care may not be required.
4. 38 to 40 weeks at birth—full-term baby

REFERENCES

Abramovici, D., Mattar, F., & Sibai, B. (1998). Conservative management of severe preeclampsia. *Contemporary Obstetrics and Gynecology,5*,1992, 80–105.

American Academy of Pediatrics, American College of Obstetrics and Gynecology (1992). *Guidelines for Perinatal Care* (3rd ed., pp. 102–108). Washington, D.C.: American College of Obstetrics and Gynecology.

American Academy of Pediatrics Committee on Fetus and Newborn. (1992). Hospital stay for healthy term newborns. *Pediatrics, 96*(4), 788–790.

Annas, G. J. (1995). Women and children first. *New England Journal of Medicine, 333*(24), 1647–1651.

Beebe, S. A., Britton, J. R., Britton, H. L., Fan, P., & Jepson, B. (1996). Neonatal mortality and length of newborn hospital stay. *Pediatrics, 98*, 231–235.

Braveman, P., Egerter, S., Pearl, M., Marchi, K., & Miller, C. (1995). Problems associated with early discharge of newborn infants—early discharge of newborns and mothers: A critical review of the literature. *Pediatrics, 96*(4), 716–726.

Cowan, M. J. (1996). Hyperemesis gravidarum: Implications for home care and infusion therapies. *Journal of Intravenous Nursing, 19*, 46–58.

Creasy, R. K. (1984). Preterm labor and delivery: Disorder of parturition. In R. Creasy & R. Resnik (Eds.), *Maternal-fetal medicine* (pp. 401–448). Philadelphia: W.B. Saunders.

Creasy, R. K. Prevention of preterm birth. *Birth Defects, 19*(5), 97.

Elliott, J. P., Flynn, M. J., Kaemmerer, E. L., & Radin, T. G. (1997). Terbutaline pump tocolysis in high-order multiple gestation. *Journal of Reproductive Medicine, 42*, 687–693.

Fangman, J. J., Mark, P. M., Pratt, L., Conway, K. K., Healey, M. L., Oswald, J. W., & Uden, D. L. (1994). Prematurity prevention programs: An analysis of successes and failures. *American Journal of Obstetrics and Gynecology, 170*(3), 744–750.

Gabbe, S., Hill, L., Schmidt, L., & Schulkin, J. (1998). Management of diabetes by obstetrician-gynecologists. *Obstetrics and Gynecology, 91*, 643–647.

Griffin, P. D. M. (1995). *The managed care resource manual for obstetrics* (pp. 1–239). Marietta, GA: Healthdyne Perinatal Services.

Johnson, K. A., & Little, G. A. (1999). State health agencies and quality improvement in perinatal care. *Pediatrics, 103*, 233–247.

Kogan, M. D., Alexancer, G. R., Jack, B. W., & Allen, M. C. (1998). The association between adequacy of prenatal care utilization and subsequent pediatric care utilization in the United States. *Pediatrics, 102*(1), 25–30.

Kotula, C. (1994). High risk pregnancy. *Continuing Care, 6*, 15–18.

Mamelle, N., Segueilla, M., Munoz, F., & Berland, M. (1997). Prevention of preterm birth in patients with symptoms of preterm labor—The benefits of psychologic support. *American Journal of Obstetrics and Gynecology, 10*, 947–952.

Matria Healthcare, Inc. (1996). *Management of preterm labor in a managed care environment*. Marietta, GA: Matria.

Matria Healthcare Inc. (1998). *Managing diabetes in pregnancy in a managed care environment*. Marietta, GA: Matria.

Matria Healthcare Inc. (1999). *Time makes a difference*. Marietta, GA: Matria.

Naef, R. W. III, Chauhan, S. P., Roach, H., Roberts, W. E., Travis, K. H., & Morrison. J. C. (1995). Treatment for hyperemesis gravidarum in the home: An alternative to hospitalization. *Journal of Perinatology, 15*, 289–292.

NIH Consensus Development Panel (1995). Effect of corticosteroids for fetal maturation on perinatal outcomes. *Journal of the American Medical Association, 273*, 413–417.

Rust, O., Perry, K., Andrew, M., Roberts. W., Martin, R., & Morrison, J. (1997). Twins and preterm labor. *Journal of Reproductive Medicine, 42*, 229–234.

Sala, D. J., & Moise, K. J. Jr. (1990). The treatment of preterm labor using portable subcutaneous terbutaline pump. *Journal of Obstetrical, Gynecologic, and Neonatal Nursing, 19*(2), 108–115.

Scialli, A. R. (1998). High risk pregnancy: Nausea and vomiting. *Contemporary Obstetrics and Gynecology, 5*, 13–16.

CHAPTER 16

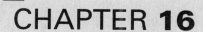

Pediatric Case Management

LORI A. DAVIS

LEARNING OBJECTIVES

Upon completion of this chapter, the reader will be able to:

1. Define the important terms and concepts relative to pediatric case management.

2. Discuss the important issues related specifically to pediatric case management.

3. Discuss the challenges and opportunities related to pediatric case management and the special issues related to this population.

IMPORTANT TERMS AND CONCEPTS

Apnea Monitor
Bronchopulmonary Dysplasia (BPD)
Caregiver
Communication
Financial Impact on the Family
Health Maintenance Organization
   (HMO)
Home Health Care
Identification of Pediatric Cases With
   Potential High-Risk Complications
Individuals With Disabilities Education
   Act (IDEA)

Medically Fragile Child
Neonatal Intensive Care Unit (NICU)
Peripherally Inserted Central Catheter
   (PICC)
Premature Infants
Prescribed Pediatric Extended Care
   (PPEC)
Technology Dependent Child
Very-Low-Birth-Weight Baby (VLBW)

■ INTRODUCTION

A. Pediatric case management is care management not of a child but of a family unit. You will discover that the issues surrounding the pediatric client encompass the entire family unit of the child.

245

B. Owing to the availability of advanced medical technologies, emergency medicine, and rapidly expanding medical knowledge, the pediatric population requiring case management has grown exponentially.

C. The primary client focus in this chapter is case management of the technology-dependent or medically fragile child.

1. Twenty million American children experience chronic conditions, and 4 million children suffer from disabling chronic conditions (Newacheck, Stein, & Walker, 1996).

2. With the capabilities within the medical community, we have begun rescuing children who would otherwise have not survived outside of the womb or who would not have survived to realize a cure for their childhood cancer.

3. With these medical miracles comes a myriad of issues to be resolved if the child is to experience any normalcy in his or her life. Twenty years ago, infants born at 24 weeks' gestation rarely survived. Today, not only do these infants survive, but in many instances they thrive—but not without the assistance of ever-changing health care technology and expertise.

■ KEY DEFINITIONS

A. Apnea monitor—An apnea monitor is used as a warning device to alert the caregiver of a decreased heart rate, decreased depth of respiration, or cessation of respiration. The cardiorespiratory monitor only warns of a problem, it does nothing to correct a problem.

B. Caregiver—The individual who is the parent, responsible party, guardian, or custodian for the pediatric client.

C. Individuals With Disabilities Education Act (IDEA)—IDEA, a federal law, defines the required educational components that must be available to all individuals with developmental disabilities.

D. Medically fragile child—The child who is medically stable but is fragile as a result of congenital disability, injury, illness, disease, or accident who requires frequent monitoring and treatment for the condition to remain in a state of satisfactory health.

E. Prescribed Pediatric Extended Care (PPEC): A day care for the medically fragile or technology-dependent child.

F. Technology-dependent child—Child who needs both a medical device to compensate for the loss of a vital body function and substantial and ongoing nursing care to avert death or further disability (U.S. Congress, 1987).

G. Very-low-birth-weight baby (VLBW)—An infant weighing less than 1500 g (3 lb, 5 oz)

■ PEDIATRIC CASE MANAGEMENT MODELS

A. The case manager—In case management of the pediatric client, there are often several case managers involved. These may include:

    1. A hospital case manager

    2. The clinic or specialty practice case manager

    3. Home health case manager

    4. A payor source case manager (Deming, 1996)

B. The facility-based and clinic-based case manager

    1. Facility-based and clinic-based case managers often are nurses with advanced degrees or certification in a particular specialty, or social workers (Deming, 1996).

    2. The facility-based case manager is responsible for the care coordination while the client is in the facility; this person may have responsibility for a particular unit or floor, whereas other facility-based case managers may have all discharge planning and case responsibilities for a particular specialty.

    3. The clinic-based case manager is often the case manager who will "know" the client for the longest period of time and have the most accurate clinical account of client history for a specific physician. Often, the clinic-based case manager is the one to alert the payor source case manager to changes in the client condition or situation once the child has left the facility.

C. The payor source case manager

    1. The payor source case manager is responsible for navigating the client through the health care system and is often the "lead" case manager directing and coordinating care.

    2. The payor source case manager is responsible for knowledge of what the health plan allows regarding service, providers, and treatment options covered by the plan. Therefore, this case manager has the ability to interpret and relay the terms of the policy to all other parties.

    3. The payor source case manager must have knowledge of the geographic area, providers, and services available within the region.

    4. The payor source case manager is often not an expert in pediatric care; therefore, he or she must rely on the expertise of those in the clinic and facility to expound on the particulars of care and treatment for the pediatric patient.

    5. Communication is a key function in this role. As important as clinical knowledge is, so is the ability to communicate effectively with all members of the case management team.

D. The home health case manager

    1. The child's care at home is extremely important, and the home health case manager must have substantial experience with pediatric care. This case manager (and other professionals in the home) are the eyes and ears to the other team members once the patient has been discharged from the facility and is cared for at home.

    2. The home health case manager's ability to assess home and social situations is very important.

        a. Environmental issues are the case manager's responsibility as well.

        b. Home safety is important whether the child is technology dependent or receiving home nursing care alone.

3. Sometimes, home health care companies and home equipment vendors subcontract services to other providers if they cannot immediately meet the home health care need of the child. As a case manager from any venue, it is important to know by whom services are being rendered at all times and that the provider is qualified and accredited to provide such services.

■ THE CASE MANAGEMENT TEAM

A. The ultimate goal of the case management team is to provide services that are uninterrupted, coordinated, developmentally and age appropriate, psychologically sound, and comprehensive (White, 1997).

B. The pediatric care management team should include:
1. The case manager or managers
2. Pediatric client
3. Caregiver
4. Primary care physician
5. Specialty physicians
6. Social services
7. Home health care provider
8. Therapists
9. Dieticians
10. Nutritionists
11. Pharmacists
12. School
13. Insurance company or others assuming financial responsibility
14. Anyone else who has an interest in the child's well-being

C. Communication throughout the team is key for a successful outcome. The child may be cared for by multiple physicians at multiple facilities or clinics.
1. Candid discussion with the parents or caregivers of the child is important.
2. Nothing will be resolved easily if decisions are made that do not involve the caregiver in the process.
3. This concept is best illustrated in the following case: A child had a private duty sitter at home. The child spilled a pitcher of red fruit drink while seated on the sofa. The parents had asked previously that he not be given the drink unless he was in the kitchen. The home care company was quick to accept responsibility and resolve the situation. They soon replaced the sofa for the client. It had been documented on the plan of care that the parents did not want him to have fruit drink unless he was in the kitchen. When the home care manager made a follow-up call to the family to evaluate their satisfaction with the problem resolution, he was stunned to find that they were still dissatisfied. The family said that they had received the new sofa and it was nice, but no one had replaced the lost pitcher of fruit drink.

■ THE CHILD

A. Age of the pediatric patient

1. Typically, pediatric case management includes children from birth to 18 years of age.
2. In some instances, there may be a perinatal or maternal–child case manager who works with children who are premature or are still in the neonatal period (the first 30 days after birth).
3. The case management responsibility of those infants would be specific to the institution or corporation policy.

B. Premature infants and those with congenital defects

1. Children requiring case management can have one problem or a multitude of problems. Prematurity and congenital defects account for a large number of children requiring case management.
2. Advanced technology in neonatal intensive care units (NICUs) has increased the number of children who survive, but it also has increased those requiring long-term or even lifetime care.
   a. Over the last 25 years, throughout the industrialized world survival for the pediatric client has dramatically improved such that about 90% of children with disabilities reach their 20th birthday (O'Shea, Klinepeter, Goldstein, Jackson, & Dillard, 1997).
   b. In 1960, only 3 out of 10 very-low-birth-weight (under 1500 g) newborns survived for at least a month (U.S. Congress, 1987).
   c. By 1980, nearly twice as many were surviving (U.S. Congress, 1987).
   d. In the 1990s, the survival rate of babies weighing less than 1lb, 10 oz was around 80% (Deming, 1996).
3. Complications of prematurity include bronchopulmonary dysplasia (BPD), necrotizing enterocolitis (NEC), intraventricular hemorrhage (IVH), hydrocephaly, and cerebral palsy.
4. Premature infants often require treatment at home with any of the following home health services: durable medical equipment, infusion services, home therapies, or home health nursing.
5. Many of these children are technology dependent. The technology-dependent child is defined as one who needs both a medical device to compensate for the loss of a vital body function and substantial and ongoing nursing care to avert death or further disability (U.S. Congress, 1987) (Table 16–1).
6. Examples:
   a. A child who has severe BPD might require an extended hospital stay, oxygen therapy at home, enteral feedings at home, and an apnea monitor.
   b. A child who lost a large part of his or her intestine owing to NEC might require multiple hospitalizations and surgeries, in addition to home total parenteral nutrition (TPN) or continuous enteral feedings.
   c. The child who has a moderate degree of cerebral palsy might not require as much "technology" as others but may require a specialized wheelchair, rehabilitation, and perhaps feeding assistance.

TABLE 16–1

Summary of Office of Technology Assessment Estimates of the Size of the Technology-Dependent Child Population

Defined Population	Estimated Number of Children
Group I	
Requiring ventilator assistance	680 to 2000
Group II	
Requiring parenteral nutrition	350 to 700
Requiring prolonged intravenous drugs	270 to 8275
Group III	
Requiring other device-based respiratory or nutritional support	1000 to 6000
Rounded subtotal (I + II + III)	**2300 to 17,000**
Group IV	
Requiring apnea monitoring	6800 to 45,000
Requiring renal dialysis	1000 to 6,000
Requiring other device-associated nursing	Unknown, perhaps 30,000 or more

(U.S. Congress, Office of Technology Assessment [1987]. *Technology-dependent children: Hospital v. home care—A technical memorandum, OTA-TM-H-38.* Washington, D.C.: U.S. Government Printing Office.)

  d. All of these situations would require services, skills, and/or equipment that might fall outside the normally covered items under a health plan.
  7. A pediatric provider for these services, and the understanding by the payor source of the needs of the child, are absolutely essential.
C. The child with illness and injury
  1. Another group of children to consider are those who have childhood cancer that might require home chemotherapy, frequent hospitalizations, frequent clinic visits, home health nursing, or perhaps a bone marrow or stem cell transplant, requiring extensive communication and coordination of the care management team for an optimum outcome.
  2. One major goal in case management for children is to allow the child to lead the most normal daily life possible. Often this includes coordinating care with the school system or day care center.
  3. Accidents and other illnesses account for another large portion of the home health or rehabilitation services the child may require.
  4. Osteomyelitis is frequently seen in children requiring case management.
    a. Depending on the location of the infection and the susceptibility and sensitivity of the organism, children with osteomyelitis often require home intravenous (IV) antibiotics.
    b. Many children require placement of a central venous catheter or a

long-dwelling device such as a peripherally inserted central catheter (PICC).

    c. The duration of care at home can be anywhere from 7 days to several months of IV antibiotic therapy.

5. Traumatic brain injury

    a. The pediatric population has seen an increase in traumatic brain injury because of the popularity of all-terrain vehicles (ATVs), motorcycles, and bicycles.

    b. Children with traumatic brain injuries need to be seen in a comprehensive facility where there is extensive expertise and services specific for the brain-injured child.

    c. The subsequent rehabilitation these children require is also vitally important to optimize the potential for a partial or complete recovery.

■ THE NUCLEAR FAMILY

A. The family

1. Several indicators should be addressed in assessing the family of the technology-dependent or medically fragile child. It is well documented that family members may experience adverse consequences as a result of the need to focus energy and resources on the child who has a chronic condition. Disposable income, employment, parental health, sibling health and adaptation, and family interaction and support levels are indicators of child health outcomes.

    a. Siblings—ratings of siblings' health status (cognitive, physical, social, and emotional)

    b. Parents—the frequency of occurrence of financially burdensome out-of-pocket expenses for child health care, including premium expenditures; the impact of child health care demands on parental employment (e.g., work out of the house, employment patterns, hours worked, and work loss days); ratings of parents' health status (cognitive, physical, social and emotional)

    c. Family unit—the nature and level of family support provided through the plan (e.g., level of informal care giving, psychological support and social support, crisis intervention, respite care) (Newacheck, Stein, & Walker, 1996).

2. As a case manager, you may not always be able to address or impact every issue surrounding your pediatric client; however, you will be able to understand more clearly the behaviors of the client and family when you are aware of the challenges they face and how they react to them.

B. The caregiver

1. When a child is sick or injured, each member of the family, whether nuclear, blended, extended, or foster, is affected to some degree.

2. Establishing the primary caregiver is crucial.

    a. Often the primary caregiver is the child's mother or father.

    b. The primary caregiver is the one who will be responsible for learning all facets of the child's care. This includes learning cardiopulmonary resuscitation (CPR), procedures, treatments, and equipment that might be necessary at home.

3. The case manager should assess the primary caregiver for the willingness and motivation to learn, as well as the ability to learn.

4. The payor source case manager is reliant on the nurses and therapists who have worked with the child and the family to relay this information as well. Home health care professionals are excellent in assessing the abilities of the caregiver; however, it would be prudent to determine caregiver abilities well in advance of discharge.

5. Case management must be performed in cooperation with the child, family, and care management team. In working with the caregiver or parents, it is vitally important to establish rapport with them.

   a. Listening is a sometimes seldom used but highly needed skill.

   b. One unwritten but widely understood rule in the pediatric care industry is "Listen to the mother (caregiver)." The mother or caregiver is with the child most often and knows better than anyone when "something is not right."

   c. Never discount what the primary caregiver is telling you about a child. He or she may not have the medical terminology or be the most eloquent in self-expression, but caregivers do very often know their child and what might be necessary.

C. Siblings

1. The siblings of a technology-dependent or medically fragile child are often deeply affected by the circumstances in the home and family. They may feel resentment, loss of attention, anger, fear, and hostility.

2. They show signs of irritability and jealousy as a result of the added attention given to the disabled or ill child. The parent may feel guilty, depressed, or helpless in the situation.

3. Family counseling or individual counseling with the child may be beneficial and could possibly prevent difficulties in the future.

D. Financial impact on the family

1. The family undergoes stress when the child is ill, not only from the disease or condition itself but also from the financial impact on the caregiver and family.

2. Family income is significantly lower in families with a child assisted by technology.

3. Reduced income is often seen because the mother is usually the primary caregiver. In homes in which the mother was required to quit work, the loss of income combined with medical expenses and supplies not covered by health insurance can be overwhelming.

■ AFTER HOSPITALIZATION

A. Prescribed Pediatric Extended Care (PPEC)

1. Traditional day care is rarely an option for the very ill child. Although many day care centers accept children with mild to moderate disabilities, caregivers are often reluctant to use them.

2. There are specialized day care centers for medically fragile or technology-dependent children in locations across the country, called PPEC. They are few in number, and reimbursement sources have been reluctant to cover the cost associated with this type of day care completely or partially (Thyen, Kuhlthau, & Perrin, 1999).

3. The benefits of PPEC for the medically fragile or technology-dependent child include:

   a. The child can receive speech, occupational, and physical therapies.

   b. Physicians often visit or make rounds in the PPEC.

   c. PPECs often offer admission to children without disabilities at a reduced rate.

   d. Technology-dependent children can model their behavior after children who are not impaired. Many children with disabilities learn a great deal by this patterning behavior.

   e. The unimpaired children also learn early in life about the acceptance of those with disabilities.

   f. The natural play therapy of being around other children rather than isolated at home or in a facility is an obvious benefit of this arrangement.

   g. The children in the PPEC also benefit from a daily nurse assessment that can include measurement of weight daily, lab work, wound care, and central line care.

   h. The caregivers and families of these children are exposed to a widened support group as well, with daily close contact with health professionals and, more important, the parents or caregivers of the other children.

   i. The family experiences some success as well, because parents are able to return to work and do not need to rely on state-funded resources for survival.

   j. Stress on the caregiver is reduced by having some respite time as well.

4. The disadvantages of PPEC include location, transportation, and expense.

   a. Location—the expense of setting up a PPEC facility that would be convenient to all is not practical. Usually, there is only one institution of this type in a major metropolitan area.

   b. Tranportation—transportation is not always an issue; more likely, it is the transporting of the child to a facility that is not convenient to the caregiver's place of employment.

C. Expense—cost of this type of care can vary from $200 to $400 per day. The cost of several home health visits, inpatient rehabilitation, or rehospitalization would be greater over the long term. If there were acceptance within the payor sources of this type of care, this concept could be quite successful and beneficial to both the health plans and the child over the long term.

B. Home health care

   1. There are many home health care companies available in every community, but most often the majority of their patients are elderly adults.

However, many agencies that focus on adults employ a few clinicians who have the appropriate pediatric experience to provide basic and sometimes even high-tech care of the child.

2. A few agencies in some larger metropolitan areas primarily focus on the home health care needs of the child.

a. When referring to an agency with which you are unfamiliar, you will need to ask regarding their capabilities. When referrals are made to a home health agency for a child, you should specifically ask whether they have pediatric-experienced clinicians available.

b. It would be a wise decision to have them fax or send you marketing materials that quote exactly what they can and cannot provide for the pediatric patient.

c. Verify the company's ability to provide pediatric equipment. Even a blood pressure cuff small enough for an infant or child might not be available. In this managed care climate, many agencies are seeking to diversify their business mix from the Medicare primary to the private insurance markets. In doing so, they are almost required contractually to provide services for patients of all ages. Be very vigilant in the care of the child.

3. Most of the same services that you can obtain in the home for adult patients can be provided to the pediatric and neonatal client as well. Available home care products and services include IV hydration fluids, TPN, IV antibiotics, chemotherapies, enteral feedings, home oxygen, pulse oximetry monitoring, home blood pressure monitoring, home ventilator care, tracheostomy care, private duty nursing, sitter services, hospice services, home apnea monitors, wound care, central venous catheter care, physical therapy, occupational therapy, speech therapy, and skilled nursing visits.

4. Other important information to know about the home health provider is whether they are JCAHO accredited and when accreditation was obtained. It is also worthwhile to know whether the agency you are working with is JCAHO accredited in pharmacy, home health services, and equipment.

5. If they are a Medicare provider, you can check with your state agencies on their current standing as a home health provider.

6. Today, severely disabled children are cared for at home rather than being institutionalized, as was done in decades past. Most often, the primary caregiver is a parent. It is crucial to know both the capabilities and the limitations of the caregiver.

a. When the child goes home, it is extremely important for all emergency numbers and plans to be clearly written out and placed in a conspicuous place near the telephone.

b. The home health care provider and hospital discharge planner or case manager can often screen the parent or caregiver before discharge. Depending on the technology that the child is given, pre-discharge home health care teaching begins early and the duration of teaching required will vary.

(i) With a ventilator-dependent child, home health care teaching might begin a full 30 days in advance of the anticipated discharge date.

(ii) A child going home with home parenteral nutrition may require a 7- to 10-day in-hospital instruction program or the option of 3 to 4 days with extensive home nursing follow-up.

7. The home health care agency caring for the child is responsible for ensuring the safety of the home regarding the home therapy or service provided.

   a. For instance, if a child is discharged with a home ventilator, the home health care agency or home equipment provider would ensure that there were adequate electrical outlets and space for the system in the home. If the home is determined to be inadequate, the provider would notify the physician and hospital immediately.

   b. Determinations should be made before the discharge decision, particularly if the service provided is life-sustaining.

   c. Most JCAHO-accredited, state-certified agencies have home safety guidelines and policies with which they must adhere. Sometimes a social worker home visit might be necessary if the situation warrants such assistance.

8. The advantages and disadvantages of home care should be weighed carefully and individually for the medically fragile or technology-dependent child.

   a. Costs of care—the cost of pediatric home health care is relatively the same as that for adult home health care. There are a few companies who sell the service as high-tech or highly specialized, but for the most part, comparable care is available at the usual home health care rates. The cost of home health care is most often significantly less than care provided in the hospital, even for the most high-tech client. If hourly nursing services are required as well, the cost can increase significantly.

   b. Often, the equipment, supplies, and personnel are billed at separate rates. When these costs are combined, the daily rate for home health care in some situations could be higher than the cost of 1 inpatient day in the hospital. For example, if there is to be 24-hour registered nurse care, with oxygen, a ventilator, multiple medications, therapies, and other ancillary equipment and supplies in the home, carefully evaluate the feasibility of discharge to home health care. This should be evaluated on a case-by-case basis.

   c. If the home care environment might aggravate problems or difficulties with care or management of the care, the choice may be to use a pediatric subacute facility, if available, or to lengthen the hospital stay; however, most managed care organizations frown on a "social admission" or keeping a child in the hospital because the home or the caregiver is not suitable for the level of care required in the home. Consider the legal implications and responsibilities.

   d. The advantages to the child are that he or she is in a familiar environment near family and friends. Usually, the child is cared for in his or her own bedroom near toys.

■ IDENTIFYING CASES WITH POTENTIAL HIGH-RISK COMPLICATIONS

A. In the current legal climate, we must be constantly vigilant to the exposure we have as professionals, particularly when children are involved. We concern ourselves with the prompt, quality care the child receives first and foremost, but we must also consider each case as if we will be called on to review it in years to come. As case managers, we are increasingly held accountable for the outcome in the cases we manage.

B. With children and obstetric cases, the statute of limitations can be endless in some states. In most states, when children are concerned the statute of limitations is 21 years.

C. Treat each case as if it were the one that you will be scrutinized for in the future. In your work as a case manager, you should always be prepared for an appointment with the legal system.

D. With issues of abuse, neglect, and guardianship, it does not take a medically negligent incident to bring the case into the legal system.

E. Documentation is critical. Many case managers who enter the practice think that perhaps by leaving the clinical bedside, charting and documentation no longer reign supreme. This is a false assumption. As a case manager, documentation is extremely important, not only for communication purposes but also for the legal implications that are present. Document as if you will have no recollection of any event or contact within 5 years. A very basic but common error in documentation is failure to put a complete date on the entry. The year is often left blank. Documentation should always be objective and factual. The case you think is not high risk is often the one that turns out to be so later on.

F. With children, conversations that you have as a case manager with the parent or caregiver are crucial. Records of the times that you telephoned the caregiver, whether or not he or she answered, are important. Copies of letters or memos sent to any part of the team should be kept. Notes regarding conversations, home visits, team conferences, calls to physician offices, and voice mail messages you receive are critical information components, even in the simplest of cases.

G. Identifying cases that are considered high risk is a judgment call on the part of the case manager in most instances. Some companies have policies or listings of what they consider to be quality issues or high-risk clients. Many of the types of cases presented in the following list may not be high risk, but it would be prudent to evaluate them and document your findings accurately. A thorough assessment at the beginning of the case management period would also be an asset. Consistent communication with other members of the care management team is also recommended.

H. Some high-risk pediatric clients or cases include:
   1. Hospital admission longer than 7 to 10 days
   2. Hospital readmission following discharge within 24 to 48 hours
   3. Birth weight of less than 1500 g
   4. Premature birth

5. Multiple births
6. Neonatal intensive care unit admission
7. Severe or multiple congenital defects
8. Normal infant admitted to hospital within 30 to 60 days of birth
9. Any intensive care admission of a child or neonate
10. Hospital stay increased owing to nosocomial infection or other complication of hospitalization
11. Accident involving any provider or facility
12. Suspected or confirmed child abuse or neglect
13. More than two hospitalizations within 12 months
14. Frequent emergency room visits
15. Cancer
16. Traumatic brain injury
17. Multiple physician specialties consulted
18. Multiple surgeries
19. Sibling of patient with sudden infant death syndrome (SIDS)
20. Any child receiving home health care services or home medical equipment
21. Suspected or known noncompliance with physician orders

■ COST–BENEFIT ANALYSIS

A. Managed care has made a huge impact on the health care delivery system. Children with chronic illnesses and disabilities are increasingly joining managed care arrangements.

B. States are actively enrolling Medicaid beneficiaries in managed care plans. By 1994, 40 states were operating or developing Medicaid-managed care plans (Newacheck, Stein, & Walker, 1996). Medicaid programs in many states have been hampered by repeated funding cuts that directly affect patient care. Theoretically, the programs save vital funds for necessary operations by allowing managed care organizations to provide utilization management for this population.

C. Managed care organizations typically operate by a system of preferred physician networks. Sometimes an independent physician association (IPA) manages the population further. The providers a child might use are further limited, and it is hoped that the primary care physician who manages the care provides only what is absolutely necessary in the way of treatment.

D. The ideal form of health care is to maintain health and prevent illness; thus, the health maintenance organization (HMO) was developed. Some critics note that the HMO or managed care system limits the availability of expert care, particularly in cases in which pediatric subspecialties are concerned.

E. It is a case manager's role to assist the family and the child in the navigation of this complex system. Whether or not a physician is a participating provider, the affiliation should not impede the quality or availability of necessary pediatric care.

F. Benefit plans do not always allow for the complexity of pediatric case management. As a case manager, it is critical that you carefully weigh the options available and measure them against the benefit plan. Sometimes, services or products are excluded from coverage and there is no "major medical" compliment to the plan. In instances such as this, a medical decision must be made by the payor about whether it is wise to uphold the policy itself or offer a prudent decision to cover a service based on its potential to prevent medical complications. Issues such as this are confronted daily in case management. Determinations should always be made with the patient's well-being and interest coming first and foremost. In situations like these, the case manager is the client advocate as well as the payor source advocate.

G. Example: It is cost effective to uphold the denial of disposable medical supplies. What if those disposable medical supplies are central catheter care supplies? Is it not more cost effective in the long run to pay for the catheter supplies than to pay for a potential hospital stay for sepsis if the care is not given? Of course, from a case management point of view the reasonable and prudent decision is to cover the supplies despite what the policy or plan dictates. The client receives quality medical care at home and avoids the possibility of contracting an infection while being hospitalized. The payor source pays a small amount of money to prevent a potential complication of central line care.

■ COMMUNITY RESOURCES

A. Technology-dependent or medically fragile children are living longer and often are outliving their resources. Case managers are constantly in search of ways to help these children, their families, and the community to take better care of them.

B. In establishing a client support system, it is important to interview the family and tap into resources of which they may be unaware, including:
1. Church groups
2. Their employer groups
3. Friends and civic groups
4. Local and national chapters of such organizations (such as The March of Dimes, Cystic Fibrosis Foundation, The American Cancer Society, The American Heart Association, The National Head Injury Foundation, The American Lung Association, Easter Seals, Make-a-Wish Foundation, Candlelighters, SIDS Foundation, United Cerebral Palsy Association, Shriners, Kiwanis, Rotary, Lions, Association for Retarded Citizens, and The Spina Bifida Association)
5. Sometimes, large corporations are willing to donate funds if they are told specifically what the monies will be used for and what is needed.
6. State-sponsored Title V programs can help families obtain specialized medical or rehabilitation services, durable medical equipment and supplies, assistive technology, rehabilitation therapies, and other types of community-based care the child may need. Specific programs vary from state to state, and eligibility for these services is sometimes, but not always, based on financial need. Programs are typically ad-

ministered through the state maternal and child health agency (American College of Emergency Physicians, 1997).

7. IDEA, a federal law, defines the required educational components that must be available to all individuals with developmental disabilities. Part H of IDEA addresses only early intervention for infants and toddlers from birth to 3 years of age and their families. Although early intervention is federally mandated, it is the responsibility of individual states to set up delivery systems that meet the needs of their youngest citizens (Berger, Holt-Turner, Cupoli, Mass, & Hageman, 1998).

8. The children's hospital in your area may also have resources and equipment that have been donated to them from children who no longer need them or who are deceased.

9. Some home health equipment companies also keep reusable items for their clients who cannot afford to purchase them. Wheelchairs often fit into this category. As children outgrow their wheelchairs, they sometimes donate them back to the hospital or company so that other children might use them.

REFERENCES

American Academy of Pediatrics, Committee on Children with Disabilities (1995). Guidelines for home care of infants, children, and adolescents with chronic disease. *Pediatrics, 96*, 161–164.

American College of Emergency Physicians, Emergency Medical Services for Children, National Task Force on Children With Special Health Care Needs (1997). EMS for children: Recommendations for coordinating care for children with special health care needs. *Annals of Emergency Medicine, 30*, 274–280.

Beebe, S. A., Britton, J. R., Britton, H. L., Fan, P., & Jepson, B. (1996). Neonatal mortality and length of newborn hospital stay. *Pediatrics, 98*, 231–235.

Berger, S. P., Holt-Turner, I., Cupoli, J. M., Mass, M., & Hageman, J. R. (1998). Caring for the graduate from the neonatal intensive care unit: At home, in the office, and in the community. *Pediatric Clinics of North America, 45*, 701–712.

Cavalier, S., Escobar, G., Fernbach, S., Quesenberry, C., & Chellino, M. (1996). Post discharge utilization of medical services by high-risk infants: Experience in a large managed care organization. *Pediatrics, 97*, 693–699.

Deming, L. (1996). Planning earlier discharge from the NICU. *The Journal of Care Management, 4*, 13–27.

Giacoia, G. P. (1997). Follow-up of school-age children with bronchopulmonary dysplasia. *Journal of Pediatrics, 130*, 400–408.

Goldberg, A. I. (1995) Pediatric home health: The need for physician education. *Pediatrics, 95*, 928–930.

Health Care Finance Administration, Children's Health Insurance Program. September 26, 1999. *www.hcfa.gov/init/children.htm*

Insure Kids Now. September 26 1999. *www.insurekidsnow.gov*

Ireys, H. T., Grason, H. A., Guyer, B. G. (1996). Assuring quality of care for children with special needs in managed care organizations: Roles for pediatricians. *Pediatrics, 98*, 178–185.

Kuhlthau, K., Perrin, J. M., Ettner, S. L., McLaughlin, T. J., & Gortmaker, S. L. (1998). High-expenditure children with supplemental security income. *Pediatrics, 102*, 610–615.

Liptak, G. S. (1998). The child who has severe neurologic impairment. *Pediatric Clinics of North America, 45*, 123–144.

Newacheck, P. W. (1996). Children's access to primary care: Differences by race, income, and insurance status. *Pediatrics, 97*, 26–32.

Newacheck, P. W., Stein, R. E. K., & Walker, D. K. (1996). Monitoring and evaluating managed care for children with chronic illnesses and disabilities. *Pediatrics, 98*, 952–958.

Osberg, J. S., Kahn, P., Rowe, K., & Brooke, M. M. (1996). Pediatric trauma: Impact on work and family finances. *Pediatrics, 98*, 890–897.

O'Shea, T. M., Klinepeter, K., Goldstein, D. J., Jackson, B. W., & Dillard, R. G. (1997). Survival and developmental disability in infants with birth weights of 501 to 800 grams, born between 1979 and 1994. *Pediatrics, 100*, 982–986.

Scholer, S. J. (1997). Predictors of injury mortality in early childhood. *Pediatrics, 100,* 324–347.

Strauss, D., Ashwal, S., Shavelle, R., & Eyman, R. (1997). Prognosis for survival and improvement in function in children with severe developmental disabilities. *Pediatrics, 131,* 712–716.

Thyen, U., Kuhlthau, K., & Perrin, J.M. (1999). Employment, child care, and mental health of mothers caring for children assisted by technology. *Pediatrics, 103,* 1225–1242.

Toder, D. S., & McBride, J. T. (1997). Home care of children dependent on respiratory technology. *Pediatrics in Review, 18,* 274–280.

U.S. Congress, Office of Technology Assessment (1987). *Technology-dependent children: Hospital v. home care—A technical memorandum, OTA-TM-H-38.* Washington, D.C.: U.S. Government Printing Office.

Westbrook, L. E. (1998). Implications for estimates of disability in children: A comparison of definitional components. *Pediatrics, 101,* 1025–1030.

White, P. H. (1997). Success on the road to adulthood: Issues and hurdles for adolescents with disabilities. *Rheumatic Diseases Clinics of North America, 23,* 696–707.

Wilson-Costello, D., Borawski, E., Friedman, H., Redline, R., Fanaroff, A. A., & Hack, M. (1998). Perinatal correlates of cerebral palsy and other neurologic impairment among very low birth weight children. *Pediatrics, 102,* 315–321.

CHAPTER 17

. . . .

Geriatric Case Management and Continuum of Care

SHERRY L. ALIOTTA

LINDA N. SCHOENBECK

LEARNING OBJECTIVES

Upon completion of this chapter, the reader will be able to:

1. List various methods of identifying high-risk geriatric patients for case management.
2. Assess for and identify common geriatric problems.
3. Assess and identify care needs of the geriatric patient.
4. List available tools to aid in assessment of geriatric patients.
5. Describe comprehensive geriatric assessment and when such assessment is useful.
6. Identify steps of the geriatric placement process.
7. Define the components of aging in place.
8. Identify levels of care available for placement of the geriatric patient.
9. Identify community resources to assist with common problems.
10. Define Medicare criteria for Medicare Part A coverage in a skilled nursing facility.
11. List common payment and insurance issues and resources.

IMPORTANT TERMS AND CONCEPTS

Aging in Place
Assessment
Assessment Tools for Geriatric
    Placement
Custodial Care
Long-Term Care (Nursing Home)
Medicare Criteria for Continued Stay
    under Medicare Part A
Nonskilled Rehabilitation Therapy or
    Restorative Nursing

PRA
PRA Plus
Screening
Screening Instruments
SF (Short Form) 36 and SF (Short
    Form) 12
Skilled Nursing Facility (Medicare)
Skilled Nursing Facility Versus
    Custodial Care (Nursing Home)
Skilled Rehabilitation Therapy

■ INTRODUCTION

A. The population that is older than 65 years of age is growing.

B. Just 4% of the population was older than 65 years at the beginning of the century; now the proportion of elderly individuals exceeds 12%.

C. Eighty-five percent of those over 65 years of age have at least one chronic condition, and 30% have three or more chronic illnesses.

D. Geriatric patients are seen by case managers in
1. Hospitals
2. Skilled nursing facilities
3. Home health agencies
4. Health maintenance organizations
5. Physician groups
6. Community agencies
7. Others

E. Expertise in the case management of geriatric patients is critical for case managers owing to
1. Numbers of patients seen in this category
2. Diversity of health care delivery sites and services attending to this group

F. Case management of the geriatric patient differs from other patient populations with whom case managers may have worked in their case management practice.

G. Demographics (Rhoades & Krauss, 1996)
1. Over 9 million Americans older than 65 years of age live alone.
2. Of that number, 2 million state that they have nowhere to turn if they need help.
3. Eighty percent of those living alone are women.
4. Nearly half of the persons aged 85 or older live alone.
5. Older women, the very old, and the minority elderly population have, on an average, the lowest incomes among the older population.

6. In 1996, there were 16,840 nursing homes with a total of 1.76 million beds.
7. Functional disability has increased. Almost 72% of 1987 nursing home residents needed help with three or more activities of daily living (ADLs). In 1996, 83% of residents needed assistance, a 15% increase.
8. More than 83.3% of nursing home residents received help with three or more ADLs, including bathing, dressing, toileting, transferring from bed to chair, feeding, and mobility.
9. About one third of all nursing home costs are paid out of pocket by individuals and their families.
10. Women compose more than two thirds (71.6%) of the total nursing home population.
11. Approximately half of all residents are age 85 and older.

■ KEY DEFINITIONS

A. PRA: A valid and reliable tool for identification of high-risk seniors (age 65 years or greater) developed by Chad Boult and associates from the University of Minnesota. PRA stands for predictor of repeat admissions, and the term identifies geriatric patients who have a statistically higher probability of repeat hospital admission.

B. Screening: The process by which a health care provider institutes specific criteria to select potential recipients of case management. A screening questionnaire can be administered to a defined population of individuals (i.e., new enrollees into a Medicare risk plan) to identify those at high risk for an adverse health event who may be candidates for case management (HMO Work Group on Care Management, 1996).

C. Abuse: The willful infliction of injury, unreasonable confinement, intimidation, or cruel punishment with resulting pain or mental anguish, or the willful depreciation by a caretaker of goods or services that are necessary to avoid physical harm, mental anguish, or mental illness (Abyad, 1996).

D. Neglect: The failure to provide the goods or services that are necessary to avoid physical harm, mental anguish, or mental illness (Abyad, 1996).

■ AGING IN PLACE

A. The process by which a person chooses to remain in his or her living environment (home) and to remain as independent as possible despite the physical or mental decline that may occur with chronic disabilities or the aging process (Callahan, 1992).
1. This independence can be maintained by contracting with any health services needed, such as
   a. Nursing care
   b. Skilled rehabilitative therapy services
2. Independence may also be maintained by contracting for other needs, such as

     a. Assistance with ADLs

     b. Incontinence care

     c. Assistance with instrumental activities of daily living (IADLs)

     d. Assistance with personal and legal affairs

B. Barriers to aging in place

  1. Financial barriers

     a. Individual may lack ability to pay

     b. Individual may not want to pay for services

  2. Lack of community services

     a. May be in rural area with no access to services

     b. May not be enough community services to meet needs

     c. Frailness of the individual may require more assistance than possible from the community

  3. Quality of care concerns

     a. Caregivers may not be properly trained

     b. Caregivers may not be licensed or supervised adequately

       (i) Possible abuse and neglect

       (ii) Lack of quality care

  4. Individual barriers

     a. Owing to physical or psychological factors

     b. Is danger to self and others

C. Programs for aging in place

  1. Federal—Older Americans Act of 1965

     a. Administration on Aging

       (i) Administers key programs to help vulnerable older Americans

       (ii) Works closely with state, regional, and Areas of Aging agencies

  2. State and community programs

     a. Provide supportive in-home and community-based services

       (i) Nutrition

       (ii) Transportation

       (iii) Senior center

       (iv) Homemaker services

     b. Emphasis on elder rights programs

       (i) Nursing Home Ombudsmen programs

       (ii) Legal and insurance counseling services

       (iii) Elder abuse prevention efforts

     c. Contracts with public or private groups

       (i) Referral, outreach, case management, escort and transportation

       (ii) In-home services for homemakers, personal care, home repair, and rehabilitation

       (iii) Educational programs

■ COMMON GERIATRIC PROBLEMS

A. Although numerous problems can occur in the geriatric population, a few deserve mention due to their

1. Frequency of occurrence
2. Underrecognition and treatment
3. Multiple causes
4. Impact on the individual's ability to function

B. This list is not all-inclusive or comprehensive but represents common issues.

1. These issues are also presented to serve as a reminder to case managers working with the geriatric population.
2. Often, other issues are also presented to serve as a reminder to case managers working with the geriatric population.
3. Many of the issues presented here can manifest themselves in a variety of ways and can also be the precipitating cause of other issues. For this reason, the case manager must be aware of these issues.
4. Many case managers do not see the individuals they are charged with managing, or they do not complete in-depth assessments.
5. The points are presented here in order to familiarize the case manager with the key points for each problem so that he or she can appropriately intervene.
6. Regardless of the case management setting, the case manager can ensure that the problems presented here are adequately assessed and the issues addressed appropriately.

C. Altered mental status

1. A great deal of elder assessment depends on the assessment of a person's mental state to some degree (Gallo, Reichel, & Anderson, 1988).
2. Changes in mental status can be very subtle and often go unrecognized.
3. There are several types and causes of cognitive decline, and dementia is not the only cause of cognitive decline.
4. Case managers who work with geriatric patients should familiarize themselves with the different causes of cognitive decline and risk factors.
5. Many, if not most, cognitively impaired older people have at least one treatable underlying or concurrent condition (Miller, 1999).
6. Altered mental status can be the cause of many other problems identified by case managers:
   a. Nonadherence to treatment plans or medications, or both
   b. Injuries such as falls and burns
   c. Nutritional deficits
   d. Agitation or aggressive behavior
   e. Depression
   f. Social isolation

7. A baseline assessment of mental status using a standardized tool can help identify and track the progression of mental status.
   a. Standardized tools
      (i) There are several tools that test mental status.
      (ii) One of the most popular is the Short Portable Mental Status Questionnaire for the Assessment of Organic Brain Disease in the elderly population (Pfeiffer, 1975).
      (iii) Another popular questionnaire is the Folstein Mini-Mental Status Examination (Folstein, Folstein, & McHugh, 1975).
      (iv) Several other tests are available to identify and quantify the presence of cognitive deficits.
      (v) The choice of instrument depends on the practice setting of the case manager.
      (vi) The case manager may not be the one who actually administers the test, but he or she should be aware of the availability of the various tools and recommend their use when appropriate.

D. Urinary incontinence
   1. Although the urinary system is affected by changes in aging, incontinence should not be thought of as an inevitable part of aging.
   2. Assessment for incontinence or the risk of incontinence should be multifaceted and cover the following factors (Miller, 1999):
      a. Risk factors influencing elimination, such as prostate surgery
      b. Social risk factors such as being able to read bathroom signs when out
      c. Signs and symptoms of actual dysfunction, such as leaking urine
      d. Whether incontinence is acknowledged. Ask when the problem began, and what has been done about it.
      e. Fears about incontinence that include changing activities because of the need to go to the toilet
      f. Behavioral signs, such as a urine odor or use of pads
      g. Environmental factors that may contribute to incontinence, such as having to go upstairs to use the bathroom
   3. Incontinence is often unreported and can have a significant impact on the life and functioning of the older adult.
   4. It is important for case managers to assess for and arrange interventions directed at resolving and/or improving the problem.

E. Safety issues
   1. Falls
      a. Multiple risk factors are associated with falls in the elderly (Miller, 1999).
         (i) Age-related changes such as:
            (a) Vision and hearing changes
            (b) Osteoporosis
            (c) Slowed reaction time
            (d) Altered gait

        (e) Postural hypotension

        (f) Nocturia

    (ii) Medical problems

    (iii) Psychosocial factors such as depression

    (iv) Medications

    (v) Environmental factors

    (vi) Any combination of the above-mentioned items

  b. The case manager should assess for the presence of the above-mentioned risk factors, especially if there is a history of previous falls.

  c. As the case manager conducts the overall assessment of the individual, he or she should think about the possibility of falls and whether any of the information collected puts the individual at greater risk.

  d. Resources are available to help the case manager with the assessment.

    (i) The physical therapist can assess the individual's gait and balance.

    (ii) A thorough home safety evaluation can identify environmental concerns.

    (iii) A thorough history from the primary care physician that includes medications and health conditions can assist with identifying medical risk factors.

  e. The case manager should tailor the interventions directed at preventing falls to the specific risk factors.

  f. Although creating a safe environment is a good overall intervention, it will not fully address the risk of falls if the medication the person is taking makes him or her dizzy.

2. Elder abuse and neglect

  a. As many as one third of victims unequivocally deny abuse (Abyad, 1996).

  b. The prevalence of abuse varies in several studies but ranges between 1% and 10% (Miller, 1999).

  c. Risk profiles (Abyad, 1996)

  d. Victims' characteristics:

    (i) Females are at a higher risk owing to the fact that they outlive men and because of gender issues.

    (ii) Advanced age

    (iii) Greater dependency

    (iv) Alcohol abuse

    (v) Intergenerational conflict

    (vi) Isolation

    (vii) Internalization of blame

    (viii) Provocative behavior

    (ix) Past history of abuse

  e. Abusers' characteristics:

  (i) Alcohol and drug abuse

  (ii) Mental illness

  (iii) Caregiver inexperience

  (iv) History of abuse as a child

  (v) Stress

  (vi) Economic dependence on elder

f. Families' characteristics:

  (i) Caregiver reluctance

  (ii) Overcrowding

  (iii) Isolation

  (iv) Marital conflict

  (v) History of past abuse

g. In assessing elders and creating care plans, it is natural for the case manager to look to the family as a large part of the caregiver equation.

h. It is critical that the case manager evaluate the potential for risk and intervene to reduce and/or eliminate the risk.

i. Some examples of interventions include:

  (i) Provide education to the caregiver about each aspect of the expected care.

  (ii) Discuss examples of situations in which the behavior of the elder patient causes frustration, anger, or feelings of helplessness in the caregiver. Help the caregiver identify appropriate responses to these feelings.

  (iii) Set realistic expectations, and frankly discuss the demands of caring for a dependent individual.

  (iv) Provide for direct observation of the home situation and the interaction between the elder family member and the caregivers. A home health nurse may be able to identify subtle signs of trouble before it occurs.

  (v) Assess the support system of the caregiver, and assist him or her in identification of support groups or respite from caregiver activities.

  (vi) Support and encourage the elderly person to continue to be as independent as his or her condition allows.

  (vii) Refer the caregiver to marital, substance abuse, or other specialized counseling services.

  (viii) Recommend different arrangements for the elderly person. Not every family can successfully provide care for the elder family member.

j. Most states have specific reporting requirements for elder abuse and neglect. Most require reporting by the health care professionals who suspect abuse.

k. The case manager should become aware of both the state and organizational reporting policies for elder abuse and neglect.

l. The case manager can recognize the possibility of elder abuse and neglect through signs such as the following:
   (i) Direct reports by the elder of incidents
   (ii) A rapid or unexplained decline in the physical condition of the elderly patient
   (iii) Malnutrition
   (iv) Suspicious injuries or conflicting reports of injury from the patient and the caregiver (Abyad, 1996).
      (a) Lacerations and bruises in multiple states of healing
      (b) Multiple fractures in various states of healing
      (c) Scald burns with demarcated immersion lines and no splash marks, involving the anterior or posterior half of extremity, or to the buttocks or genitals
      (d) Cigarette burns
      (e) Rope burns or marks
m. Many case managers may not see the patient or examine them for these types of injuries.
n. Although most health care professionals are trained to recognize abuse, it is still possible for them to miss the signs.
o. Case managers may be the first to complete the picture and recognize abuse. This is especially true if the caregiver takes the patient to multiple providers and the case manager is the only constant of the health care team.
p. Case managers will want to act as an advocate for the patient and take immediate steps to ensure the patient's safety.

F. Depression
1. Depression is underreported and undertreated in the elderly population.
2. Depression can be the root cause of many other observed problems in the elderly, such as:
   a. Nonadherence to treatment
   b. Social isolation
   c. Cognitive impairment
   d. Malnutrition
   e. Alcohol abuse
3. There are tools available to detect unrecognized depression in the geriatric individual.
4. Again, even though the case manager may not be responsible for the administration of such tests, he or she should be aware of their existence and recommend them as appropriate.
5. The Geriatric Depression Scale (Yesavage, 1983), developed by Yesavage and colleagues, was used in one geriatric program with good reported success.
6. Case managers using the scale believed that they were able to refer geriatric patients who might be suffering from depression for further evaluation.

7. The Beck Depression Inventory (Gallo, Reichel, & Anderson, 1988) is another tool for detecting depression.

8. The Beck Inventory is administered by an interviewer but has been adapted for self-administration.

9. Regardless of what tool is used, if any, case managers should be aware of the potential for depression.

10. Appropriate referrals should be arranged if depression (actual or potential) is detected.

G. Constipation

1. Individuals older than the age of 55 are at increased risk for constipation.

2. Other risk factors include (University of Iowa, 1998):
   a. Recent abdominal surgery
   b. Limited physical activity
   c. Inadequate diet, with fiber less than 15 g per day
   d. Intake of medications known to contribute to constipation
   e. History of chronic constipation
   f. Laxative abuse history
   g. Other co-morbidities known to cause constipation

3. Interventions include diet, exercise, fluid intake, and laxative use, according to the individual situation.

H. Polypharmacy

1. Over 50% of individuals older than the age of 65 years take four or more medications on a routine basis.

2. The normal physiologic changes associated with aging cause the elderly individual to be more prone to medication-related problems.

3. The combination of several medications and the aging process can cause issues in the elderly.

4. All of the problems mentioned earlier in this section can be triggered by medications.

5. Adherence issues increase in proportion to the complexity of the regimen (Council for Case Management Accountability—Hamilton, 1999).

6. A thorough assessment of the individual's prescription and nonprescription medications is essential to the case management assessment of the elderly.

7. Case managers can enlist the aid of the physician or the pharmacist to review the medications used by the older person and can make recommendations for changes.

8. Case managers can remember to consider medications in relation to other issues presenting in the case.

■ IDENTIFICATION OF HIGH-RISK GERIATRIC PATIENTS

A. A brief history of early identification efforts:

1. In the early days of case management, cases were identified primarily

through diagnostic criteria or through an event such as a worker's compensation injury.

2. Most of the cases were identified after the diagnosis or event had already occurred.

3. With the advent of the managed Medicare programs, health maintenance organizations (HMOs) found themselves at financial risk for large populations of geriatric members.

4. Once a geriatric member became ill, costs were greater and the illnesses were often more severe.

5. The added burden of co-morbidities in this population made interventions by case managers more difficult.

6. There was an increasing demand for methods to identify geriatric patients before the onset of illness or a major decline in health status. Two reasons propelled the need for earlier identification:

   a. Once a geriatric member became ill, he or she consumed two to four times more resources than a healthy geriatric member. This problem increased costs of care.

   b. The more reactive style of case management that relied on a diagnosis or event did not fulfill the potential for case management impact in this population.

7. Early efforts at identification and prediction of risks were intuitive and based primarily on the case manager's or medical director's knowledge and experience.

8. Questionnaires of varying lengths, some up to 12 pages, were mailed to geriatric health plan members, and trigger criteria were established to help identify geriatric patients who were, or could be, at high risk.

9. There were several pitfalls to the early use of questionnaires:

   a. Intuition has its limits. Some questions that a practitioner believes would be useful in predicting risk are not useful.

   b. Without a specific method of scoring the questionnaires, case managers were left to use their judgment regarding which geriatric members were at risk and should be contacted.

      (i) In one informal comparison, one group of case management staff contacted approximately 40% of the members returning a questionnaire, and another group of staff contacted approximately 6% of the members returning the identical questionnaire.

      (ii) The emphasis and focus of the two groups varied significantly and resulted in different rates of follow-up.

      (iii) There was no way to determine whether either group was actually focusing on the group of patients that could most benefit from case management.

   c. Without a scoring methodology, case managers were still required to review each questionnaire. This did not yield any real efficiency or accuracy in the identification of high-risk geriatric patients.

B. Screening versus assessment

1. It is important to differentiate screening from assessment. Without a clear differentiation of these two concepts, case managers will spend time and resources where they are not necessary.
2. When individuals are identified primarily because of a diagnosis or event, most of those individuals are ultimately deemed appropriate for case management.
3. In the circumstance in which the overwhelming majority of the individuals who are referred to case managers actually need case management, assessment by the case manager is a logical first step.
4. When the goal is to identify individuals who are at risk or in the very early stages of decline, different strategies are necessary.
5. One method of addressing the issues of earlier identification and increasing the objectivity in follow-up was the development of screening tools that are valid and reliable in predicting risk.
6. Use the example of a health fair, in which random blood glucose levels are obtained via finger stick. This is illustrative of several key principles of screening:
   a. The screening is aimed at a broad group of individuals to identify as many as possible and as early as possible.
   b. Individuals other than health care professionals can do the screening.
   c. The screening does not positively determine that the individual meets the criteria or diagnosis and requires further assessment by a health care professional.
7. Screening accomplished the objectives of:
   a. Identifying those geriatric patients who may be at risk before an adverse event without using case management resources
   b. Providing an objective method of determining which of the members required assessment by a case manager
8. Assessment also differs from screening in several ways. Unlike screening,
   a. An assessment is reserved for those who have met some initial criteria and not broadly applied.
   b. A qualified case manager should perform a comprehensive case management assessment.
   c. An assessment can determine wheter the individual actually needs further follow-up.
9. Goals of assessment include:
   a. Collection of data in order to identify problems or issues
   b. Determination of whether the problems or issues identified may be impacted by case management interventions
   c. Creation of an individualized plan of care

C. Development of the Predictor of Repeat Admission (PRA)
   1. The first widely used screening questionnaire was the PRA.
   2. In 1994, Chad Boult and his associates at University of Minnesota published information on the PRA (Boult, Dowd, McCaffery, et al., 1994).

3. The PRA was brief (seven questions) and allowed for scoring that placed geriatric members into high-risk, medium-risk, and low-risk groups.

4. This allowed case managers to focus interventions based on the actual risk of the member being hospitalized.

5. Although it is efficient and accurate, the original PRA was somewhat unsatisfactory to case managers.

   a. The questions that were used to calculate the risk score did not always equate with the data case managers used to judge the individual to be at risk.

   b. The answers to the questions and the score provided the case manager with little information as to where to focus the assessment. For example, were there issues with medication compliance?

6. The PRA Plus (HMO Work Group on Care Management, 1996) added a set of bridging questions.

   a. The bridging questions were not a part of the scoring.

   b. The questions provided a bridge from the screening of individuals to the assessment of individuals for case management.

   c. Items such as functional status, which allowed the case manager the opportunity to focus in on potential problem areas, were added.

D. SF (Short Form) 36: This document is a comprehensive short form with only 36 questions.

1. It yields an 8-scale health profile, as well as summary measures of health-related quality of life.

2. As documented in more than 750 publications, the SF-36 has proved useful in monitoring general and specific populations, comparing the burden of different diseases, differentiating the health benefits produced by different treatments, and screening individual patients.

3. Development of the SF-36 Health Survey and collection of norms for the general U.S. population were supported by grants to the Health Assessment Lab at the Health Institute, New England Medical Center (Boston, Massachusetts) from the Henry J. Kaiser Family Foundation (John E. Ware Jr., principal investigator).

4. The SF-36 is an excellent baseline measure, as is the SF-12 (a shorter version of the SF-36), which can be administered as part of the screening process to allow for comparison of outcomes after case management intervention.

■ COMPREHENSIVE GERIATRIC ASSESSMENT

A. A small number of geriatric patients should receive a comprehensive geriatric assessment.

B. The assessment is usually conducted by a team of geriatric experts from multiple disciplines and encompasses all aspects of the individual's health and functioning.

C. Usually connected with an academic medical center or veteran's hospital, the assessment is conducted on referral.

D. The elements of the geriatric assessment include:
1. Physical
2. Functional
3. Social
4. Financial
5. Cognitive
6. Nutritional
7. Environmental
8. Medications

E. Geriatric assessment is recommended when there are multiple problems (recognized or unrecognized) and when the current plans are not addressing the identified problems or issues.

■ GERIATRIC ASSESSMENT FOR PLACEMENT OF THE GERIATRIC PATIENT

A. Functional ability assessment: ADLs
1. Assessment categories:
   a. Bathing
   b. Dressing
   c. Toileting
   d. Transferring
   e. Continence
   f. Feeding
2. Scoring
   a. The individual receives a point for every function that he or she is able to do independently.
      (i) A score of 6 indicates full function.
      (ii) A score of 4 indicates moderate impairment.
      (iii) A score of 2 indicates severe impairment.

B. Functional ability assessment: IADLs
1. Assessment categories assesses the following:
   a. Use of the telephone
   b. Getting to places beyond walking distance
   c. Going shopping for groceries
   d. Preparing own meals
   e. Doing own housework
   f. Doing own handyman work
   g. Doing own laundry
   h. Taking own medication
   i. Managing own money
2. Scoring
   a. These items can be made gender specific by the interviewer.

b. The score range is 9 (poor) to 27 (good).
c. Scores are patient specific only.

C. Psychological health assessment: Folstein Mini-Mental State Examination
1. Categories of assessment:
a. Orientation to time, place, and date
b. Registration: name three objects
c. Attention and calculation
d. Recall
e. Language: repetition, commands, read, and repeat
f. Draw a clock
g. Assess level of consciousness
2. Scoring
a. The score range is 0 (poor) to 30 (good).
b. Scores are patient specific only.

D. Psychological health assessment: Yesavage Geriatric Depression Scale
1. The short form addresses various moods with 15 questions.
2. Scoring is cumulative, based on a "yes or no" response.

E. Physical health assessment
1. Compiles a traditional list of defined diagnoses and symptom complexes
2. Documentation of the number of days of hospitalization and disability can define the severity of health problems.
3. May use New York Heart Association Four Point Functional Disability Scale for clarification of degree of disability if the disorder is due to a cardiac problem
a. A subjective assessment to determine the severity of congestive heart failure
b. Scoring system with problem history of last 30 days

■ LEVELS OF CARE FOR THE GERIATRIC PATIENT

A. History
1. Almshouses: institutions to house the poor, aged, and mentally ill: regulation 1873.
2. County homes: result of regulation; historically, terrible conditions for the older adult.
3. 1935—Social Security Act: provided catalyst for privately funded institutions for the aged.
4. 1965—Medicare and Medicaid reimbursement allowed expansion of this industry.
5. 1965—Older Americans Act created primary vehicle for organizing, coordinating, and providing community-based services and opportunities for older Americans and their families.

6. Office of Nursing Home Affairs of 1971 and Nursing Reform Act of 1987 established minimum requirements for nursing assistants, created a resident rights statement, and implemented a single standard for 24-hour care for all residents in the nursing homes.

B. Long-term care
1. Definition
   a. Long-term care provides medical care, nursing care, or all assistance needed for those with a chronic illness or disability that prevents the individual from caring for himself or herself for an extended period of time.
   b. Long-term care can be provided in the home setting, community setting, or nursing home.
      (i) Home setting using home health aides, visiting nurses, and home-delivered meals
      (ii) Adult day care centers
      (iii) Respite services to give caregivers a break from daily responsibilities
2. Long-term care in the nursing home
   a. Nursing homes primarily exist to serve a small portion of the elderly population with severe medical and disability problems that require 24-hour care.
      (i) This population cannot stay in the home for financial reasons, because caregivers and resources are unavailable, or by personal choice.
      (ii) The intensity of home services is no longer possible.
      (iii) The resident is no longer safe in a home environment.
      (iv) The resident may require skilled care but has exhausted Medicare Part A benefits or is not eligible for Medicare Part A benefits.
   b. Provides rehabilitation services (restorative nursing) to *maintain* function in the geriatric patient
      (i) Walking the patient on a daily basis
      (ii) Passive range-of-motion exercises
      (iii) Help with feeding activities
   c. Functional characteristics may contribute to the decision to place a patient in a nursing home for long-term care.
      (i) Difficulty with toileting and incontinence
      (ii) Memory or orientation problems
      (iii) Behavior problems
      (iv) Sensory and communication problems

C. Skilled nursing facility (Medicare)
1. Definition
   a. Provides skilled nursing care and other medical services on a 24-hour basis to those who are age 65 or older or who are disabled.
   b. Has been certified under the Medicare Act to have high standards of care.

    c. Paid for by Medicare, following a qualifying hospitalization.

    d. Provides the necessary level of medical care around the clock for the patient who no longer meets acute criteria or specialized care of the hospital, at a greatly reduced cost.

2. Services

    a. Physicians on call at all times to cover any emergency

    b. Qualified nursing personnel on duty at all times

    c. Rehabilitation services to *restore* function in the geriatric patient

    d. Dental care

    e. Drugs and any related laboratory or x-ray study services

    f. Maintain a separate, confidential clinical record

    g. Room and board

    h. Activities to encourage self-care and the patient's return to the normal routine of life in the community

    i. Social services to provide discharge planning

        (i) Return individual to prior living arrangement or the most appropriate level of care required.

        (ii) Accommodate individual and families in planning for needed care.

        (iii) Coordinate care needed at next place of residence for discharging individual.

3. Qualifications for continued stay in a skilled nursing facility (Medicare)

    a. Diagnosis is related to condition that was treated in the hospital.

    b. The individual requires skilled nursing services on a daily basis.

        (i) Skilled nursing care is defined as services provided by qualified technical or professional health personnel to ensure the safety of the patient and the desired result.

        (ii) Owing to the inherent complexity of the skilled service, it can be performed safely or effectively only by or under the general supervision of skilled nursing.

    c. Examples of direct skilled nursing services:

        (i) Intravenous, intramuscular, or subcutaneous injections

        (ii) Nasopharyngeal and tracheotomy aspiration

        (iii) Insertion, sterile irrigation, and replacement of catheters

        (iv) Application of dressings

        (v) Treatment of decubitus ulcers of Grade 3 or worse

    d. The individual requires skilled rehabilitation services on a daily basis.

        (i) Skilled rehabilitation service is defined as services by qualified technical or professional health personnel to ensure the safety of the patient and the desired result.

        (ii) Owing to the inherent complexity of the skilled service, it can be performed safely and/or effectively only by or under the general supervision of skilled rehabilitation professionals.

        (iii) Services must be reasonable and necessary for the treatment of the patient's condition.

        (iv) Patient must have the potential for improvement or return to prior level of function in a reasonable amount of time.

    e. Examples of direct skilled rehabilitative services:

        (i) Physical therapy: does not include maintenance or restorative therapies

        (ii) Occupational therapy: does not include vocational or recreational programs

        (iii) Speech therapy: does not include restorative speech programs

D. Custodial care

  1. Level of care mainly for the purpose of performing ADLs.

  2. May be provided by persons without professional skills or training.

  3. This level of care is intended to:

    a. Maintain and support the patient's existing level of health

    b. Preserve health from further decline

  4. May be provided in a long-term care (nursing home) setting

E. Skilled nursing facility (Medicare) versus long-term care (skilled care and custodial care)

  1. Medicare Part A coverage (skilled nursing facility)

    a. Allows only up to 100 days of skilled care during a benefit period, only if the strict skilled criteria are met.

    b. Is not intended for chronic illness or disabilities.

    c. All skilled services must be reasonable and necessary.

    d. The individual must have potential for improvement or ability to return to prior level of function in a reasonable amount of time.

    e. Skilled service does not mean that the individual cannot care for himself or herself.

    f. It is not intended to provide maintenance therapies to maintain function (restorative nursing).

  2. Long-term care (skilled care)

    a. The individual may require skilled care but has exhausted Medicare Part A benefit period or is not eligible for benefits.

    b. The individual can no longer care for himself or herself and requires assistance in ADLs, taking medication, or skilled treatments.

  3. Long-term care (custodial care)

    a. The individual can no longer perform daily tasks necessary to maintain health and safety.

      (i) Cannot safely perform ADLs

      (ii) Cannot preserve health from further decline

    b. Individual by choice or circumstance has decided to reside in the nursing home as primary residence.

    c. Individual may receive nonskilled physical therapy services (restorative nursing by nursing assistants) to maintain function.

■ INSURANCE COVERAGE

A. According to a report by the American Association of Retired Persons (AARP Public Policy Institute & The Lewin Group, 1997):

1. 62% (21,234,000) of Medicare beneficiaries have private supplemental insurance.
2. 13% (4,477,000) belong to a Medicare HMO.
3. 14% (4,633,000) have Medicare only.
4. 10% (3,265,000) were on Medicaid for a full year.
5. 2% (724,000) were on Medicaid for part of a year.

B. This report further projects that these beneficiaries will spend an average of 19% of their incomes on out-of-pocket expenses, and individuals with incomes below the poverty level will spend as much as 35% of their incomes on out-of-pocket costs.

C. These numbers are provided to demonstrate the limitations of insurance coverage for this group and to highlight the need for case managers to assess the individual's financial status carefully, regardless of insurance coverage.

■ FINANCIAL ASSESSMENT

A. Inquiries regarding finances are often difficult to initiate.

B. In general, individuals are not comfortable providing information about their finances. This is especially true if the inquiries are over the telephone.

C. However, economic issues can have a direct impact on the health of an elderly individual.

D. The Older Americans Resources and Services Multidimensional Functional Assessment Questionnaire (OARS) contains an assessment of financial resources.

E. The case manager can arrange for this type of in-depth assessment of finances via the social worker or, depending on the practice setting, may complete the assessment personally.

F. Even without the complete assessment, the case manager should identify whether finances may be the root cause of other issues:

1. Does the person fail to follow his or her special diet because of lack of funds?
2. Does he or she ever alter the medication schedule to prolong the interval between refills to save money, or not take the medication at all?
3. Does the patient miss doctor's appointments for health maintenance or chronic illness management owing to insufficient funds?
4. Is the patient's housing substandard or unsafe owing to lack of funding for a more suitable living situation?

G. Case managers may be able to intervene in any of the above-mentioned situations (or others) to limit the impact of financial issues on the health and well-being of the older adult.

■ RESOURCES

A. The American Association of Retired Persons has information on virtually every aspect of successful aging and serves as a resource for case managers and patients.

B. The American Society on Aging has an extensive library of educational materials aimed at case managers and patients. In addition, it sponsors numerous conferences throughout the year for those working with older adults.

C. The Area Agency on Aging (AAA) offers a variety of programs, from information and referral to hands-on support programs. This is a number that should be in every case manager's telephone book. New or seasoned case managers should contact the AAA in their area and familiarize themselves with the services available.

D. Local public health departments often provide for in-home visits by public health nurses for health promotion activities. This is especially valuable for low-income elderly.

E. Service organizations such as the Salvation Army or St. Vincent DePaul Society often offer a variety of programs for the elderly population, such as:
   1. Adult day health programs
   2. Friendly visitor programs (on the phone or in person)
   3. Equipment loan programs
   4. Free or low-cost transportation

F. Churches and religious groups often offer services to their members or the community at large.

REFERENCES

AARP Public Policy Institute (Gross, D., Gibson, M. J., Caplan, C. F., & Brangan, N.) & The Lewin Group (Alecxih, L. & Corea, J.) (1997). *Out of pocket health spending by Medicare beneficiaries age 65 and over: 1997 projections.* Publication #9705, December 1997. AARP @ www.aarp.org

Abyad, A. (1996) Elder abuse: Diagnosis, management, and prevention. *Medical Interface,* October, 97–101.

The Administration on Aging and the Older Americans Act (1999). *Aging In America,* November, 1–5. *http://www.aoa.dhhs.gov/aoa/pages/aoafact.html.*

American Nurses Association and Association of Rehabilitation Nurses (1986). *Standards of rehabilitation nursing practices.* MO: American Nurses Association.

Boult, C., Dowd, B., McCaffery, D., et al. (1994). Screening elders at risk for hospitalization. *Journal of the American Geriatrics Society, 42,* 456–470.

Burke, M., & Walsh, M. (1992). *Gerontological nursing: Care of the frail elderly.* St. Louis: Mosby–Year Book.

Bushnell, F. K. (1992). Self-care teaching for the congestive heart failure patient. *Journal of Gerontological Nursing, 10,* 27–32.

Callahan, J. (1992). Aging in place. *Generations: Journal of the American Society of Aging,* Spring.

Carlson, R. (1988). Adult rehabilitation: Attitudes and implications. *Journal of Gerontological Nursing, 14,* 24–30.

Case Management Society of America (CMSA). (1996). *Code of professional conduct for case managers.* Rolling Meadows, IL: Commission for Case Manager Certification.

Council for Case Management Accountability—Hamilton, G. A. (1999). Patient adherence outcome indicators and measurement in case management and health care. A state of the science paper. 8.

Folstein, M., Folstein & McHugh. (1975) Mini-mental state: A practical method for grading the cognitive state of patients for the clinician. *Journal of Psychiatric Resources, 12,* 189–198.

Frolik, L. E. (1992). Charlottesville, VA: Mitchie Company.

Gallo, J., Reichel, W., & Andersen, L. (1988). *Handbook of geriatric assessment.* Gaithersburg, MD: Aspen.

Gurland, B. (1997). The assessment of the mental health status of older adults. In *Handbook of mental health and aging.* New York: Prentice Hall.

Hankes, D. (1984). Self-care: Assessing the aged client's need for independence. *Journal of Gerontological Nursing, 18,* 26–31.

HIAA guide to long-term care insurance (1999). *Consumer Information,* December, 1–13; http://www.hiaa.org/cons/guideltc.html.

HMO Work Group on Care Management (1996). *Identifying high-risk Medicare HMO members: A report from the HMO Work Group on Care Management: Chronic care initiatives in HMOs.* Washington, D.C.: Group Health Foundation.

Hoenig, H., et al. (1994). Adult rehabilitation: What do physicians know about it and how should they use it? *Journal of American Geriatrics, 42,* 341–347.

How to translate terminology used by therapists into MDS lingo. (1998). *National Report on Subacute Care, 16,* 5–8.

Kane, R. (1981). *Assessing the elderly: A practical guide to measurement.* New York: Lexington Books.

The Merck manual of geriatrics (1995–1999). Whitehouse Station, NJ: Merck.

Miller, C. A. (1999). *Nursing care of older adults: Theory and practice* (3rd ed.). Philadelphia: Lippincott Williams & Wilkins.

NebGuide. (1999). *Nursing home insights.* December, 1–7; *http://www.unl.edu/pubs/homemgt/g1013.htm.*

Norris, J. N., et al. (1997). *Quality of care in the nursing home.* St Louis: Mosby–Year Book, Inc.

Pfeiffer, E. (1975). A short portable mental status questionnaire for the assessment of organic brain deficit in the older adult patient. *Journal of American Geriatrics, 23,* 433.

Rehabilitation of geriatric patients (1999). *Scientific American,* March, 1–8.

Rhoades, J. A., & Krauss, N. A. (1996). *Nursing Home Trends, 1987 and 1996: MEPS Chartbook No. 3.* October, 1–5; *http://www.meps.ahcpr.gov/papaers/chartbk3a.htm.*

University of Iowa. (1998). *Research based protocols no.* June 49 Obtained from National Guideline Clearing House via Internet at *www.guidelines.gov*

Uris, P., & Kearns, J. M. (1990). *Essentials of quality nursing care for the elderly.* Boulder, CO: Western Institute of Nursing.

US care. (1999). Glossary of long-term care terms. April; *http://www.uscare.com/glossary.html.*

U.S. Bureau of the Census (1996). *Statistical abstract of the United States: 1996* (116th edition). Washington, D.C.: U.S. Government printing Office.

U.S. Department of Health and Human Services (1991). *Aging America: Trends and projections.* Washington, D.C.: U.S. Government Printing Office.

Van Nostrand, J. F., Clark, R. F., & Romoren, T. I. (1993). Nursing home care in five nations. *Aging International,* June, 1–5.

Whitman Group (1993). *Gerontological nursing specialist professional nursing update.* Huntingdon Valley, PA: The Whitman Group.

Wilson, J. (1987). *Partial history of long term care regulation.* Salem, OR: Senior Disabled Services Division.

Yesavage, J. A., & Brink, T. L. (1983). Development and validation of a geriatric depression screening scale: A preliminary report. *Journal of Psychiatric Research, 17,* 4.

CHAPTER **18**

. . . .

Leadership Skills and Concepts

SUZANNE K. POWELL

DONNA IGNATAVICIUS

LEARNING OBJECTIVES

Upon completion of this chapter, the reader will be able to:

1. Define important terms and concepts relative to leadership.
2. List the essential components of effective leadership.
3. Differentiate between aggressive and cooperative negotiation.
4. Identify key critical thinking strategies and skills for case managers.
5. Describe the role of the case manager in delegation and supervision.
6. Compare and contrast hard and soft savings.
7. List considerations for developing budgets.
8. Discuss the role of the case manager as an agent of change.

IMPORTANT TERMS AND CONCEPTS

Empowerment
Conflict Management
Critical Thinking
Delegation
Negotiation

Cost–Benefit Analysis
Hard Savings
Soft Savings
Change Agent

■ INTRODUCTION

A. Case management requires a wide array of management skills: delegation, conflict resolution, crisis intervention, collaboration, consultation, coordination, identification, and documentation. However, case managers are no longer just managers of care; they are leaders, and there is a difference. *Managers manage systems; leaders lead people.* Case managers do both; they manage cases and lead, or guide, people. Leadership is one step up on the ladder of professional growth. As case management continues to grow in responsibility, leadership qualities will necessarily be presumed (Powell, 2000a).

B. Leadership is about the ability to influence people to accomplish goals. Leaders can be formal (by position in the organization or society) or informal (by amount of influence they have on others).

■ KEY DEFINITIONS

A. *Negotiation* is essentially a communication exchange for the purpose of reaching agreement.

B. *Critical thinking* is purposeful, outcome-directed thinking that aims to make judgments based on facts and is based on scientific principles (Alfaro-LeFevre, 1999).

C. *Empowerment* is allowing employees or subordinates to make decisions with support by the leader or manager.

D. *Delegation* is the process of assigning tasks to a qualified person and supervising that individual as needed.

■ LEADERSHIP SKILLS

A. The jury is still out about whether leaders are born or made. However, experts have noticed specific actions that successful leaders share, regardless of the type of organization they lead.

B. Effective leaders
   1. *Promote empowerment.* They emphasize the strengths and use the talents of others in the organization. Leaders share decision-making with others, allowing those people at the point of care or service to be the key decision-makers. Then they share in the success and give credit where it is due.
   2. *Promote a vision.* People need a vision of where they are going. Leaders provide that vision (*Manager's Intelligence Report*, 1997).
   3. *Follow the golden rule.* Anyone who has been demeaned or treated with disrespect knows what effect that treatment has on the work (*Manager's Intelligence Report*, 1997).
   4. *Admit mistakes.*
   5. *Praise others in public. Criticize others only in private.*
   6. *Stay close to the action.* In case management, this is the administrator who goes to the "front lines" occasionally to stay in touch with the re-

ality of the working situation. This also means that the leader is visible and accessible.

7. *Say, "I don't know"* when confronted with a case management problem, then assist with a solution.
8. Focus on *what* is right, not *who* is right.
9. *Motivate others* by
   a. Establishing credibility
   b. Improving communication skills
   c. Being a role model
   d. Taking an interest in others
   e. Rewarding positive behaviors
   f. Sharing decision-making
   g. Offering constructive criticism (Ellis & Hartley, 1995)

C. Conflict management is an important skill for leaders. Five strategies can be employed, from less desirable to most desirable:
1. Avoidance
2. Competition ("I win, you lose")
3. Accommodation ("You win, I lose")
4. Negotiation (also known as compromise) (see next section)
5. Collaboration ("You win, I win") (the best strategy)
   a. Takes more time to use
   b. Save for complex or emotional issues

■ NEGOTIATION SKILLS

A. In the current health care environment of scarce resource availability and declining benefits, the art of negotiation is extremely important.

B. Negotiation serves several important purposes (Powell, 2000a):
1. It has the capacity to control costs. This is one of the primary reasons case managers negotiate.
2. It has the capacity to gain medically necessary benefits for the patient that otherwise the patient would not receive. This is the other primary reason case managers negotiate.
3. It can avoid chaos (Jones et al., 1998). Many case managers have lived through the frustration and chaos when the patient deteriorated, at least partly because the negotiation for the requested service or equipment was denied.
4. Negotiation can be a learning experience. Case managers may learn why the request is denied (sometimes there is a valid reason). They may also reveal weaknesses in the "No!" argument that could lead to further strengths in the case manager's negotiation stance.

C. Successful negotiation steps
1. Be optimally prepared. Before negotiation begins, it is wise to do some research; understand the other side before negotiation.
2. Negotiation starts by stating the problem or problems and the goal,

and stating what is needed to solve the problem. State the request in a positive and thorough way. Areas in which there is agreement can be put aside; then begin to search for a mutual compromise (Rehberg & Sullivan, 1997).

3. Use the three Cs—communicate, communicate, and communicate. Common mistakes can create a defensive environment that is not conducive to negotiation. Some behaviors that may be problematic include poor listening skills, poor use of questions, improper disclosure of ideas, mismanagement of issues, inappropriate stress reactions, rejecting alternatives too quickly, misusing a negotiating team member, not disclosing true feelings, improper timing, and being aggressive rather than assertive (Hein & Nicholson, 1994).

4. Be realistic. Attempting to negotiate for a service or a price that absolutely will not be covered or met wastes everyone's time and energy.

5. Put it in writing. Once an agreement has been reached, write it down and have all parties sign it.

D. There are two types of negotiators: aggressive and cooperative. Aggressive negotiators use psychological maneuvers such as intimidation and threats to make their "opponent" feel disparaged. Cooperative negotiators try to establish trust.

1. The aggressive negotiator (Jones et al., 1998):
   a. Moves psychologically against his or her opponent. Note the key word psychologically. If the case manager feels that something is amiss, that is, that he or she is being toyed with, bring the case back to facts.
   b. Common tactics include intimidation, accusation, threats, sarcasm, and ridicule.
   c. There is a overt or covert claim that the aggressive negotiator is superior.
   d. The aggressive negotiator will make extreme demands and few concessions.
   e. There will be frequent threats to terminate negotiations.
   f. False issues will be brought up time and again. This is another time to bring the case back to facts.

2. Weaknesses of the aggressive method (Jones et al., 1998):
   a. It is more difficult to be a successful aggressive.
   b. Tension and mistrust that develop may increase the likelihood of misunderstandings.
   c. Deadlock over one trivial issue may escalate other issues.
   d. The opponent may develop righteous indignation and pursue the case with more vengeance.
   e. The reputation as an aggressive hurts future negotiations.
   f. Aggressive tactics increase the number of failed negotiations.
   g. The trial rate for aggressive negotiators is more than double.

3. The cooperative negotiator (Jones et al., 1998):
   a. Moves psychologically toward his or her opponent.

b. This negotiator establishes a common ground. For case managers, the common ground is the patient.

c. This negotiator is trustworthy, fair, objective, and reasonable. This is very important. Respect and trustworthiness are critical for negotiations and for self-respect as a case management professional.

d. This negotiator works to establish credibility and unilateral concessions. The attitude is one of "win-win."

e. This negotiator seeks to obtain the best joint outcome for everyone. This requires respect, empathy, and active listening, as described in other sections of this text.

f. Future negotiations are made easier.

4. Strengths of the cooperative method (Jones et al., 1998):
   a. Promotes mutual understanding.
   b. Generally produces agreement in less time than the aggressive approach.
   c. Produces agreements in a larger percentage of cases than aggressives.
   d. Often produces a better outcome than aggressive strategies.
   e. There is a much higher percentage of "successful" negotiations.

5. Weaknesses of the cooperative method (Jones et al., 1998):
   a. Aggressive negotiators view cooperative negotiators as weak, so they push harder.
   b. Cooperative negotiators risk being manipulative or exploitive because of the assumption that, "if I am fair and trustworthy and make decisions with all parties in mind, then the other side will feel an irresistible moral obligation to reciprocate."

■ CRITICAL THINKING AND DECISION-MAKING

A. Critical thinking (CT) is broader than problem solving. It is more than finding a single solution to a problem (Alfaro-LeFavre, 1999).

B. In health care, CT may be referred to as clinical reasoning; in nursing, it is sometimes equated to the nursing process. However, CT is not exactly synonymous with these terms.

C. CT is being creative and thinking outside the box or "connecting the dots." In general, it is the ability to
   1. Put together the known components of the problem or situation
   2. Research all possible solutions
   3. Find a way to improve the condition (Powell, 2000a)

D. CT is focused on outcomes, not tasks. It is purposeful, outcome-directed thinking that aims to make judgments based on facts. It is reflective and reasonable thinking about client problems without a single solution and is focused on deciding what to believe and do.

E. Characteristics of a good critical thinker
   1. Flexible
   2. Creative

    3. Communicator, especially listening

    4. Open-minded

    5. Willing to change

    6. Outcome focused

    7. Able to see "the big picture"

    8. Caring

F. Variables that affect critical thinking (Ignatavicius, 1999)

    1. Thinking styles

    2. Personal factors, such as age, gender, and education

    3. Situational factors, such as available time, resources, peer support, and administrative support

G. Levels of critical thinking

    1. Basic level: knowing right from wrong

    2. Complex level: identifying all possible alternatives or solutions ("It depends")

    3. Committed level: selecting the most reasonable alternative ("Plan A") and having one or more backup plans in case Plan A is unsuccessful

H. Critical thinking strategies and cognitive skills based on American Philosophical Association (APA) study (Facione & Facione, 1995)

    1. Interpretation (clarifying meaning)

    2. Analysis (examining ideas, data)

    3. Evaluation (assessing outcomes)

    4. Inference (drawing conclusions)

    5. Explanation (justifying actions)

    6. Self-regulation (self-examination and correction)

I. Critical thinking process

    1. Analyze all of the problems.

    2. Determine the expected outcomes.

    3. List all possible alternatives and solutions to the problems.

    4. Select the best or highest-priority alternative.

    5. Determine if the plan worked (Were the outcomes met?).

■ DELEGATION SKILLS

A. Some case managers see delegation as a loss of power and control.

B. Some case managers simply do not trust others to do the job correctly. They live by the credo that if you want something done correctly, do it yourself.

C. Some case managers feel a legal liability when delegating responsibility.

D. Delegation standards that will minimize risk (Powell, 2000a):

    1. Always act in a reasonable and prudent manner.

    2. Ensure that the delegate is qualified to perform the tasks.

    3. Assign tasks that are within the person's scope of practice.

4. Provide proper supervision (guidance and monitoring) to the person to whom the task was delegated.

E. Effective delegation recommendations

1. Stress results, not details. Make it clear that you are more concerned with the final outcome than with all of the day-to-day details. This provides autonomy to the one who is responsible for the results.

2. Do not always become the solution to everyone's problems. Teach others how to solve problems, rather than just providing the answer. Again, this builds confidence and independence and provides autonomy.

3. When an employee or coworker comes to you with a problem and a question, ask him or her for possible solutions. Be there to brainstorm when needed.

4. Establish measurable and concrete objectives. Make them clear and specific. This is the road map that others can follow.

5. Develop reporting systems. Obtain feedback from written reports, statistical data, and planned face-to-face meetings. This does not always work in case management if a particularly tough problem arises; teach employees when to come to you with details, and when to come to you after exhausting other avenues.

6. When appropriate, give strict but realistic deadlines. This gives the task credibility and gives the person accountability.

7. Keep a delegation log. This is especially important for very busy people or those with many employees.

8. Recognize and use the talents and personalities of the people you work with. Being a good delegator is very much like being a good coach.

■ COST–BENEFIT ANALYSIS

A. In 1996, the Health Insurance Association of America (HIAA) reported that case managers save $30 for every case management dollar spent.

B. Many case managers will be asked to conduct a cost analysis of a case or parts of a case. For example:

1. Occasionally, family members need comparative financial information.

2. Insurance companies, who are inclined to refuse payment for a requested plan if they believe that a less cost-intensive solution is available, may request prices.

3. Many case managers are required to make a formal documentation of savings per case for accounting purposes.

4. Disease management case managers may be required to contribute to the savings information for an entire population of disease-specific patients.

C. Many case managers shun this responsibility. There may be several reasons for the dislike (Powell, 2000b), such as the following:

1. We did not go into the helping professions to do accounting work. We are case managers to improve the quality of a patient's life.

2. We already know that we improve quality and decrease costs per case; justifying our existence is another's responsibility.

3. It is difficult to understand accounting and budgeting concepts.
4. It is often tedious and time-consuming to address and report financial details.

D. Case managers are as real an expense to the payers and facilities who hire us as physician services, hospital costs, and medications. Cost analysis is one method used to prove our worth in the business world.

E. Hard savings or avoided costs—when costs were measurably saved or avoided.

F. Examples of hard savings include (Powell, 2000b):
1. Change in the level of care facilitated by the case manager
2. Change in the patient's length of stay facilitated by the case manager
3. Change to a contracted PPO provider facilitated by the case manager
4. Negotiation of price of services, supplies, equipment, or per diem rates facilitated by the case manager
5. Negotiation of frequency of services facilitated by the case manager
6. Negotiation of duration of services facilitated by the case manager
7. Prevention of unnecessary bed days, supplies, equipment, services, or charges facilitated by the case manager
8. Finding nonauthorized charges that are not warranted

G. Soft savings or potential savings (or potential costs or charges) are less tangibly measurable than hard savings. If no case manager was assigned to this patient, the potential costs incurred could have been much higher than with case management; they represent costs that were avoided most likely because of case management intervention.

H. Examples of soft savings include (Powell, 2000b):
1. Avoidance of potential hospital readmissions
2. Avoidance of potential emergency department visits
3. Avoidance of potential medical complications
4. Avoidance of potential legal exposure
5. Avoidance of potential costs, equipment, and supplies
6. Avoidance of potential acute care days
7. Avoidance of potential home health visits
8. Other soft savings relate to quality and satisfaction. It is difficult to put a dollar amount on the following:
   a. Improved quality of care
   b. Improved patient and family satisfaction with case management
   c. Improved patient compliance
   d. Improved quality of life

■ CASE MANAGEMENT OUTCOMES AND BUDGETARY ISSUES

A. First attempts at measuring outcomes should be easily and concretely measurable.
1. Begin by looking at only one or two outcomes.

2. Cost savings have been the most common measurement used for case management outcomes.
   a. Hard savings are more tangible and easily measured; soft savings are more obscure.
   b. Quality of life issues are also more nebulous and will require careful consideration when turning them into something that is measurable (Powell, 2000b).

B. Defining a budget when beginning an outcomes management program
   1. Measuring outcomes is an important marketing tool, but the process requires resources of time, money, and personnel.
   2. It is important to assess what resources will be needed and to define a budget for the project that is acceptable to the organization. Consider the following (Powell, 2000b):
      a. What resources are available to plan, select, modify or develop, and implement an effective case management intervention?
      b. What resources are required to plan, select, modify or develop, and implement a case management intervention?
      c. In some projects, other people or organizations are asked to commit resources to the project. In those instances, determine what resources will be required of others. Are they willing and able to provide the resources? Some resources to consider are provider staffing, physician time, and beneficiary co-payments or deductibles.
      d. Can the improved outcome be translated into projected cost savings? If the cost of the case management intervention exceeds the amount of projected cost savings, is this still acceptable to the organization?
      e. Data collection and analysis is complex and costly. Does the case management organization have the necessary resources and information systems to execute these tasks, or can the organization secure appropriate data elements from other avenues that will provide the information necessary to record outcome measurements? Put a dollar amount on this and assess whether it is feasible.

■ CASE MANAGERS AS CHANGE AGENTS

A. Although some people embrace change, most find it intimidating. Because of the unpredictable nature of change, some people respond to it with fear. Change is at the core of stress.

B. New and fast-changing managed care and financial constraints must be managed.

C. Case management is more important than ever before in order to manage these changes in the best interests of the patients; case managers are essentially change agents.

D. The three components of the change process are
   1. Unfreezing the current behavior or situation
      a. Determine driving forces (supportive forces for the change).
      b. Determine restraining forces (opposing forces for the change).

      c. Develop plan to overcome resistance to change.

  2. Implementing the change

      a. Enabling the change

      b. Monitoring the change

  3. Freezing the new change

      a. Sustaining and supporting the change

      b. Evaluating the change

E. Attitudes to help agents of change cope:

  1. Sometimes these methods fail. You have worked hard with the case and used the clinical pathways. Then it seems the case is falling off the path at every turn, and variances are winning. There is no shortage of problems.

      a. First, assess whether you could have done anything differently for a better outcome.

      b. If so, learn from it.

      c. If not, realize that sometimes these methods fail.

  2. Choose your battles carefully. Many aspects of case management are completely out of the case manager's realm of control. Assess whether the problem is something that you can make an impact on.

  3. Remember this wise adage. Robert Eliot, a cardiologist at the University of Nebraska, had developed two rules for keeping things in perspective (Charlesworth & Nathan, 1984):

      a. Don't sweat the small stuff.

      b. It's all small stuff.

  4. Remember that change is risk.

  5. It's OK to disagree. Not everyone has to be in agreement to move forward. Use the continuous quality improvement (CQI) tool of consensus.

  6. Anticipate changes. Don't wait for changes to happen. Be proactive with other possiblities.

REFERENCES

Alfaro-LeFevre, R. (1999). *Critical thinking in nursing*. Philadelphia: W.B. Saunders.

Charlesworth, E., & Nathan, R. (1984). *Stress management: A comprehensive guide to wellness*. New York: Atheneum.

Ellis, J. R., & Hartley, C. L. (1995). *Managing and coordinating nursing care*. Philadelphia: J.B. Lippincott.

Facione, N. C., & Facione, P. A. (1996). Externalizing the critical thinking in knowledge development and clinical judgment. *Nursing Outlook, 44*(3), 129–136.

Hein, E. C., & Nicholson, M. J. (1994). *Contemporary leadership behavior*. Philadelphia: J.B. Lippincott.

Ignatavicius, D. D. (1999). Critical Thinking Workshops.

Jones, Skelton, & Hochuli. (1998). Seminar in Phoenix, Az.

The manager's intelligence report. (1997). Chicago: Lawrence Ragan Communications, Inc.

Powell, S. K. (2000a). *Case management: A practical guide to success in managed care*. Philadelphia: Lippincott Williams & Wilkins.

Powell, S. K. (2000b). *Advanced case management: Outcomes and beyond*. Philadelphia: Lippincott Williams & Wilkins.

Rehberg, C., & Sullivan, G. (1997). The art of negotiation: A delicate balance. *Nursing Case Management, 2*(4), 177–179.

■

CHAPTER **19**

• • • • • • • • • • • • • •

Outcomes Management

SHERRY L. ALIOTTA

LEARNING OBJECTIVES

Upon completion of this chapter, the reader will be able to:

1. Define outcomes.
2. List reasons why outcomes management is important.
3. Describe the common categories of outcomes.
4. List the characteristics of effective outcome measures.
5. Describe methods of incorporating outcomes measurement into practice.
6. Identify resources for outcomes measurement.
7. Identify outcomes initiatives.
8. Identify key issues in reporting outcomes.

IMPORTANT TERM AND CONCEPTS

Benchmarks
Direct Outcomes
End Outcomes
External Validity
Indicators
Intermediate Outcomes
Internal Validity

Outcomes
Outcomes Measurement
Process Measures
Reliability
Risk Adjustment
Variation

■ INTRODUCTION

A. For several years, case managers have used outcome information from providers to make referral decisions.

B. Case managers are now being called on to measure and report outcomes of case management.

C. Although there have been numerous anecdotal descriptions of case management outcomes, objective, scientific evidence is sparse.

D. Several issues have contributed to the lack of valid, reliable outcomes data:

1. Inconsistent definitions of case management and the interventions performed by case managers.

2. Inconsistent methods of measurement. For example, one group calculates cost savings using one method, and another group calculates cost savings in a different way.

3. Organizations maintaining their methods of measuring outcomes as proprietary to their program and process.

4. The initial acceptance of case management as a tool to reduce costs reduced the need for case managers to define, document, and measure carefully the results of their activities except via cost savings.

■ KEY DEFINITIONS

A. Outcomes are the qualitative measures or results of a process and performance (Rieve, 1997).

B. External validity—the degree to which the results of a study can be generalized to settings or samples other than the one studied (Polit & Hungler, 1989)

C. Internal validity—the degree to which it can be inferred that the experimental treatment or independent variable, rather than the uncontrolled extraneous factors, is responsible for observed effects on the dependent variable (Polit & Hungler, 1989)

D. Reliability—the degree of consistency or accuracy with which an instrument measures the attribute it is designed to measure (Polit & Hungler, 1989)

E. Direct (intermediate) case management outcomes—the measurement or results of those activities and interventions that are within the scope of the case manager's practice and control.

F. End health system outcomes—those performance indicators measured for the health care system overall and including the following:

1. Cost of care

2. Quality of care

3. Health status outcomes achieved

G. Indicator—a quantitative measure that allows for demonstrating achievement.

H. Process measures—used primarily to determine the degree to which the process is being executed as planned. For example, "The number of patients receiving a case management assessment within two business days."

I. Benchmarks—established by the leaders or toughest competitors in the field; used by others to measure their performance continuously with these leaders (Powell, 2000).

J. Variation—the stability (or lack thereof) in a process. If the process has a large amount of variation (instability), it is more difficult to manage than a process with only a slight degree of variation (Powell, 2000).

K. Risk adjustment—a process for introducing an allowance for factors that would introduce bias. For example, in one health plan, Medicare-aged patients may be counted as 1.5 patients when establishing caseload numbers. This "risk adjustment" (counting one person as if he or she were one and a half) is meant to account for the additional time that these more complex patients require from a case manager.

■ DEFINING OUTCOME MEASUREMENT

A. In addition to the technical definition, outcomes are a result of a process.

B. When selecting outcome measures, we are attempting to determine in advance the potential effects, side effects, or consequences of our actions.

C. Outcome measurement can assist in the demonstration of value by validating:
   1. What is effective
   2. What is not effective
   3. The costs of an intervention
   4. Whether the cost of the intervention is substantiated by the return on the investment

D. Outcomes have often been discussed in terms of outcomes management.

E. Outcomes cannot be managed: the structure and process that produced the outcome must be managed, and the outcome measured.

F. It has been said that, "A system is perfectly designed to produce the outcome it produces."

G. If you want different outcomes, you must change your structure or process.

H. Therefore, outcomes measurement must incorporate the structure and the process to ensure reliability and validity.

■ THE RATIONALE FOR OUTCOMES MEASUREMENT

A. Measuring outcomes allows us to base improvement on measurement.

B. Without effective outcome measurements, we are unable to track improvements or declines in performance objectively.

C. Measurement of outcomes provides a method for demonstrating value to the customers of a process.

D. The ability to verify positive outcomes provides a powerful rationale for a service.

E. Outcome measurement allows us to determine which processes and interventions are effective and which are not.

F. With appropriate outcomes, data stakeholders can be educated regarding the value or potential value of the process or intervention.

G. Finally, outcome data provide information to allow us to determine whether the results of the process or intervention yield the desired return on investment.

■ COMMON CATEGORIES OF OUTCOME INDICATORS

A. Clinical outcomes are demonstrated through various indicators, such as
  1. Morbidity
  2. Mortality
  3. Improvement or deterioration in symptoms
  4. Absence of complications

B. Functional indicators include the ability to
  1. Maintain one's lifestyle
  2. Complete the required health-related activities
  3. Return to gainful activities
  4. Perform vocational tasks (return to work)

C. Financial indicators focus on costs, such as
  1. Costs of care
  2. Savings
     a. Per year
     b. Per episode
  3. Recidivism and the cost of job-related injuries or disease

D. Satisfaction with care

E. Many times, indicators measure the outcome of the process itself (process measures) and not the impact of the process (outcome measures).

F. Process measures are important because they allow us to understand what we are doing.

G. Understanding what we are doing is key to improving our processes and linking processes with the impact of the processes.

H. It is critical that case management move beyond what we do to why what we do matters.

I. Each of the indicators mentioned earlier provides the opportunity to demonstrate impact (outcome measures) as well as process (process measures).

■ CHARACTERISTICS OF EFFECTIVE OUTCOME MEASURES

A. The following characteristics were adapted from Neil Power and are a part of a presentation given by Sherry L. Aliotta and Marlys Severson at the Disease Management Congress in February, 1999.

B. Effective outcome measurements are

1. Valid, which means that the effect seen is actually related to the intervention and is not a random occurrence.
2. Reliable, which is defined as measuring what it is actually intended to measure.
3. Not easy to manipulate, as objective and quantifiable as possible.
4. Comprehensive, covering most or all aspects of the process being measured.
5. Dynamic, which means that the measure can change to reflect changes in practice.
6. Flexible, which means that if an outcome measure can demonstrate outcomes for more than one process or be used to demonstrate multiple outcomes, this is a positive attribute.
7. Cogent, which means that the outcome measure must make sense to the user.

■ INCORPORATING OUTCOME MEASUREMENT INTO PRACTICE

A. Build outcome measures into any new intervention, process, or program.

1. Consider the goals that led you to begin the intervention, process, or program.
   a. List the problems you are trying to solve.
   b. Describe exactly what you want to improve.
2. List the method you will use to determine whether you have reached your goal.
   a. Describe what things will occur when you have achieved the desired outcome (e.g., no patients will be re-hospitalized in the first 60 days after discharge for the same or a related diagnosis, or Mrs. Smith will schedule doctor's appointments at least one time per month and keep the scheduled appointments).
   b. Be as specific and as descriptive as possible.
3. Determine how you can measure that achievement using different research designs.
   a. Before-and-after comparison—for example, how many appointments were scheduled and kept before case management, or before case management 90% of patients returned to the hospital within 60 days past discharge, and after case management re-hospitalization within 60 days occurred with only 20% of patients.
   b. Randomized comparison—for example, a group of patients who are statistically similar is chosen. The group is randomly assigned to one of two groups before the intervention is tested. One group receives the intervention, and the other group does not receive the intervention. The two groups are compared and the impact of the intervention is evaluated.
   c. Comparison groups—for example, a group of patients receiving an intervention is compared with a statistically similar group of patients who do no receive the intervention. This differs from the randomized comparison in that the groups may not have been selected

in advance of the comparison, and the groups may have differing reasons for why an intervention was not given.

   d. Other methods of measuring impact include:
      (i) Comparison with established benchmarks (e.g., recommendations for hemoglobin A_1C testing in diabetics).
      (ii) Progress toward an established goal. (This could include increasing or decreasing a particular measurement. For example, admissions for congestive heart failure patients have declined 15%, and we expect to reach our goal of 45% reduction in 3 months.)

4. Identify the best reporting method.
   a. Use of a data base can allow you to report in multiple ways and from multiple perspectives.
      (i) Depending on their needs, different perspectives are requested by different people.
      (ii) If you are unable to show the results in a way that will allow your audience to identify the value of the results to them or to those for whom they are responsible, your results may not receive the attention they deserve.
   b. Identify people who are the stakeholders in the process.
      (i) When establishing a report, it is important to know who will be receiving the report and why the report is needed.
      (ii) Determine what you know or understand about the stakeholders in order to gain insight into the problem from their perspective. For example, physicians may need to know which of their patients have not had a recommended test or treatment in order to ensure that the patient gets the needed service, and the unit manager may want to know the test or treatment that is most frequently missed in order to examine interventions that may be used to remind practitioners to complete the service.
   c. Make sure your report addresses the needs of the stakeholders.
   d. Become familiar with the use of graphs, charts, and diagrams that will provide an interesting and illustrative visual representation of the data.

5. Ask and answer the "so what?" question.
   a. Quantify or describe the impact or final outcome of the process.
   b. If you increased or improved something, what changed other than the process? For example, if the patient keeps all of his or her doctor's appointments, what happens as a result? If readmissions decline, were costs decreased or were patients more satisfied?

B. Think in terms of quantifying and measuring.
   1. Instead of describing and explaining, think of objective ways to count or measure the event.
   2. Collect baseline measurements to use as a comparison for improvement. It is difficult to judge progress without recording your starting point.
   3. Ask yourself how you will know whether your plans or programs are working and how you can demonstrate that success to others.

C. Learn how to use data bases and other computer programs.
   1. Data bases can store information in a format that allows it to be retrieved in various ways.
   2. This flexibility allows the case manager to look at all of the available information in several ways.
      a. Sorted by different factors such as age, diagnosis, and interventions
      b. Sorted by common factors, such as all those with "x, y, and z"
      c. Sorted by different elements, such as all those with "x but not y or z"
   3. Looking at the data in different ways can help identify outcomes or suggest other areas for study.
D. Review statistical principles.
   1. Know the key statistical tools to be used in simple comparisons.
   2. Familiarize yourself with the methods of critically reading and evaluating research papers and findings.
E. Review the continuous quality improvement (CQI) processes and tools:
   1. Develop an understanding of key CQI principles.
   2. Be familiar with CQI tools for process improvement.

■ RESOURCES AND INITIATIVES FOR OUTCOME MEASURES

A. The Council for Case Management Accountability (CCMA)
   1. Sponsored by the Case Management Society of America (CMSA)
   2. The council was formed in 1996.
   3. Its formation was begun in response to the increasing demand for accountability in health care through outcomes reporting.
   4. The first "product" of the council was the "Dimensions of Accountability" (CMSA, 1997).
   5. The CCMA sought opinions from numerous stakeholders, including:
      a. Business leaders
      b. Accrediting bodies
      c. National health care—related organizations
      d. Case managers from
         (i) Academic centers
         (ii) Hospitals
         (iii) Managed care
         (iv) Worker's compensation
         (v) Home care
         (vi) Rehabilitation centers
      e. Legislators
   6. The goals established for the CCMA include:
      a. Establishing a framework for accountability and defining consistent mechanisms for reporting and comparing performance measurements industry wide

    b. Dispersing the findings of the CCMA to the key stakeholders

    c. Identifying existing measures and indicators that can be linked to those available and used at present, and identifying where there are gaps or no measurements exist

    d. Demonstrating the Dimensions of Accountability

        (i) The Dimensions of Accountability provide a framework for the core model and concepts.

        (ii) With this model, case managers acknowledge that the end outcomes of the health care system are multifactorial. This means that to achieve the end outcomes, factors other than effective case management must occur.

        (iii) The Dimensions of Accountability model states that "This is what case managers do to contribute to the final outcome."

        (iv) By demonstrating the effectiveness of the case manager's ability to achieve the direct outcomes, and by demonstrating the impact on the final outcome, case managers can document their impact.

        (v) The Dimensions of Accountability model links the core functions of case management as established in the *Standards of Practice for Case Managers* (CMSA, 1995):

            (a) Assessment

            (b) Planning

            (c) Facilitation

            (d) Advocacy

        (vi) The core functions produce and are linked to the direct outcomes of case management:

            (a) Patient knowledge

            (b) Patient involvement in care

            (c) Patient empowerment

            (d) Patient adherence

            (e) Coordination of care

        (vii) The direct outcomes produce and are linked to the end outcomes of

            (a) Improved health status

            (b) Increased quality of care

            (c) Decreased costs

B. Disease management

    1. Because disease management focuses on specific disease states and specific interventions, the outcomes have been more precisely defined and documented than general case management activities.

    2. The structure of the outcomes measurement and reporting in disease management is a resource to those functioning in a more general case management role.

    3. Disease management has done a good job of implementing outcomes into practice, as has been described in the early section of this chapter.

C. The Internet
1. From journal articles on-line to web sites, the Internet has changed how information is located and retrieved.
2. *http://www.guidelines.gov* is the web site for the National Guideline Clearinghouse (NGC).
    a. The site contains 200 evidence-based clinical practice guidelines with the hope of having close to 400 by 1999. The goal for the first 5 years is 3500 guidelines.
    b. The site can be searched by
        (i) Disease or condition
        (ii) Treatment or intervention
        (iii) Submitting organization
3. Internet sites, such as the one mentioned earlier and others, can help in the construction of effective outcomes measures.
4. Journal articles regarding outcomes are becoming more numerous, and many make specific recommendations for implementation.
5. Conferences are featuring an increasing number of presentations specifically related to outcomes, and other presentations feature outcomes reporting on the project presented.

■ KEY ISSUES IN OUTCOMES REPORTING

A. Varying definitions
1. For effective comparisons, definitions need to be exact.
2. Even if there are similarities, minute differences can alter the results of a comparison.
3. For example, compare a Granny Smith apple with a Red Delicious. Both are apples, but evaluation would reveal distinct differences.
4. For case management to compare outcomes across the industry, definitions must be precise.
5. Definitions are clearer than in the past owing to the *Standards of Practice for Case Managers,* the *Ethics Statement,* and other such documents.
6. More work needs to be done with everyday practice and interventions to develop concise definitions.

B. Varying methodologies
1. In addition to definitions, the methods for calculating and reporting results must be consistent.
2. In one organization, there were several different methods of calculating cost savings.
3. It is impossible to complete a valid comparison of results if the methodology used to determine the results is different.
4. It is a key issue for future outcomes comparison to use the same methodologies for calculating and reporting outcomes.

C. Sharing of outcomes methodologies
1. Some organizations believe that the definitions, methodologies, and reporting practices are proprietary to them.

2. For this reason, they do not wish to share these details with the industry at large.

3. In order to create an opportunity for the growth of outcomes methodology and reporting, organizations on the forefront of case management should gain recognition for setting the standard in outcomes methodology rather than for being the only one with good outcomes methodology.

REFERENCES

Case Management Society of America (1995). *Standards of practice for case managers.* Little Rock, AR: CMSA.

Case Management Society of America (1997). *White paper.* Little Rock, AR: CMSA.

Polit, D. F. (1989). *Essentials of nursing research: Methods, appraisal and utilization* (2nd ed., p. 395). Philadelphia: J.B. Lippincott.

Powell, S. (2000). *Advanced case management: Outcomes and beyond.* Philadelphia: Lippincott Williams & Wilkins.

Rieve, J. A. (1997). Benchmarking and using outcomes data. *Case Manager,* July/August, 55–62.

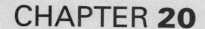

CHAPTER 20

• • • • • • • • • • • • • •

Continuous Quality Improvement

SUZANNE K. POWELL

LEARNING OBJECTIVES

Upon completion of this chapter, the reader will be able to:

1. Define important terms and concepts related to continuous quality improvement (CQI).

2. Articulate the uses for some major CQI tools for process improvement.

3. Discuss important problem-solving cycles and methodologies for case managers.

4. Identify different types of teams, team developmental stages, and team roles.

5. Describe decision-making techniques for process improvement.

IMPORTANT TERMS AND CONCEPTS

Bar Chart
Brainstorming
Cause-and-Effect Diagram
CASE © PDCA
Common Cause
Consensus
Continuous Quality Improvement (CQI)
Control Chart
CQI Tools for Process Improvement
Deming's "Fourteen Points"
Edward Deming
Facilitator

Fishbone Diagram
Flowchart
Force Field Analysis
Ishikawa Diagram
Joseph Juran
Lower Control Limits (LCL)
Multidisciplinary Patient Care Team
Multivoting
Negative Correlation
Nominal Group Technique
Outlier
Pareto Diagram

PDCA Cycle	Scatter Diagram
Philip Crosby	Special Cause
Pie Chart	Stages of Team Development
Positive Correlation	Statistical Process Control Chart
Process Flow Diagrams	(SPCC)
Project Team	Shewhart Cycle
Quality Advisor	Stephen Covey
Quality Council	Trend Chart
Root Cause Analysis	Upper Control Limits (UCL)
Run Chart	Variation

■ INTRODUCTION

A. Continuous quality improvement (CQI) tools and techniques are used to analyze and assess the impact of case and disease management processes, pathways, and protocols; this is how we can "prove our worth" in a language business people and CEOs understand. "Case managers have been instrumental in the creation and utilization of critical/clinical pathways, protocols, guidelines, and other interventions to improve health care quality. The next step, as leaders, is to self-evaluate our profession using statistically valid methods" (Powell, 2000b, p. 131).

B. CQI contributes tools to aid the case manager in evaluating, organizing, and presenting the outcomes. CQI applies tools of process improvement and believes that if you can measure it, you can improve it.

■ KEY DEFINITIONS

A. Continuous quality improvement (CQI)—CQI is a cyclical process; thus, the word "continuous." The foundational problem-solving method, the PDCA cycle, is also cyclical. CQI is a process that continuously and cyclically seeks to improve performance in order to enhance quality, efficiency, and efficacy.

B. CQI tools for process improvement—It has been said that one cannot improve what cannot be measured. An organization must know how to assess, measure, and evaluate its processes systematically in order to improve the outcomes, that is, the results of those processes. CQI methods and tools provide the foundation for this work.

C. PDCA cycle—This problem-solving cycle, also called the Shewhart cycle, is an acronym that stands for *plan-do-check-act*.

D. CASE © PDCA cycle—CASE © PDCA is an acronym that can be used by case managers to assess, plan, test, evaluate, and put into action efforts of quality improvement. The acronym "CASE" is actually imbedded in the planning phase of the PDCA cycle (Powell, 2000b).

E. Team—A team is a group of people who have come together for a specific purpose; ideally, teams are empowered to assess problems, initiate changes, and evaluate the impact of those changes.

■ THE CQI GURUS

A. W. Edwards Deming—The 14 Points (Gibbons, 1994)
1. Create constancy of purpose for improvement of product and service.
2. Adopt the new philosophy.
3. Cease dependence on mass inspection.
4. End the practice of awarding business on price tag alone.
5. Improve constantly and forever the system of production and service.
6. Institute training on the job.
7. Institute leadership.
8. Drive out fear.
9. Break down barriers between staff areas.
10. Eliminate slogans, exhortations, and targets for the workforce.
11. Eliminate numerical factors.
    a. Eliminate numerical quotas for the workforce.
    b. Eliminate numerical goals for people in management.
12. Remove barriers to pride of workmanship.
13. Encourage education and self-improvement for everyone.
14. Take action to accomplish the transformation.

B. Joseph M. Juran—10-Step Quality Improvement Process (Gibbons, 1994)
1. Build awareness of the need and opportunity for improvement.
2. Set goals for improvement.
3. Organize to reach the goals (e.g., establish a quality council, identify problems, select processes that need improvement, appoint teams, and train facilitators and team members).
4. Provide training throughout the organization.
5. Carry out projects to solve problems.
6. Report progress.
7. Give recognition.
8. Communicate results.
9. Keep score.
10. Maintain momentum by making annual improvement part of the regular systems and processes of the company.

C. Philip B. Crosby—14-Step Improvement Plan (Gibbons, 1994)
1. Management commitment is defined, created, and exhibited.
2. Quality improvement teams are formed.
3. Measurement to determine areas for improvement.
4. Cost of quality measures is developed as a stimulus.
5. Quality awareness is created in everyone.
6. Corrective action is taken on problems previously identified.
7. Zero defects planning.
8. Employee education of all employees in the company.
9. Zero defects day is held to let all employees know there has been a change.

10. Goal setting for individuals and groups.
11. Error cause removal by employees sharing with management the obstacles they face in attaining goals.
12. Recognition for those who participated.
13. Quality councils to communicate regularly.
14. Do it all over again to emphasize that quality improvement never ends.

D. Stephen R. Covey—Seven Habits of Highly Successful People (Covey, 1989)
   1. Habit #1. Be proactive.
   2. Habit #2. Begin with the end in mind.
   3. Habit #3. Put first things first. The goal of Habit #3 is to decrease urgency and crises. Covey states that people spend their time doing one of four activities:
      a. Urgent/Important—These are important, crisis tasks that must be attended to. They are necessary and must be managed.
      b. Not Urgent/Important—Covey states that as one spends more time in this quadrant of planning and clarifying, less time will be spent in the urgent/crisis quadrant.
      c. Urgent/Not Important—This quadrant can be reduced with good planning.
      d. Not Urgent/Not Important—This quadrant can be eliminated almost entirely.
   4. Habit #4. Think win-win.
   5. Habit #5. Seek first to understand, then to be understood.
   6. Habit #6. Synergize. The basis for synergy is valuing people's differences. Here, the whole is greater than the sum of its parts.
   7. Habit #7. Sharpen the saw.

■ TOOLS FOR PROCESS IMPROVEMENT

A. Three fundamental questions should be asked before starting any improvement process (Langley et al., 1992):
   1. What are we trying to accomplish?
   2. How will we know that a change is an improvement?
   3. What changes can we make that will result in improvement?

B. CQI tools for process improvement help answer these questions. The CQI tools for process improvement that will be examined in this chapter include flowcharts, run (trend) charts, statistical process control charts (SPCC), pie charts, bar charts, Pareto charts, cause and effect diagrams (fishbone or Ishikawa diagram), and scatter diagrams (Table 20–1).

C. Software is available to help map out the various tools. Some examples are provided; other examples of the tools for process improvement can be found in various books listed in the references for this chapter.
   1. Flowcharts
      a. Flowcharts, also called process flow diagrams, are pictorial repre-

TABLE 20–1
CQI Tools and Techniques

The Chart	Primary Function	Use To
Flowcharts	Displays the process	• Increase understanding of problems • Analyze processes • Identify gaps between current and desired situation • Identify opportunities to improve • Plan for change
Run charts	Displays data trends over time	• Increase understanding of problems • Identify gaps between current and desired situation • Identify opportunities to improve • Analyze processes
Control charts	Determines stability of data trends over time	• Increase understanding of problems • Identify gaps between current and desired situation • Monitor process performance • Identify opportunities to improve • Analyze processes • Evaluate tasks
Pie charts	Displays the percent each variable contributes to the whole	• Increase understanding of problems • Identify gaps between current and desired situation • Identify variables affecting process • Identify opportunities to improve
Bar charts	Compares categories of data at one point in time	• Increase understanding of problems • Identify variables affecting process • Identify opportunities to improve
Pareto charts	Determines the most frequent causes of a problem (i.e., the most important problems of a process)	• Increase understanding of problems • Identify and list problems • Indicate reasons likely to yield the most improvement • Separate the "vital few" from the "trivial many" • Identify variables affecting process

continued

TABLE 20–1
CQI Tools and Techniques (*Continued*)

The Chart	Primary Function	Use To
Cause-and-effect charts	Displays multiple causes of a problem	• Identify opportunities to improve • Analyze processes • Evaluate tasks • Increase understanding of problems • Identify and list problems • Identify root causes • Identify variables affecting process • Identify opportunities to improve • Analyze processes • Plan for change
Scatter diagram	Displays the relationship between two variables	• Increase understanding of problems • Identify opportunities to improve • Analyze processes • Plan for change • Evaluate tasks

(Powell, S. K.; [2000]. *Advanced case management: Outcomes and beyond*. Philadelphia: Lippincott Williams & Wilkins. Reprinted with permission.)

sentations of the steps in a process. Although each team member may be fully knowledgeable about his or her segment of the work being done, he or she may not be clear about the complete process or system. Flowcharts take complicated routines, jobs, and events and display them so that they can be analyzed by individuals inside and outside that area of expertise (Box 20–1).

   b. A high-level flowchart is a basic flowchart with an general overview of all the steps. It does not include detailed processes.

   c. A low-level flowchart is more detailed and includes more steps.

2. Run (trend) charts

   a. A run chart, also referred to as a trend chart, is a basic line graph that displays similar data over a period of time. This type of graph monitors processes or occurrences in order to identify trends.

   b. The vertical axis (the y axis) displays the variable that is being measured.

   c. The horizontal axis (the x axis) displays the time units.

   d. Run charts present a good visual representation of such case management issues as utilization management data, infection rates, and patient satisfaction scores.

BOX 20–1

Commonly Used Flowchart Symbols

• •

SYMBOL	USE THIS FLOWCHARTING SYMBOL
Circle or oblong	• To show the beginning of a process • To show the end of a process
Square or rectangle	• To show a step in the process being flowcharted
Diamond shape	• To show a decision point: there are always two arrows coming from a diamond shape, each showing the options that may be chosen (such as "yes" or "no")
Arrow	• Arrows point to the direction of the process or flow; if too many arrows point upward, this may indicate an opportunity for improvement in the process

---

3. Statistical Process Control Charts (SPCCs)

   a. A control chart, also known as a statistical quality control (SQC) chart or SPCC, is similar to a run chart in that it shows trends of data over time.

   b. In addition, control charts exhibit control limits. These control limits define the acceptable range of the data being monitored.

       (i) Upper control limits (UCLs)

       (ii) Lower control limits (LCLs)

   c. Understanding variation is germane to the appreciation of control charts. A variation is simply a change in the data. It is critical to know whether a variation is from a stable common cause or from an unstable special cause.

       (i) Common causes hover in the midrange between the UCLs and the LCLs; they are considered an inherent part of the system, are predictable, and are under control.

       (ii) Special causes fall outside of the UCLs and LCLs; they are considered unpredictable and out of control.

   d. One application that has proved to be effective is for the purpose of patient self-monitoring. Case management applications for control charts include the following (Powell, 2000b):

       (i) Diabetes patients—blood sugar monitoring and education

       (ii) Congestive heart failure—weight monitoring and education*

       (iii) Renal patients—weight monitoring and education*

---

*The control chart for patients with renal failure and congestive heart failure would require a chart tailored to the patient's specific weight prescription.

    (iv) Patients taking warfarin (Coumadin)—monitoring International Normalized Ratio (INR) levels

    (v) Asthma patients—monitoring peak flow meter results

    (vi) Pain management—charting pain levels and pain medication administration

4. Pie charts

    a. Pie charts are used to display the percentage that a category contributes to the total of all categories.

    b. An application (Powell, 2000b): If a case management agency or department wants to see immediately where the case management referrals are coming from, they may collect data on all referrals (the whole pie). The various referral sources would become the different slices of the pie. (See Figure 20–1 for an example of a pie chart.)

5. Bar charts

    a. A bar chart, at its simplest level, is used to compare data at one point in time. From the pictorial diagram, data analysis efforts can be enhanced.

    b. Histograms and Pareto charts are more advanced forms of bar charts. (See Figure 20–2 for an example of a bar chart.)

6. Pareto chart

    a. A Pareto chart consists of a series of bars (as in a bar graph) that are displayed from tallest (most frequent contributing factor) to smallest (least frequent contributing factor); it also has a line graph component that displays a cumulative percentage.

    b. In health care, it is estimated that 20% of the patients account for approximately 80% of the health care dollars. It was Joseph Juran who coined the famous 80/20 rule, when he observed through test-

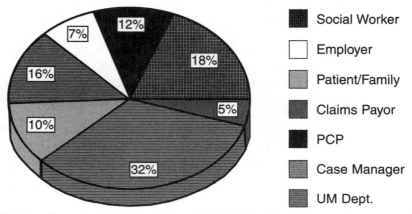

Case Management Referral Sources

Social Worker

Employer

Patient/Family

Claims Payor

PCP

Case Manager

UM Dept.

FIGURE 20–1   Example of a pie chart. (Powell, S.K. [2000]. *Advanced case management: Outcomes and beyond.* Philadelphia: Lippincott Williams & Wilkins. Reprinted with permission.)

Reasons for Case Management Closure

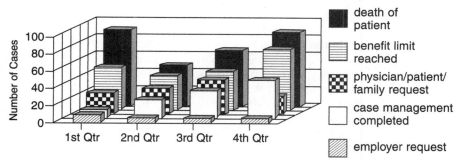

FIGURE 20–2. Example of a bar chart. (Powell, S.K. [2000]. *Advanced case management: Outcomes and beyond.* Philadelphia: Lippincott Williams & Wilkins. Reprinted with permission.)

    ing that 80% of the problems typically are caused by 20% of the contributing factors.

    c. The Pareto Principle separates "the vital few from the trivial many" (Vilfredo Pareto); it states that whenever a quality problem has multiple causes, a relative few of those causes account for most of the incidents (McLaughlin & Kaluzny, 1994).

7. Cause-and-effect diagram (Fishbone or Ishikawa diagram)

    a. Cause-and-effect diagrams are used to explore all of the factors that influence a process or situation.

    b. Before a team can "fix" a problem, they must first identify and understand the multiple causes of the problem.

    c. Cause-and-effect diagrams are also known as the Ishikawa diagram after its originator, Kaoru Ishikawa, or as a "fishbone" diagram because of its shape.

    d. Advantages of cause-and-effect diagrams:

      (i) The creation of the diagram itself is educational and motivates important players to speak to each other about the problem process.

      (ii) It helps focus the discussion; irrelevant discussion and complaints are reduced.

      (iii) It is an active process with a goal: to uncover the root cause of a problem.

      (iv) Data usually must be collected with this tool. This increases objectivity and reduces personal opinion.

      (v) It demonstrates the level of the staff's understanding of the process. The more complex the diagram is, the more the workers know about the process.

      (vi) It can be used for a large variety of problems.

8. Scatter diagrams (scattergrams)

    a. Scatter diagrams display the relationship, or correlation, between two variables; they are useful because they display all of the data as a whole rather than individually. Any time two case management variables intersect, a scattergram is the tool of choice to determine whether a relationship exists between them. It is a good idea to at least suspect that the two variables affect each other.

  b. Interpretation of scatter diagrams—in general:

    (i) Positive correlation: The points run in a linear fashion, from the lower left corner to the upper right corner. "Higher" scores of one variable correlate with "lower" scores of the other variable. Improving one variable will likely improve the other variable (Schroeder, 1994).

    (ii) Negative correlation: The points run in a linear fashion from the upper cleft corner to the lower right corner. "Higher" scores of one variable correlate with "lower" scores of the other variable. Increasing one variable will likely decrease the other variable (Schroeder, 1994).

    (iii) No correlation: The points are scattered all over the plot with no obvious pattern. There is no definite relationship between the two variables.

    (iv) If in a positive or negative plot structure there is a group of points in one quadrant, this group is known as "outliers" and may represent "special causes" (Executive Learning, 1997b).

    (v) If the pattern in the positive or negative correlation scatter diagram is "tight," the factors being studied are probably responsible for most of the variation; if the pattern is "loose," there may be other factors affecting the data.

■ CONTINUOUS QUALITY IMPROVEMENT PROBLEM-SOLVING METHODOLOGIES

  A. The PDCA cycle

    1. Called the Shewhart cycle after its originator, or the PDCA cycle.

    2. PDCA stands for *plan-do-check-act*.

      a. Plan a change or a test aimed at improvement.

      b. Do the change; carry it out (preferably on a small scale).

      c. Study the results. What was learned?

      d. Act. Depending on what was learned in the study phase, one has three options:

        (i) Adopt the change.

        (ii) Abandon the change.

        (iii) Run through the cycle again, possibly under different environmental conditions.

  B. The CASE © PDCA cycle (Powell, 2000b)

    1. This problem-solving methodology was modified from the PDCA cycle specifically because of the intensive planning phase that must go on while planning a case management project.

    2. The acronym CASE is actually imbedded in the planning phase of the PDCA cycle (Powell, 2000b) (Box 20–2).

BOX 20–2
The Case Management Continuous Quality Improvement Process

• •

Plan the improvement and the
data collection
 Clarify case management opportunities for improvement
 Assess the data
 Strategize the target interventions
  for improvement
 Evaluate for feasibility and plan
  the pilot test

**Useful Tools and Techniques
in the *Plan Phase***
Force field analysis
Pareto chart
Brainstorming
Flowcharts
Check sheets
Control charts
Nominal group technique/
 Multivoting
Cause-and-effect diagram
Run charts

Do the improvement and the data
collection on a small scale

**Useful Tools and Techniques
in the *Do Phase***

Check sheets	Surveys
Run charts	Control charts
Flowcharts	Pareto charts
Scatter diagram	Histograms
Cause-and-effect diagrams	

Check the results of the pilot project

**Useful Tools and Techniques
in the *Check Phase***

Control charts	Run charts
Histograms	Pareto charts
Cause-and-effect diagram	

Act to continue improving the
process

**Useful Tools and Techniques
in the *Act Phase***

Flowcharts	Check sheets
Control charts	Pareto charts
Brainstorming	
Cause-and-effect diagrams	
Nominal group technique/ multivoting	

CASE © PDCA is an acronym that can be used by case managers to assess, plan, test, evaluate, and put into action efforts of quality improvement. The acronym CASE is actually embedded in the "planning" phase of the PDCA cycle.

(Powell, S. K. [2000]. *Advanced case management: Outcomes and beyond.* Philadelphia: Lippincott Williams & Wilkins. Reprinted with permission.)

3. CASE © PDCA cycle stands for
   a. **Plan**
      (i) Clarify the case management opportunities for improvement.
      (ii) Assess the data.
      (iii) Strategize the target interventions for improvement.
      (iv) Evaluate the feasibility and plan the pilot test.
   b. **Do**
   c. **Check**
   d. **Act**

■ CASE MANAGERS WORKING IN PROJECT TEAMS

A. Types of teams
   1. Multidisciplinary patient care team—may be planned for weekly or biweekly meetings or may be impromptu. The agenda and purpose is focused on patient care.
   2. CQI cross-functional team—most often has a set schedule, a specific goal or goals, and an assigned group of team members (with occasional experts called in) that changes infrequently.
   3. Improvement teams—exist to improve processes, products, services, and morale. Typically, these teams are not permanent. Once the improvement is completed, they are disbanded (unless another round of continuous improvement will commence).
   4. Steering team or council—major function is to coordinate and support improvement in the organization. This team plans, organizes, and facilitates other teams. A quality council is a type of steering team; it assesses the organization and initiates and "steers" the improvement team in the right direction.

B. Stages of team development—"Teams go through fairly predictable stages before reaching maturity and synergy. Understanding these stages as normal may keep groups from overreacting or setting unrealistic expectations too soon in the team process" (Powell, 2000b, p. 192). The four stages are:
   1. Forming
   2. Storming
   3. Norming
   4. Performing

C. Team roles and responsibilities—i.e., team "job descriptions"
   1. Quality advisor
      a. Often a member of the quality council
      b. Acts as a team advisor or consultant
      c. Has expertise in the quality improvement process
      d. The goal of the quality advisor is to move the team toward self-sufficiency in working together as a group and in use of the process improvement tools.

2. Team leader
   a. Coordinates and directs the work of the team
   b. May often facilitate the team meetings (when teams are self-sufficient
   c. Are also team members who contribute ideas, help interpret data, and participate in all team decisions
3. Team members
   a. Should consider their participation as a priority responsibility, rather than an intrusion on their "real jobs"
   b. Are the functional core of any team
4. Recorder
   a. Records the team's mission, as defined by the consensus process
   b. Summarizes and records the work and decisions of the team
   c. Composes the minutes of each meeting and distributes to the team and quality advisor
5. Scribe
   a. Keeps ideas "visible" during the meetings (e.g., on flipcharts)
   b. Organizes the team's key ideas, questions, agreements, etc.
   c. Gives the flipcharts to the recorder at the end of the meeting to include in the minutes
6. Timekeeper
   a. Keeps the team on track according to the time set on the agenda
   b. Calls out the time remaining on each agenda item at intervals determined by the team

D. Characteristics of effective teams
   1. Team members are clear about the team mission and goals.
   2. Team members have clearly defined roles and responsibilities.
   3. Communication is direct and succinct, and there is free expression; criticism is constructive.
   4. Team members actively listen to one another; input from all members is valued.
   5. Only one person speaks at a time; interruptions are minimal.
   6. All team members participate in discussions in balanced doses.
   7. A cooperative, friendly, supportive climate exists; members seem to enjoy each other.
   8. Team members are committed and complete assignments, working toward common goal.
   9. Team members use an agenda; the agenda is adhered to most of the time.
   10. The team has well-defined decision-making procedures that are understood by members.
   11. The team agrees on and adheres to a set of "team ground rules."
   12. Good minutes are kept so that past decisions are easily found.
   13. Periodically, the team stops to assess its own performance.

14. Team members share knowledge for the benefit of the project.
15. The team uses a scientific approach to drawing conclusions about causes/solutions.
16. Members feel free to express disagreement during discussions; conflicts are worked out.
17. Team members make every attempt to attend meetings; it is a priority for them.
18. Team decisions reflect a consensus; this is facilitated by the team leader.
19. The work of the team is accepted and used; management supports the team's recommendations or changes.
20. The whole team is given credit and recognized for accomplishments; success is shared.

E. Characteristics of effective team meetings
    1. Use of ground rules
    2. Use of agendas
    3. Fill key meeting roles
    4. Take minutes
    5. Adhere to the "100 mile rule"—no one should be called from a meeting unless it is so important that the disruption would occur even if the meeting was 100 miles away from the workplace.
    6. Summarize the meeting at the end
    7. Draft the next meeting agenda
    8. Compute cost of the meeting
    9. Project closure

■ **DECISION-MAKING TECHNIQUES FOR PROCESS IMPROVEMENT** (Table 20–2)

A. Brainstorming
    1. An easy way to generate a wide variety of ideas from all participants in a short period of time. Any time there is dissension among the case management ranks, brainstorming can be used to calm the storm.
    2. Focus on processes, not people; this is critical.
    3. Types of brainstorming sessions:
       a. In round-robin brainstorming, everyone in the team presents an idea in turn around the group until all finally "pass."
       b. Popcorn is when anyone can call out an idea, in no order, until all ideas are out.
       c. Paperstorming is when the ideas are committed to paper or e-mail. This approach saves time and can be more private, although it does not allow for "hitchhiking," which is a powerful method of squeezing out more ideas.

B. Multivoting
    1. Designed to reduce a list of more than 10 ideas to a manageable number, with limited discussion and difficulty.

TABLE 20–2

Decision-Making Techniques for Process Improvement

The Chart	Primary Function	Use To
Brainstorming	Generates multiple ideas in a short time	• Increase understanding of problems • Identify and list problems • Clarify customer (internal or external) expectations • Consider multiple solutions • Identify root causes • Identify variables affecting process • Identify opportunities to improve • Analyze processes • Plan for change • Evaluate tasks
Multivoting	Narrows long lists of ideas or variables	• Increase understanding/priorities of problems • Evaluate tasks
Nominal group technique	Generates multiple ideas, then narrows and prioritizes the list	• Increase understanding of problems • Identify and list problems • Consider multiple solutions • Identify root causes • Identify variables affecting process • Identify opportunities to improve • Analyze processes • Plan for change
Force field analysis	Depicts driving and restraining forces that impact a proposed change	• Increase understanding of problems • Identify and list problems • Identify variables affecting process • Analyze processes • Plan for change
Root cause analysis	Identifies the root cause(s) of a problem	• Increase understanding of problems • Identify and list problems • Identify root causes • Identify variables affecting process • Identify opportunities to improve • Plan for change
Consensus	Generates agreement among members	• Increase understanding of problems • Plan for change • Evaluate tasks

(Powell, S. K. [2000]. *Advanced case management: Outcomes and beyond.* Philadelphia: Lippincott Williams & Wilkins. Reprinted with permission.)

2. This is accomplished through a series of votes; each vote will cut the list more.

3. Multivoting often follows a brainstorming session.

C. Nominal group technique

1. A structured method of generating a list and then narrowing it down.

2. Two phases:
   a. The first phase is silent brainstorming (paperstorming).
   b. The second phase is voting to reduce the list.
3. There is a relatively low level of interaction of the group members during phase one; therefore, it is good for highly controversial issues.

D. Force field analysis
  1. A force field analysis can be considered one of the tools for process improvement; however, it is also useful in the decision-making process. After the team has developed a control chart and has decided on what the variances are, a force field analysis is a method used to find out what forces are causing problems in the process.
  2. This tool is based on the supposition that all events are the result of two forces:
     a. Driving forces—forces that push for change
     b. Restraining forces—forces that restrict change

E. Root cause analysis
  1. A root cause analysis is another tool for process improvement. After a control chart has demonstrated what the variances are, a root cause analysis is an investigative method to get to the root, or cause, of a problem.
  2. In many ways, this technique holds the key to successful change efforts. Improvement requires change; however, the change made must correspond to the true cause (or root) of the problem. A root cause analysis uncovers the bottlenecks that impede the free flow of a process; this bottleneck is often the cause of poor performance.
  3. This tool is required for some accreditation applications, such as the Joint Commission on Accreditation of Healthcare Organizations (JCAHO).
  4. How to perform a root cause analysis—the simplest method to get to the underlying cause of the problem is by merely asking the team "Why." Some CQI experts say that a series of "five whys" will usually suffice.

F. Consensus
  1. Consensus is a decision in which all of the team members find a common ground that is acceptable enough for everyone to support the decision. The key word is "support." In other words, no member actively opposes it. The members believe that the decision was reached fairly and openly and represents the best solution at the time.
  2. Consensus is not a unanimous vote that represents everyone's first choice, nor is consensus a majority vote, in which only the majority get something they are happy with, whereas the minority get something they do not want at all. It does not mean that everyone is totally satisfied. Consensus does not represent a compromise; a creative solution can still be achieved with consensus. Finally, consensus is not a product of a passive mentality; creativity cannot be achieved with "group think."

REFERENCES

Brassard, M., & Ritter, D. (1994). *Memory jogger II.* Goal/QPC—Methuen: Joiner Associates.

Covey, S. (1989). *Seven habits of highly effective people.* New York: Simon & Schuster.

Covey, S. (1992). *Principle-centered leadership.* New York: Simon & Schuster.

Covey, S. (1994). *First things first.* New York: Simon & Schuster.

Deming, E. (1986). *Out of the crisis.* Cambridge, MA: MIT Center for Advanced Engineering Study.

Executive Learning (1997a). *FAST PDCA—leaders guide.* Brentwood: Executive Learning, Inc.

Executive Learning (1997b). *Handbook for improvement: A reference guide for tools and concepts* (2nd ed.). Brentwood: Executive Learning, Inc.

Fisher, R., & Ury, W. (1991). *Getting to yes: Negotiating agreement without giving in.* New York: Viking Press.

Gibbons, S. (1994). Three paths, one journey. *Journal for Quality and Participation,* Oct/Nov, 36–45.

Ishikawa, K. (1990). *Introduction to quality control.* Tokyo: 3A Corporation.

Joiner, B. (1994). *Fourth generation management: The new business consciousness.* New York: McGraw-Hill.

Juran, J. (1989). *Juran on leadership for quality: An executive handbook.* New York: The Free Press.

Langley, G. J., Nolan, K. M., et al. (1992). *The foundation of improvement.* Silver Spring, MD: API Publishing.

McLaughlin, C., & Kaluzny, A. (1994). *Continuous quality improvement in health care: Theory, implementation, and applications.* Gaithersburg, MD: Aspen.

National Association for Health Care Quality (NAHQ) (1997). *NAHQ guide to quality management* (7th ed.). Glenview, IL: NAHQ.

National Association for Health care Quality (NAHQ) (1998). *NAHQ guide to quality management* (8th ed.). Glenview, IL: NAHQ.

Powell, S. K. (2000a). *Case management: A practical guide to success in managed care* (2nd ed.). Philadelphia: Lippincott Williams & Wilkins.

Powell, S. K. (2000b). *Advanced case management: Outcomes and beyond.* Philadelphia: Lippincott Williams & Wilkins.

Scholtes, P.R., Joiner, B., & Streibel, B.J. (1996). *The team handbook* (2nd ed.). Madison, WI: Joiner Associates.

Schroeder, P. (1994). *Improving quality and performance: Concepts, programs, and techniques.* St. Louis: Mosby–Year Book.

Senge, P. (1990). *The fifth discipline.* New York: Doubleday/Currency.

Temme, J. (1996). *Team power.* Mission, KS: Skillpath Publications.

CHAPTER 21

· · · · · · · · · · · · · ·

Complementary and Alternative Medicine (CAM)

JANICE E. BENJAMIN

LEARNING OBJECTIVES

Upon completion of this chapter, the reader will be able to:

1. Describe the current impact of CAM on the health care industry and its potential to change the delivery of health care.
2. Define underlying concepts and terms relative to CAM.
3. Discuss briefly a variety of CAM modalities, along with the indications and contraindications for their use.
4. Discuss the differences between CAM and allopathic medicine, as well as the areas in which they complement each other.
5. Identify barriers to third-party reimbursement and HMO benefits for CAM, and the CAM modalities most often considered for inclusion.
6. Discuss issues related to research into CAM modalities and the challenges to the conventional scientific model CAM poses.
7. Identify ways in which case management can integrate CAM into treatment plans, and the challenges and opportunities it presents.

IMPORTANT TERMS AND CONCEPTS

Acupuncture
Alexander Technique
Allopathic Medicine
Aromatherapy

Auric Field
Autogenic Training
Ayurvedic Medicine
Bioenergy Therapies

Biofeedback	Mind-Body Medicine
CAM (Complementary and Alternative Medicine)	Musculoskeletal Therapies
	Naturopathic Medicine
Chiropractic Manipulation	National Institutes of Health (NIH)
Craniosacral Therapy	Neurolinguistic Programming (NLP)
Creative Visualization	Nutritional Supplementation
Doshas (Vata, Pitta, Kapha)	Physiotherapy
Feldenkrais Therapy	Polarity Therapy
Flower Essences	Preventive Medicine
Guided Imagery	Qi
Hatha Yoga	Reflexology
Herbal Medicine/Herbology	Relaxation Response
Homeopathy	Rolfing
Hydrotherapy	Sound Healing
Hypnosis	Structural Integration
Law of Similars	Therapeutic Touch
Magnetic Therapy	Traditional Chinese Medicine
Meditation	Yin/Yang

■ INTRODUCTION

A. Definitions of complementary and alternative medicine (CAM) and its historical roots

B. Brief history of CAM in the United States and the impact of consumer initiatives in bringing CAM into the mainstream of health care delivery

C. Current efforts toward creating integrative medicine and incorporating CAM into the health care delivery system

D. Theoretical contrasts between CAM and allopathic medicine:

1. The biomedical model of cellular pathology as the root of disease compared with the model of a disruption of bioenergetic pathways as the root of disease

2. Prevention and wellness interventions as the model for treatment compared with acute care interventions and symptom management as the model for treatment

3. Treatment focused on building the body's own immunity and reparative systems compared with treatment focused on disease processes

E. Broad categories of CAM modalities available in the United States:

1. Whole health care systems, which have theoretical foundations, diagnostic guidelines, and treatment protocols for addressing the full range of health care conditions

2. Mind-body medicine therapies, which effect health through accessing and strengthening the relationship between the mind and body

3. Musculoskeletal therapies, which work by restoring and maintaining the functions of the body's skeletal and muscular systems

4. Bioenergy therapies, which work on the bioelectrical and biomagnetic fields of the body

5. Herbal medicine, which uses whole plants to treat disease and maintain health
6. Nutritional supplementation, which prescribes megadoses of vitamins and minerals to treat disease and maintain health

■ ALTERNATIVE WHOLE HEALTH CARE SYSTEMS

A. Traditional Chinese medicine (TCM)
   1. TCM definition of health and the historical foundation of TCM in the Chinese culture's relationship with nature
      a. The view of humans as the place where Heaven (Yang) and Earth (Yin) come together, so that health is the balance of these forces in the body-mind-spirit
      b. The importance of the patient's relationship to the environment and the seasons, and living in harmony with the changes in nature
   2. Theoretical concepts upon which clinical practice is based
      a. Qi as bioenergy flow through defined meridians, or pathways, in the body
      b. Yin/Yang and their inter-relationships and interplay within the body
      c. The six organ systems (lung, kidney, liver, heart, pericardium, spleen) and their interrelated functions
      d. Theories on the progression of disease [Six Stages, Four Levels, San Jiao progression]
   3. Modalities used in treatment, including acupuncture, herbal medicine, diet therapy, heat, cupping, and massage
   4. Theoretical and clinical research into the biological mechanisms of action for effecting change with TCM, including neural, biochemical, and bioelectrical theories
   5. Conditions that can be treated and research supporting the effectiveness of TCM, including the 1998 National Institutes of Health (NIH) consensus conference outcomes and the recommendations of the World Health Organization (WHO)
   6. Education and licensure requirements for practice

B. Ayurvedic medicine
   1. Theoretical foundations for diagnosis and treatment, and Ayurveda's historical roots in the spiritual culture of India
   2. Identifying the patient's constitutional type, or dosha, as the basis for maintaining health and designing treatment during illness
      a. Vata, which represents the aspects of thinness, dryness, cold, activity, imagination, and the respiratory and circulatory systems
      b. Pitta, which represents the aspects of heat, a medium build, strong appetite, emotionality, and the digestive system
      c. Kapha, which represents the aspects of heaviness, slow movement, sweet and salty tastes, good memory, and the physical structures of the body

3. Modalities for clinical treatment, including diet, massage, herbs, meditation, yoga, detoxification, and breathing exercises
4. The role of the mind and spiritual practice in healing
5. Conditions that can be treated by Ayurvedic medicine, and contraindications for its use
6. Current research and educational requirements for practice

C. Naturopathic medicine
  1. History of naturopathy in the United States, and its historical roots in European natural cure movements
  2. Six principles of practice that define naturopathic medicine:
     a. The body has the ability to heal itself, and treatment is designed to support the innate wisdom of the body.
     b. Treat the underlying cause, rather than just suppress the symptoms.
     c. Do no harm; thus, use only natural means and substances.
     d. Treat the whole person, body, mind and spirit.
     e. The physician is a teacher to empower the patient.
     f. Prevention is the best medicine.
  3. Naturopathic philosophy of disease cause and progression, and the importance of not suppressing natural body processes, such as fever, by which the body attempts to restore homeostasis
  4. Modalities used in treatment, including diet, vitamin/mineral therapy, herbal medicine, hydrotherapy, spinal manipulation, homeopathy, and massage
  5. Educational and licensure requirements for practice

D. Homeopathic medicine
  1. Discovery and development of homeopathy by the German physician, Hahnemann, in the 1700s
     a. "Provings," or the testing of substances on health persons to determine their indications for treatment
     b. Creating remedies based on the results of the provings
  2. How homeopathic remedies work on the energetic body, rather than the cellular body, to stimulate the body's own healing processes
  3. Three principles upon which homeopathy is based:
     a. Law of Similars, which is based upon the principle that "like cures like"
     b. Law of Infinitesimal Doses, which is based upon the principle that the more dilute the homeopathic remedy, the stronger its effect
     c. Law of Holism, which is based on the principle that treatment directed to the whole person, not just the symptom, is more effective
  4. Making a uniquely detailed and thorough assessment and choosing a homeopathic remedy
     a. Constitutional remedies
     b. Treating acute and chronic illness
     c. Treating psycho-emotional conditions

5. Current research explaining the mechanisms of action based on the electromolecular structure of water

6. Educational and licensure requirements for practice

■ MIND-BODY MEDICINE

A. History of the role of the mind-body relationship in medicine in multiple cultures, from Hippocrates to Descartes to the present

B. Definition and basic concepts of mind-body medicine and the intimate connections between both

1. Herbert Benson's work on the impact of stress on the body, and his discovery of and research on the "relaxation response"

   a. Activation of the parasympathic nervous system to induce relaxation

   b. Comparisons to meditative states and similar physiological changes

2. Candace Pert's recent research on the biochemical basis for mind-body medicine and her findings that neurochemical markers found on cells outside of the nervous system allow for pathways of communication between multiple body systems

C. Guided imagery/creative visualization

1. Directed or self-initiated use of mental images to create change in the patient's health

   a. Engaging all the senses in creating a mental image

   b. Patients allowed to create images of significance to them, enhancing the process and effect

2. Conditions that can be treated, including pain reduction, reduction in nausea associated with chemotherapy, and reduction of perceived stress

3. Certification requirements for practice, or lack thereof

D. Hypnosis

1. Guided imagery directed by a therapist to implant a subconscious suggestion that promotes healing on a physical or emotional level

2. Conditions that can be treated, including phobias, insomnia, chronic pain, and depression

3. Certification or licensure requirements for practitioners

E. Meditation

1. Based on ancient Hindu practices for spiritual awakening by controlling the flow of thoughts through the mind

   a. The physiological impact of random and unconscious thoughts

   b. Research that has been done on meditative states and biological changes induced in this state

2. Mindfulness meditation, one of several styles of meditation, and its use in medical clinics for pain management

3. Meditation as compared with Benson's "relaxation response"

F. Biofeedback
1. The use of technology to reinforce the patient's efforts to regulate the body's autonomic systems through the use of the mind
2. How it works and conditions it can treat, including insomnia, asthma, hypertension, irritable bowel syndrome, and migraine headaches
3. Training requirements and potential for insurance reimbursement as it varies from state to state

G. Autogenic training
1. Mental exercises taught to reduce the physiological impacts of stress
2. Unique from other techniques in the very detailed script used to induce relaxation
3. Conditions it can treat, including high blood pressure, insomnia, and palpations, and contraindications for its use

H. Neurolinguistic programming (NLP)
1. History of the development of NLP in the 1970s through the study of popular psychotherapy techniques
2. How NLP works to access the mind-body connection through changing the relationship between the patient's nervous system, thought processing, and patterns of behavior
3. Description of how a typical session might progress, using questioning and suggestions for redefining one's images and thoughts about a health condition

■ MUSCULOSKELETAL THERAPIES

A. A broad category of treatments that bring the patient's awareness to posture and movement, and manipulate the physical body to facilitate the flow of blood and energy throughout the body

B. Alexander technique
1. History of its development in the late 1800s in Australia by an actor motivated to restore the loss of his voice
2. Therapist seen as a teacher, and what to expect in a typical session
3. The goal of Alexander to coordinate the functions of the muscle and skeletal systems for maximum efficiency

C. Feldenkrais therapy
1. History of its development in the 1940s by Moshe Feldenkrais to facilitate his recovery from an injury
2. The underlying goal to change dysfunctional postural and movement habits that are contributing to illness or pain, and how that is achieved in a session
3. The two approaches to therapy, either in a group setting (called "Awareness through Movement") or one-on-one (called "Functional Integration"), with the therapist in the role of teacher in both cases

D. Craniosacral therapy
1. Manipulation of the bones of the skull to treat a range of conditions,

including headaches, strokes, ear infections, insomnia, high blood pressure, autism, and chronic pain

2. Garner Sutherland's technique versus John Upledger's technique:
   a. Sutherland's technique developed in the early 1900s to restore and maintain spinal fluid pressure changes and electromagnetic field patterns
   b. Upledger's approach developed in the 1970s to release restrictions in the meningeal tissues and fascia within the craniosacral system
3. The overall goal to release constricted movement or adhesions in order to reduce intercranial pressure
4. Educational requirements for practitioners

E. Rolfing/structural integration
   1. Deep tissue massage developed over a period of 25 years and introduced in the 1950s by Ida Rolf
   2. Offered as a series of 10 sessions to manipulate and stretch the body's fascial tissue in order to release adhesions and relieve restricted muscle and joints
   3. Educational requirements for practitioners

F. Hatha yoga
   1. 2,000- to 4,000-year history in Hindu traditions
   2. Exercises that coordinate movement with breathing, done in a meditative state, in order to balance the nervous and endocrine systems
   3. Benefits, including enhanced blood oxygenation, balanced glucose metabolism, stimulation of the immune system, and emotional balance
   4. The current use of yoga in pain clinics and cardiac rehabilitation clinics

G. Therapeutic massage
   1. The use of touch to manipulate soft tissues of the body to relieve muscle tension and promote blood circulation
   2. Contrasting of various styles:
      a. Swedish massage, the oldest technique, to promote circulation
      b. Sports massage to improve flexibility and recover from injury
      c. Neuromuscular massage for rehabilitation
      d. Lymphatic massage for detoxification
      e. Esalen massage for inducing meditative states
   3. Licensure requirements for practitioners

H. Reflexology
   1. Massage of painful points on the hands and feet to stimulate glands, neuromuscular systems, and organs in the whole body
   2. Key benefits of treatment and indications for its use
   3. Proposed mechanisms of action:
      a. Stimulation of the nervous system
      b. The microsystem of the hands and feet reflecting the body as a whole

■ **CHIROPRACTIC MANIPULATION**

A. History of the chiropractic profession in the United States
B. Underlying theories for its effectiveness:
1. Spinal column alignment necessary for proper functioning of the nervous system
2. Stimulating the innate intelligence of the body to heal itself
C. Conditions treated, including chronic sinus infections, chronic pain, asthma, and digestive disorders
D. Educational and licensure requirements for practitioners

■ **BIO-ENERGY THERAPIES**

A. A broad category of therapies that work on balancing the patient's bio-energy and bio-magnetic fields to promote healing of the emotional and physical body
B. Polarity therapy
1. Developed in the 1940s by Dr. Randolph Stone based on his studies of Oriental and Ayurvedic medicine concepts of the body's energy fields
2. Recognizing that humans have a magnetic field around their body, with a positive and negative pole that can be disrupted (leading to illness) and subsequently restored (leading to healing)
3. Promotes the smooth flow of energy in the patient's energy field by the therapist placing her hands in designated positions on the patient's body so that negative and positive poles are joined
4. Criteria and education required for the practitioner, and the necessity for the therapist to have a balanced energy field so as not to do harm to the patient
C. Therapeutic touch (TT)
1. Developed by Dolores Krieger as a tool for health care professionals to do hands-on healing
2. The goals of TT to restore balance in the patient's energy field and to promote homeostatic changes in biochemical processes
3. Clinical research demonstrating biochemical changes in the body following this procedure, and subsequent challenges to those results
4. Description and demonstration of a TT session
D. Magnet therapy
1. History of its use throughout many cultures
2. Research on the use of magnets to promote healing of bone and to relieve pain
3. Proposed mechanisms of action:
a. Improves blood circulation
b. Affects chemical processes within and between cells
c. Affects nerve signals
d. Stimulates acupuncture points

    4. Contraindications or precautions for the use of magnets

E. Sound therapy

    1. The use of singing, chanting, and percussion instruments to promote healing

    2. The effects of sound on the human body:

        a. Rhythmic entrainment, which occurs when the human body matches its internal rhythms to the tempo of an external rhythm

        b. Resonance, which is the transmission of vibrations from one medium, such as beating drums, to another, such as the beating of the human heart

    3. The effects of sound on human brain waves occurs by activating different brain wave states of electrical activity

    4. Research in the area of sound therapy

F. Flower essences

    1. Dr. Edward Bach's work in developing flower essences as a gentler form of healing

    2. Illness seen as a reflection of imbalance in the energy field of a patient

    3. Techniques for capturing the energetic pattern of flowers in tincture form

    4. The effect of the flower's energetics on the energetic pattern of the human field, thus effecting changes in the cellular structure of the body

G. Aromatherapy

    1. The effect of the aroma of essential flower oils to stimulate the brain and effect a healing response in the whole body

    2. The importance of using food grade oils, and how to use the oils—topically, with a diffuser, and internally

    3. Indications and contraindications for their use

■ HERBAL MEDICINE

A. The use of whole plants for the treatment of disease and the maintenance of health

B. The oldest form of medicine, and still the only form of medicine for many cultures

C. Part of TCM, Ayurvedic medicine, naturopathic medicine, and many indigenous medicines

D. The preparation of herbs versus allopathic drugs, and the subsequent reduction of potential side effects

E. Recent increase of interest among consumers and the health care industry

F. Need to keep current on recent research to prevent potential complications from self-prescribed use of herbs

G. Some of the most commonly used herbs—ginseng, echinacea, gingko, milk thistle—and their indications

   H. Current publications that are addressing the correct use of herbs and potential complications

■ NUTRITIONAL SUPPLEMENTATION

   A. Recommended Daily Allowance (RDA) established by the government's council, and disputed by recent research as too low for many supplements

   B. Vitamin therapy to prevent and treat illness through the use of megadoses and the need for close supervision

   C. Brief review of how vitamins and minerals work in the body, and their therapeutic use

   D. Need for education and knowledge on current research to prevent potential side effects from improper use

■ CLINICAL INTEGRATION OF CAM

   A. Eisenberg's 1990 and 1993 surveys on consumer use of CAM and its impact on the health care industry

   B. Reasons for consumer interest in CAM:
     1. Dissatisfaction with limited allopathic options
     2. Impersonal treatment by medical doctors
     3. Increased research pointing to the benefits of CAM
     4. CAM's emphasis on wellness
     5. Concern with side effects of allopathic treatments
     6. The increased availability of health-related information and options to consumers

   C. An evaluation of the issues related to the integration of CAM and the allopathic model in a clinical setting
     1. Exploring significant differences between the two
     2. Objections by medicine and alternative practitioners to integration
     3. Consumer interest in having an integrated medical system
     4. Assessing what will be lost or gained with integration of both models—alternative health care and conventional health care

   D. Measures necessary for integrating CAM into the health care system:
     1. Acceptance by doctors and hospitals
     2. Education of doctors in CAM philosophies and modalities
     3. Credentialing of CAM providers
     4. Studies of and development of CAM outcomes
     5. Insurance coverage of CAM
     6. Education of consumers about indications and contraindications of CAM modalities
     7. Education of CAM practitioners about maneuvering through the health care delivery system and insurance systems

E. Medical centers that have successfully integrated CAM, and problems they have encountered and solved

1. Oxford Health Plans, the first major health plan to offer CAM benefits:
   a. CAM integrated into their health plan in response to member demand
   b. Internal advisory board developed standards and credentialing guidelines for a variety of CAM modalities
   c. Network of community CAM practitioners established
   d. Consumer education resources developed

2. Columbia Presbyterian Medical Center:
   a. First introduced non-invasive procedures that research indicated were effective in improving quality of life, including yoga, meditation, and guided imagery
   b. CAM seen as tools for disease management, and departments within the hospital are regularly consulted for input concerning their needs and their recommendations
   c. Focus is maintained on research and clinical trial outcomes as the basis for making decisions regarding the use of CAM
   d. Quality assurance (QA) is in place to minimize risks and ensure acceptance by allopathic care providers
   e. Obstacles identified were lack of insurance coverage and lack of consumers' and doctors' knowledge about CAM

3. Presbyterian Hospital's Health Plan:
   a. Uses acupuncturists and chiropractors because state licensure criteria are already in place; also uses in-house credentialing.
   b. Services were initiated because of consumer demand.
   c. Director of the program is involved in national efforts to facilitate integration of CAM into mainstream medicine.
   d. CAM providers are accessed on referral from the primary care provider.
   e. As further research supports the efficacy of other modalities, they will consider adding them to their treatment options.

4. Mind-Body Institute at St. Joseph's Medical Center:
   a. CAM first offered in their pain management clinic in 1974, because of the director's personal interest in CAM.
   b. Recent organization-wide decisions were made to incorporate CAM into the whole facility, following visits to various facilities already successful in their integration efforts.
   c. They designed their program on Harvard's Mind-Body Center, where much research is being done on mind-body medicine.
   d. Physician and consumer acceptance and interest were surveyed prior to initiating the program.

F. Insurance issues and concerns about the integration and coverage of CAM modalities

1. Lack of scientific proof of the efficacy of so many CAM modalities
2. Concern about incurring higher costs rather than saving money

3. Appropriate credentialing of CAM providers to assure competency
4. Lack of standards and appropriate CPT codes
5. Problems in establishing standardized fees
6. Motivation for insurance coverage:
   a. High consumer demand
   b. Some studies showing CAM less expensive
   c. Surveys indicating people attracted to CAM are healthier
   d. Preventive medicine can potentially be cost effective
7. Therapies found to be covered in a survey of 18 health plans were, in order of frequency, chiropractic manipulation, acupuncture, biofeedback, preventive medicine, nutritional counseling, massage therapy, hypnosis, acupressure, homeopathy, and naturopathy.

G. Research issues
   1. National Center for Complementary and Alternative Medicine (NC-CAM) at the National Institutes of Health (NIH)
      a. A $50 million budget for 1999, representing a 250% increase over 1998
      b. Thirteen medical centers being supported in conducting research on CAM
      c. Increased authority within the medical community with the development of the Center and its increased budget
      d. The National Cancer Institute's (NCI) creation of its own research department to do research on CAM treatments for cancer
   2. Research being done with CAM in the areas of geriatrics, HIV/AIDS, asthma, cancer, cardiovascular disease, addictions, pediatrics, allergy and immunologic disorders, women's health, stroke, and pain management through the NCCAM budget allocations
   3. Need for unique study designs for research on CAM because some theories about health and illness in CAM cannot be measured with today's models
      a. Alteration of energy fields by many CAM modalities cannot be measured with today's technology
      b. Difficulty in measuring, and thus doing research, in preventive medicine
      c. The impact of thoughts in mind-body medicine difficult to measure
   4. CAM providers often object to the current double-blind, placebo-controlled model for research because it is too impersonal, does not take into account the whole person, or appreciate the value of a "placebo" effect in treating disease
   5. The November 11, 1998 issue of the *Journal of the American Medical Association (JAMA)* wholly devoted to research on CAM, and many other indications that mainstream medicine is ready to take CAM seriously
   6. With consumer interest and willingness to pay out-of-pocket, there is a strong financial incentive to do research on and integrate CAM into mainstream medicine

H. Legal issues
1. A newly emerging concern not yet challenged or shaped
2. How to assign liability when there are no standards for practice for many of the CAM modalities
3. What is a medical facility's liability if it does not offer a CAM modality that has some research to show its effectiveness

I. Milbank Memorial Funds 1998 report offers recommendations to assure successful integration of CAM into conventional medicine.
1. Consumers need to keep well informed.
2. Physician need to keep well informed.
3. Physicians incorporating CAM into their practice need to advise their patients of their changing role.
4. CAM practitioners need to allow for scientific scrutiny.
5. Medical educators need to keep themselves current on research in CAM.
6. Health plans need to clarify their decisions regarding coverage of CAM.
7. State licensing boards need to be more accountable for the regulation of CAM.

■ IMPLICATIONS FOR NURSE CASE MANAGERS

A. Nursing care can bring stability into the health care delivery system, and empower patients in making decisions and staying informed regarding their care.

B. The process for integration of CAM into a treatment plan includes:
1. Identify who originated the request for a CAM intervention.
2. Clarify the rationale and expectations for the requested treatment and its potential to impact on patient outcomes.
3. Educate the patient and the medical team about the specific modality being considered.
4. Locate appropriate resources and reliable CAM practitioners.

C. Challenges and opportunities for nurses providing care:
1. Lack of availability of practice guidelines and standards of practice for CAM practitioners:
   a. Not enough professional documentation and discussion of clinical outcomes by CAM providers
   b. Lack of QA and utilization review for CAM modalities
2. Lack of scientific evidence originating in the United States supporting the efficacy of most CAM modalities:
   a. Resources out of the European medical professions demonstrate efficacy of many CAM modalities because it has been part of accepted medical practice for many years
   b. NIH as a reliable resource for case managers with questions about scientific evidence for CAM.

    c. Insurance companies identifying lack of research evidence as an obstacle to coverage

3. Finding a reliable source for understanding the indications and contraindications for CAM:
    a. National associations exist for most CAM modalities and can provide information.
    b. Literature searches and Internet searches can generate information for making a more informed decision.
    c. CAM research centers are increasing, and the NCCAM is now generating good research on efficacy.

4. Locating credentialing guidelines and services for CAM providers:
    a. State licensing boards set standards for their practitioners and can provide lists of qualified providers.
    b. Check with the insurance plan or HMO offering CAM coverage, as they may have credentialing guidelines for their provider list.
    c. More independent credentialing services are being created to address this need, but these services can vary from state to state.
    d. Standards set by Oxford Health Plans include meeting licensing or certification requirements, undergoing a site visit, having minimal malpractice coverage, and committing to continuing education.

5. Locating or creating outcome measures for evaluating treatments with CAM:
    a. Work closely with CAM providers and use their expected outcomes based on the professional standards and experience.
    b. Check with national associations to see what outcome measures they may have developed for that profession.
    c. Do a literature search and determine what outcomes can reasonably be expected for your patient when using a specific CAM modality.

6. Facilitating acceptance of CAM by insurance companies, physicians, and other health care providers:
    a. Be well informed about the efficacy and limitations of the CAM modality you and the patient are considering.
    b. Contact other case managers or health plans with supporting evidence of successful use of CAM.
    c. Support your patient in his or her efforts to seek support from other health care team members and in applying for coverage.

7. Educating CAM providers about managed care and insurance concepts:
    a. Think about writing an article for the state or national association newsletters for CAM associations.
    b. Become a consultant for CAM providers in your area.
    c. Keep yourself well informed and current on research on CAM so that you can constructively exchange information with CAM practitioners in your area.

8. Educating consumers about the indications and contraindications of using CAM:

    a. First, keep yourself well informed and current on research in this area.

    b. Understand that alternative and natural is not always better, especially in emergent or acute situations.

    c. Encourage the patient to become well informed.

    d. Teach a class at a local community college once you have educated yourself, and develop handouts for your patients.

    e. Familiarize yourself with CAM providers in your area.

9. Educating consumers about insurance coverage issues:

    a. Clarify what type of CAM coverage the patient's insurance company or plan offers.

    b. If they are fully committed and informed about a specific modality, direct them to the appropriate channels for appealing a decision regarding coverage of that modality.

10. Identifying which of the many CAM modalities are appropriate for each patient:

    a. Stay current on research in this area.

    b. Ask the CAM provider thorough questions and be sure you are comfortable with his or her role in caring for the patient.

    c. Consult national associations for CAM.

C. Discussion points between the patient and practitioner regarding the incorporation of CAM into their treatment care plan:

1. Ask the patient to identify his or her principal symptom, to better understand which CAM modality is appropriate.

2. Have the patient maintain a symptom diary to track outcomes.

3. Discuss the patient's preferences, level of knowledge, and expectations.

4. Review issues of safety and efficacy.

5. Identify a licensed or certified provider, using national associations as resources.

6. Provide key questions for the alternative therapy provider during initial consultation.

7. Schedule a follow-up visit or telephone call to review the treatment plan with the patient.

8. Follow up to review the response to treatment after a reasonable period of time.

9. Provide documentation.

D. The case management process and CAM

1. Case selection:

    a. Many patients are referring themselves to CAM.

    b. Many physicians are making themselves knowledgeable and referring patients to CAM.

    c. As personal knowledge increases, the case manager can identify when a CAM modality might offer a better outcome and make a recommendation.

2. Assessment/problem identification:
   a. Identify all modalities, herbs, or supplements currently used by the patient.
   b. Identify the primary care provider's support for and knowledge of CAM.
   c. Identify community providers, their educational level, licensing requirements, and credentialing status.
   d. Clarify insurance benefits and what, if any, the patient is willing to pay out-of-pocket.
   e. Proceed with assessment and problem identification as with any case management patient.
3. Development and coordination of the case management plan:
   a. Identify the patient's expectations and level of knowledge.
   b. Review issues of safety and efficacy.
   c. Coordinate with other members of the health care team.
4. Implementation of the plan:
   a. Maintain communication with the CAM provider and request regular reports.
   b. Have the patient maintain a symptom diary to evaluate changes of symptoms in his or her response to treatment.
   c. Provide regular reports to the primary care provider.
5. Evaluation and follow-up:
   a. Realize that sometimes CAM modalities show a slower response rate than allopathic interventions.
   b. Document all contacts and outcomes.

E. Share case studies and personal experience with the class.

REFERENCES

Burton Goldberg Group (1997). *Alternative medicine: The definitive guide.* Tiburon, CA: Future Medicine Publishing.

Eisenberg, D., Kessler, R., & Foster, C. (1993). Unconventional medicine in the United States: Prevalence, costs, and patterns of use. *New England Journal of Medicine, 328*(4), 246–252.

Gerber, R. (1996). *Vibrational medicine.* Santa Fe, NM: Bear & Co.

The Integrative Medicine Consult: The Essential Guide to Integrating Conventional and Complementary Medicine [monthly newsletter]; *www.onemedicine.com.*

Jonas, W.B., & Levin, J.S. (1999). *Essentials of complementary and alternative medicine.* Philadelphia: Lippincott Williams & Wilkens.

Milbank Memorial Fund Report (1998). *Enhancing the accountability of alternative medicine.* New York: Milbank Memorial Fund.

Powell, S. (2000). *Advanced case management: Outcomes and beyond.* Philadelphia: Lippincott Williams & Wilkens.

Index

Note: Page numbers followed by *f* indicate figures; those followed by *t* indicate tables; those followed by *b* indicate boxed material.